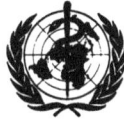

WORLD HEALTH ORGANIZATION

INTERNATIONAL AGENCY FOR RESEARCH ON CANCER

IARC MONOGRAPHS
ON THE
EVALUATION OF THE
CARCINOGENIC RISK
OF CHEMICALS TO HUMANS

The Rubber Industry

VOLUME 28

This publication represents the views and expert opinions
of an IARC Working Group on the
Evaluation of the Carcinogenic Risk of Chemicals to Humans
which met in Lyon,
16-23 February 1981

April 1982

INTERNATIONAL AGENCY FOR RESEARCH ON CANCER

IARC MONOGRAPHS

In 1971, the International Agency for Research on Cancer (IARC) initiated a programme on the evaluation of the carcinogenic risk of chemicals to humans involving the production of critically evaluated monographs on individual chemicals. In 1980, the programme was expanded to include the evaluation of the carcinogenic risk associated with employment in specific occupations.

The objective of the programme is to elaborate and publish in the form of monographs critical reviews of data on carcinogenicity for chemicals and complex mixtures to which humans are known to be exposed, and on specific occupational exposures, to evaluate these data in terms of human risk with the help of international working groups of experts in chemical carcinogenesis and related fields, and to indicate where additional research efforts are needed.

International Agency for Research on Cancer 1982
ISBN 13: 978-9-2832152-88

IARC MONOGRAPHS ON THE EVALUATION
OF THE
CARCINOGENIC RISK OF CHEMICALS TO HUMANS
Volume 28 (1982) The Rubber Industry

ERRATUM

Page 1: (Title page):   ....IARC Working Group on
the Evaluation of the Carcinogenic
Risk of Chemicals to Humans........
met in Lyon,
16-23 June 1981

CONTENTS   3

THE RUBBER INDUSTRY

Lyon, 16-23 June 1981

Members[1]

E. Boyland, London School of Hygiene & Tropical Medicine, Keppel Street (Gower Street) London WC1 7HT, UK

D. Brustein, Industrial Hygienist, United Robber, Cork, Linoleum & Plastic Workers of America, 87 South High Street, Akron, OH 44308, USA

P. Cole, University of Alabama, Department of Epidemiology, Tidwell Hall 203, Birmingham, AL 35294, USA (Vice-Chairman)

T. Fajen, National Institute for Occupational Safety and Health, Industrial Hygiene Section, Robert A. Taft Laboratories, 4676 Columbia Parkway, Cincinnati, OH 45226, USA

W.D. Harris, Industrial Toxicologist, Uniroyal, Inc., World Headquarters, Middlebury, CT 06749, USA

J.T. Hodgson, Medical Statistics Survey Unit, Health & Safety Executive, Baynards House, 1 Chepstow Place, London W2 4TF, UK

B. Holmberg, National Board of Occupational Safety & Health, Unit of Occupational Toxicology, 17184 Solna, Sweden

---

[1] Unable to attend: L. Beliczky, Director, Industrial Hygiene, United Rubber, Cork, Linoleum & Plastic Workers of America, 87 South High Street, Akron, OH 44308, USA; J.M. Peters, Director, Division of Occupational Health, Department of Family and Preventive Medicine, University of Southern California, School of Medicine, 2025 Zonal Avenue, Los Angeles, CA 90033, USA

R.A. Lemen, Director, Division of Criteria Documentation and Standards Development and Division of Technical Services, National Institute for Occupational Safety and Health, 5600 Fishers Lane, Rockville, MD 29857, USA (rapporteur sections II, III, IV)

A.J. McMichael, CSIRO, Division of Human Nutrition, Kintore Avenue, Adelaide, SA 5000, Australia

R.R. Monson, Professor, Harvard University, Department of Epidemiology, School of Public Health, 677 Huntington Avenue, Boston, MA 02115, USA (rapporteur section VII)

N. Nelson, Professor and Chairman, Institute of Environmental Medicine, New York University Medical Center, 550 First Avenue, New York, NY 10016, USA (Chairman)

A.R. Nutt, Company Health and Safety Adviser, Dunlop Ltd., Technology Division, Kingsbury Road, Birmingham B24 9QU, UK

H.G. Parkes, Medical Director, British Rubber Manufacturers' Association Ltd, Health Research Unit, Scala House, Holloway Circus, Birmingham B1 1EQ, UK

N. Segnan, Base Unit, Office of Hygiene, via della Consolata 10, 10100 Turin, Italy

B. Spiegelhalder, German Cancer Research Centre, Institute for Toxicology and Chemotherapy, Im Neuenheimer Feld 280, Postfach 101949, 6900 Heidelberg 1, Federal Republic of Germany

B. Teichmann, Academy of Sciences of the DDR, Central Institute for Cancer Research, Lindenberger Weg 80, 1115 Berlin Buch, German Democractic Republic

H. Vainio, Chief, Department of Industrial Hygiene and Toxicology, Institute of Occupational Health, Haartmaninkatu 1, 00290 Helsinki 29, Finland (rapporteur section VI)

C.A. Veys, Chief Medical Officer, Michelin Tyre Company Ltd, Head Office and Factory, Stoke-on-Trent ST4 4EY, UK

E.A. Walker, 62 Rennie Court, Upper Ground, Blackfriars, London SE1, UK

Representative from the US National Cancer Institute

T.P. Cameron, Assistant Scientific Coordinator for Environmental Cancer, Division of Cancer Cause and Prevention, National Cancer Institute, Bethesda, MD 20205, USA

Representative from SRI International

J.L. Allport, Research Analyst, Chemical-Environmental Department, SRI International, 333 Ravenswood Avenue, Menlo Park, CA 94025, USA (rapporteur section IV)

Secretariat

A. Aitio, Division of Environmental Carcinogenesis
C. Agthe, Division of Epidemiology and Biostatistics
H. Bartsch, Division of Environmental Carcinogenesis
J. Cabral, Division of Environmental Carcinogenesis
M. Friesen, Division of Environmental Carcinogenesis
L. Haroun, Division of Environmental Carcinogenesis (co-secretary)
E. Heseltine, Charost, France (editor)
D. Mietton, Division of Environmental Carcinogenesis (library assistant)
R. Montesano, Division of Environmental Carcinogenesis
I. O'Neill, Division of Environmental Carcinogenesis
C. Partensky, Division of Environmental Carcinogenesis (technical officer)
I. Peterschmitt, Division of Environmental Carcinogenesis, Geneva (bibliographic researcher)
R. Saracci, Division of Epidemiology and Biostatistics
L. Simonato, Division of Epidemiology and Biostatistics
L. Tomatis, Director, Division of Environmental Carcinogenesis (head of the programme)

J. Wahrendorf, Division of Epidemiology and Biostatistics
J. Wilbourn, Division of Environmental Carcinogenesis (<u>co</u>-
    <u>secretary</u>)
H. Yamasaki, Division of Environmental Carcinogenesis

<u>Secretarial assistance</u>

M.-J. Ghess
S. Reynaud
J. Smith
A. Zitouni

NOTE TO THE READER

The term 'carcinogenic risk' in the <u>IARC Monograph</u> series is taken to mean the probability that exposure to a chemical or complex mixture or employment in a particular occupation will lead to cancer in humans.

The fact that a monograph has been prepared on a chemical, complex mixture or occupation does not imply that a carcinogenic hazard is associated with the exposure, only that the published data have been examined. Equally, the fact that a chemical, complex mixture or occupation has not yet been evaluated in a monograph does not mean that it does not represent a carcinogenic hazard.

Anyone who is aware of published data that may alter an evaluation of the carcinogenic risk of a chemical, complex mixture or employment in an occupation is encouraged to make this information available to the Division of Environmental Carcinogenesis, International Agency for Research on Cancer, Lyon, France, in order that the chemical, complex mixture or occupation may be considered for re-evaluation by a future Working Group.

Although every effort is made to prepare the monographs as accurately as possible, mistakes may occur. Readers are requested to communicate any errors to the Division of Environmental Carcinogenesis, so that corrections can be reported in future volumes.

PREAMBLE

BACKGROUND

In 1971, the International Agency for Research on Cancer (IARC) initiated a programme on the evaluation of the carcinogenic risk of chemicals to humans with the object of producing monographs on individual chemicals. Since 1972, the programme has undergone considerable expansion, primarily with the scientific collaboration and financial support of the US National Cancer Institute.

The criteria used to evaluate the carcinogenic risk of chemicals to humans were established in 1971 and were adopted in essence by the various Working Groups whose deliberations resulted in volumes 1-16 of the IARC Monographs. In October 1977, a joint IARC/WHO ad hoc Working Group met to re-evaluate these criteria. The cardinal aim of this Working Group was to update and rewrite the Preamble to the IARC Monographs, which sets forth the criteria for their preparation. The Preamble which subsequently reflected the results of their deliberations(1), together with those of a further ad hoc Working Group which met in April 1978(2), was first adopted by the Working Group which met to evaluate some N-nitroso compounds and whose deliberations resulted in volume 17 of the IARC Monographs. Since that time, the criteria have been used by individual Working Groups whose deliberations resulted in volumes 18-24 and 26-27 of the IARC Monographs.

In June 1980, an IARC Working Group met to evaluate for the first time the carcinogenic risk of exposures to complex mixtures. Occupational situations are a typical, although by no means unique example of such exposures, and those occurring in the wood, leather and associated industries were the subject of the first volume in this expansion of the programme. The deliberations of that Working Group were published as Volume 25 of the IARC Monographs.

OBJECTIVE AND SCOPE

The objective of the programme is to elaborate and publish in the form of monographs critical reviews of data on carcinogenicity for groups of chemicals to which humans are known to be exposed, to evaluate those data in terms of human risk with the help of international working groups of experts in chemical carcinogenesis and related fields, and to indicate where additional research efforts are needed.

These monographs summarize the evidence for the carcinogenicity of the chemicals and other relevant information. The critical analyses of the data are intended to assist national and international authorities in formulating decisions concerning preventive measures. No recommendations are given concerning legislation, since this depends on risk-benefit evaluations, which seem best made by individual governments and/or other international agencies. In this connection, WHO recommendations on food additives(4), drugs(5), pesticides and contaminants(6) and occupational carcinogens(7) are particularly informative.

An ad hoc Working Group which met in Lyon in April 1979 to prepare criteria to select chemicals for IARC Monographs(8) recommended that the Monograph programme be expanded to include consideration of human exposures in selected occupations. The objective of the programme has therefore now been broadened to include the consideration of mixtures of chemicals which result in complex exposures, as they often occur in human populations. These monographs attempt to describe the industries in such a way as to indicate exposures to all known exogenous and endogenous chemicals involved in the processing or use of a material, and review all available epidemiological data in specific occupations within the selected industries. One additional aim of the deliberations of such Working Groups is to identify chemicals that should be evaluated individually for their carcinogenic risk to humans at future IARC Working Group meetings.

Up to October 1981, 28 volumes of the IARC Monographs on the Evaluation of the Carcinogenic Risk of Chemicals to Humans had been published or were in press(7). In these volumes, a total of 572 chemicals, groups of chemicals, industrial processes or occupational exposures were evaluated or re-evaluated. For 43 chemicals, groups of chemicals, industrial processes or industrial exposures, a positive association or a strong suspicion of an association with human cancer has been found. For the remaining 529 chemicals, industrial processes or occupational exposures, epidemiological data were either inadequate or unavailable to evaluate the carcinogenicity to humans – except in the case of fluorides used in drinking-water and dental preparations, for which no evidence of carcinogenic effect was found. However, 523 of the chemicals or groups of chemicals had been tested in experimental animals; there is <u>sufficient evidence</u> that 141 of these are carcinogenic in animals. There is <u>limited evidence</u> of carcinogenicity in experimental animals for a further 153 of these chemicals. The data were inadequate to evaluate the presence or absence of a carcinogenic effect for the remaining 229 chemicals.

SELECTION OF COMPLEX MIXTURES AND OF OCCUPATIONAL EXPOSURES FOR MONOGRAPHS

The complex exposures (mixtures of chemicals) are selected for evaluation on the basis of two main criteria: (a) there is evidence of human exposure, and (b) there are some data relating the exposure to cancer in humans. The occupations to be considered by IARC Working Groups are chosen on the basis that some epidemiological data have suggested that they result in increased cancer risks at various sites. As new data on complex exposures for which monographs have been prepared and new principles for evaluating carcinogenic risk receive acceptance, re-evaluations will be made at subsequent meetings, and revised monographs will be published as necessary.

WORKING PROCEDURES

Approximately one year in advance of a meeting of a working group on individual chemicals, complex mixtures, or occupational exposures, a list is prepared by IARC staff in consultation with other experts. Subsequently, as many chemical, biological and epidemiological data as possible are collected by IARC; in addition to searching the published literature, other recognized information sources on chemical carcinogenesis and related fields such as CANCERLINE, MEDLINE and TOXLINE have been used.

Six to nine months before the meeting, reprints of articles containing relevant data are sent to experts, or are used by the IARC staff, for the preparation of first drafts of the monographs. These drafts are edited by IARC staff and are sent prior to the meeting to all participants of the Working Group for their comments. The Working Group then meets in Lyon for seven to eight days to discuss and finalize the texts of the monographs and to formulate the evaluations. After the meeting, the master copy of each monograph is verified by consulting the original literature, then edited by a professional editor and prepared for reproduction. The monographs are usually published within six to nine months after the Working Group meeting.

Each volume of monographs is printed in 4000 copies, 2500 in soft covers and 1500 in hard covers, and distributed by the WHO distribution and sales service.

DATA FOR EVALUATIONS

With regard to experimental and epidemiological data, only reports that have been published or accepted for publication are reviewed by the working groups, although a few exceptions have been made. The monographs do not cite all of the literature on a particular chemical, complex mixture or occupational exposure; only those data considered by the Working Group to be relevant to the evaluation of the carcinogenic risk to humans are included.

Anyone who is aware of additional data that have been published or are in press which are relevant to the evaluation of the carcinogenic risk to humans of chemicals, complex mixtures or occupational exposures for which monographs have appeared is urged to make them available to the Division of Environmental Carcinogenesis, International Agency for Research on Cancer, Lyon, France.

THE WORKING GROUP

The tasks of the Working Group are five-fold: (a) to ascertain that all data have been collected; (b) to select the data relevant for the evaluation; (c) to ensure that the summaries of the data enable the reader to follow the reasoning of the committee; (d) to judge the significance of the results of experimental and epidemiological studies; and (e) to make an evaluation of the carcinogenic risk of the chemical, complex mixture or occupational exposure.

Working Group participants who contributed to a particular volume are listed, with their addresses, at the beginning of each publication. Each member serves as an individual scientist and not as a representative of any organization or government. In addition, observers are often invited from national and international agencies, organizations and industrial associations.

GENERAL PRINCIPLES FOR EVALUATING THE CARCINOGENIC RISK OF EXPOSURES IN OCCUPATIONS

Evidence of carcinogenicity in humans

Evidence of carcinogenicity in humans, whether it relates to an individual chemical, to a complex exposure or to an occupational exposure, can be derived from three types of study, the first two of which usually provide only suggestive evidence: (1) reports on individual cancer patients (case reports), including a history of exposure to the supposed carcinogenic agent or agents; (2) descriptive epidemiological studies in which the incidence of cancer in human populations is found to vary (spatially or temporally) with exposure to the agent(s); and (3) analytical epidemiological studies (e.g., case–control or cohort studies) in which individual exposure to the agent(s) is found to be associated with an increased risk of cancer. Since occupation is typically recorded on death certificates, routine or specially tabulated reviews of mortality by occupational category often provide a means of generating or testing hypotheses about cancer in occupational or industrial groups. Death certificate statements, however, provide no information on duration, change or details of employment, and may not include data on other factors (e.g., cigarette smoking) that may be related to cancer risk.

An analytical study that shows a positive association between exposure and a cancer may be interpreted as implying causality to a greater or lesser extent if the following criteria are met: (a) There is no identifiable positive bias. (By 'positive bias' is meant the operation of factors in study design or execution which lead erroneously to a more strongly positive association between an agent(s) and disease than in fact exists.

Examples of positive bias include, in case-control studies, better documentation of exposure to the agent(s) for cases than for controls, and, in cohort studies, the use of better means of detecting cancer in individuals exposed to the agent(s) than in individuals not exposed.) (b) The possibility of positive confounding has been considered. (By 'positive confounding' is meant a situation in which the relationship between an agent and a disease is rendered more strongly positive than it truly is as a result of an association between the agent and another agent which either causes or prevents the disease. An example of positive confounding is the association between coffee consumption and lung cancer, which results from their joint association with cigarette smoking.) (c) The association is unlikely to be due to chance alone. (d) The association is strong. (e) There is a dose-response relationship.

In some instances, a single epidemiological study may be strongly indicative of a cause-effect relationship; however, the most convincing evidence of causality comes when several independent studies done under different circumstances result in 'positive' findings.

Analytical epidemiological studies that show no association between exposure and cancer ('negative' studies) should be interpreted according to criteria analogous to those listed above: (a) There is no identifiable negative bias. (b) The possibility of negative confounding has been considered. (c) The possible effects of misclassification of exposure or outcome have been weighed.

In addition, it must be recognized that in any study there are confidence limits around the estimate of association or relative risk. In a study regarded as 'negative', the upper confidence limit may indicate a relative risk substantially greater than unity; in that case, the study excludes only relative risks that are above its upper limit. This usually means that a 'negative' study must be large to be confincing. Confidence in a 'negative' result is increased when several independent studies of sufficient size carried out under different circumstances are in agreement.

Finally, a 'negative' study may be considered to be relevant only to dose levels within or below the range of those observed in the study and is pertinent only if sufficient time has elapsed since first human exposure to the agent(s). Experience with human cancers of known etiology suggests that the period from first exposure to a chemical carcinogen to development of clinically observed cancer is usually measured in decades and may be in excess of 30 years. This also implies that the analysis of data from epidemiological studies must explicitly take into account time from first exposure according to life-table principles.

Experimental Evidence

There are few experimental data from long-term and/or short-term tests on complex mixtures (e.g., soot and tar, smoke condensate) or on exposures to a variety of chemicals that mimic those of humans in occupational environments. Such data are limited in general to the effect of a single chemical and refer in only a few instances to more than one identified chemical.

The evaluation made in the present monograph therefore relies almost entirely on epidemiological data which take into account the effects of the entire spectrum of human exposures in a given situation. One of the aims of the present monograph is to identify the possible contributing roles of individual chemicals in the carcinogenic effect of a known or suspected exposure to a complex mixture.

If experimental data on chemicals so identified exist, they will either already have been considered in an IARC Monograph, in which case suitable reference is made, or they will be included for consideration in future monographs. If, however, no experimental data exist, recommendation will be made that the chemical suspected of playing a role in the causation of human cancer be submitted to carcinogenicity testing.

The criteria used in analysing experimental data and in assessing their relevance to the evaluation of carcinogenic risk to humans(8) are described in detail in the preambles to volumes 17-24 and 26-27 of the Monographs(7).

REFERENCES

1.   IARC (1977) IARC Monograph Programme on the Evaluation of
     the Carcinogenic Risk of Chemicals to Humans. Preamble.
     IARC intern. tech. Rep. No. 77/002

2.   IARC (1978) Chemicals with sufficient evidence of carcino-
     genicity in experimental animals – IARC Monographs
     volumes 1-17. IARC intern. tech. Rep. No. 78/003

3.   WHO (1961) Fifth Report of the Joint FAO/WHO Expert
     Committee on Food Additives. Evaluation of carcinogenic
     hazard of food additives. WHO tech. Rep. Ser., No. 220,
     pp. 5, 18, 19

4.   WHO (1969) Report of a WHO Scientific Group. Principles for
     the testing and evaluation of drugs for carcinogenic-
     ity. WHO tech. Rep. Ser., No. 426, pp. 19, 21, 22

5.   WHO (1974) Report of a WHO Scientific Group. Assessment of
     the carcinogenicity and mutagenicity of chemicals. WHO
     tech. Rep. Ser., No. 546

6.   WHO (1964) Report of a WHO Expert Committee. Prevention of
     cancer. WHO tech. Rep. Ser., No. 276, pp. 29, 30

7.   IARC (1972-1981) IARC Monographs on the Evaluation of the
     Carcinogenic Risk of Chemicals to Humans, Volumes 1-28,
     Lyon, France

     Volume 1 (1972) Some Inorganic Substances, Chlorinated
        Hydrocarbons, Aromatic Amines, N-Nitroso Compounds and
        Natural Products (19 monographs), 184 pages

     Volume 2 (1973) Some Inorganic and Organometallic Compounds
        (7 monographs), 181 pages

     Volume 3 (1973) Certain Polycyclic Aromatic Hydrocarbons and
        Heterocyclic Compounds (17 monographs), 271 pages

     Volume 4 (1974) Some Aromatic Amines, Hydrazine and Related
        Substances, N-Nitroso Compounds and Miscellaneous
        Alkylating Agents (28 monographs), 286 pages

Volume 5 (1974) Some Organochlorine Pesticides (12 monographs), 241 pages

Volume 6 (1974) Sex Hormones (15 monographs), 243 pages

Volume 7 (1974) Some Anti-thyroid and Related Substances, Nitrofurans and Industrial Chemicals (23 monographs), 326 pages

Volume 8 (1975) Some Aromatic Azo Compounds (32 monographs), 357 pages

Volume 9 (1975) Some Aziridines, N-, S- and O-Mustards and Selenium (24 monographs), 268 pages

Volume 10 (1976) Some Naturally Occurring Substances (32 monographs), 353 pages

Volume 11 (1976) Cadmium, Nickel, Some Epoxides, Miscellaneous Industrial Chemicals and General Considerations on Volatile Anaesthetics (24 monographs), 306 pages

Volume 12 (1976) Some Carbamates, Thiocarbamates and Carbazides (24 monographs), 282 pages

Volume 13 (1977) Some Miscellaneous Pharmaceutical Substances (17 monographs), 255 pages

Volume 14 (1977) Asbestos (1 monograph), 106 pages

Volume 15 (1977) Some Fumigants, the Herbicides, 2,4-D and 2,4,5-T, Chlorinated Dibenzodioxins and Miscellaneous Industrial Chemicals (18 monographs), 354 pages

Volume 16 (1978) Some Aromatic Amines and Related Nitro Compounds - Hair Dyes, Colouring Agents, and Miscellaneous Industrial Chemicals (32 monographs), 400 pages

Volume 17 (1978) Some N-Nitroso Compounds (17 monographs), 365 pages

Volume 18 (1978) Polychlorinated Biphenyls and Polybrominated Biphenyls (2 monographs), 140 pages

Volume 19 (1979) Some Monomers, Plastics and Synthetic Elastomers, and Acrolein (17 monographs), 513 pages

Volume 20 (1979) Some Halogenated Hydrocarbons (25 monographs), 609 pages

Volume 21 (1979) Sex Hormones (II) (22 monographs), 583 pages

Volume 22 (1980) Some Non-Nutritive Sweetening Agents (2 monographs), 208 pages

Volume 23 (1980) Some Metals and Metallic Compounds (4 monographs), 438 pages

Volume 24 (1980) Some Pharmaceutical Drugs (16 monographs), 337 pages

Volume 25 (1981) Wood, Leather and Some Associated Industries (7 monographs), 412 pages

Volume 26 (1981) Some Antineoplastic and Immunosuppressive Agents (18 monographs), 411 pages

Volume 27 (1981) Some Aromatic Amines, Anthraquinones and Nitroso Compounds, and Fluorides Used in Drinking-Water and Dental Preparations (18 monographs), 344 pages

Volume 28 (1982) The Rubber Manufacturing Industry (1 monograph), 486 pages

8. IARC (1979)   Criteria to select chemicals for IARC Monographs. IARC intern. tech. Rep. No. 79/003

THE RUBBER INDUSTRY

1.   Choice of industry and outline

This twenty-eighth volume of IARC Monographs is devoted to an evaluation of the carcinogenic risks of exposures in the rubber industry, and is the second in a series in which mixtures of chemicals that result in complex exposures are considered. Although it is not only in occupational settings that such exposures occur, the first volumes in this expansion of the IARC Monographs programme concerned wood, leather and associated industries and the rubber industry, since there are epidemiological studies, some supported by Industry and Labour, that point to elevated cancer risks in those industries.

The present volume is concerned with the tyre manufacturing and repair sector, the cable-making sector and the manufacture of other rubber goods. Natural rubber, synthetic rubber and chemical additives are used in the industry; however, the Working Group considered only those exposures incident to the mixing of elastomers with chemicals and their subsequent conversion into finished products. Exposures occurring during the manufacture of monomers, synthetic elastomers and chemicals were not considered. (Monographs on many of the monomers used appeared in volume 19 of the series [IARC, 1979]). It is nevertheless recognized that some level of exposure to monomers, such as chloroprene, butadiene, acrylonitrile, etc., does undoubtedly occur during certain aspects of the rubber manufacturing process; and although such levels are substantially lower than those encountered in polymer production, they may nevertheless represent a significant exposure factor.

Appendix 1 is a list of some chemicals that have been used in the rubber industry and of some formed as by-products during manufacturing processes. For the chemicals used in the industry, synonyms and trade names, when available, production figures and exposure levels are given. (Exposure levels are also discussed in Section V.) Workplace levels and occupational standards are also given when available. Some of the salient biological properties of selected compounds are described in the body of the text; and brief summaries of evaluations of carcinogenicity made by previous IARC working groups for chemicals used or by-products formed in the rubber industry are given in Appendix 2.

FIG. 1.   CONSUMPTION OF NATURAL AND SYNTHETIC RUBBER
           IN VARIOUS COUNTRIES, 1979
           (From the International Rubber Study Group, 1981)

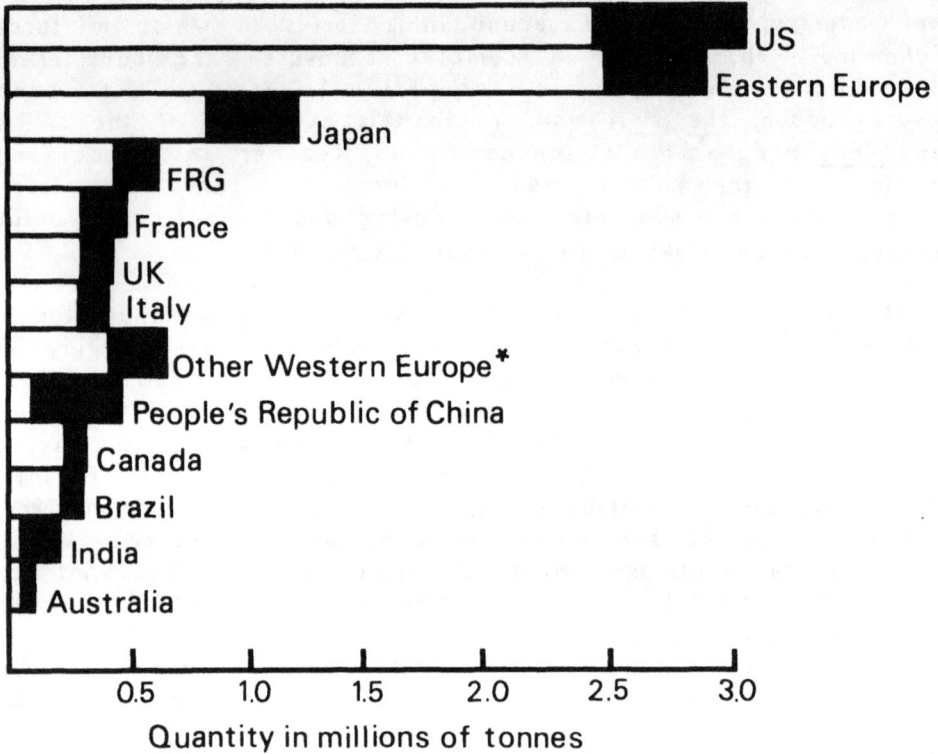

Quantity in millions of tonnes

*non-members of the European Economic Communities

2.   Estimates of use and employment

In 1980, total world consumption of natural rubber was 3.85
million tonnes, and that of synthetic rubber was 8.6 million
tonnes (The International Rubber Study Group, 1981). Figure 1
provides estimates of rubber use in various parts of the world;
and Table 1 shows the breakdown by product.

Table 1. Rubber use in western Europe by end-user industry[a]

	1978 (actual) %	1985 (forecast) %	Non-tyre use only, 1978 %
Tyres	51	45	–
Non-tyre			
Automotive	16	15	33
Mechanical engineering[b]	8	10	16
Building	7	6	14
Footwear	5	5	10
Furniture, textile	3	5	6
Electrical	3	3	6
Sports, leisure	2	4	4
Miscellaneous	5	7	10

[a] From Scabell (1978)

[b] Described as 'construction' in text, but believed to refer to mechanical engineering

The United Nations Yearbook of Industrial Statistics (1977) provides some data on the numbers of workers employed in various sectors of the industry. In various countries, data are available in which the rubber products industry is broken down according to the number of establishments, average number of persons employed, average number of operatives and gross output. Such employment figures can provide crude estimates of the total working population; however, it must be borne in mind that not all workers experience hazardous exposure(s).

3.   Variations in technology within the rubber industry

Industries are not unique, well-defined entities, i.e., there may be more than one way to manufacture a particular product, and industries usually change over time as products change or new technology is introduced. The rubber industry provides a striking example of this observation. With a complex technology that has been evolving, developing and diversifying for more than a century, it is virtually impossible either to define or to describe 'a typical rubber manufacturing operation', in terms either of the end product or of the process by which that product is made.

Currently, the product range of the rubber industry includes not only the more obvious items, such as car and truck tyres, electric cables, industrial hose and belting of all types, but also inflatable boats and life rafts, harbour protection booms, aircraft de-icing equipment, and nuclear reactor access platforms. For the domestic market, such familiar items as footwear, sports goods, toys, furniture and surgical rubber goods illustrate the extent of diversification.

The process and technology that are involved in the manufacture of this comprehensive range are almost as varied as the products themselves. The nature of the final product determines at the outset the selection of an appropriate compounding formulation from the wide range of polymers – natural or synthetic – and the numerous rubber chemicals now available; and their subsequent processing involves much potential for human exposure. This includes exposure to chemical dusts during the mixing stage, to fume arising from unvulcanized rubber compound in the milling, extruding and calendering stages, to solvents and solvent adhesives in component assembly and to curing fume given off during vulcanization, finishing and inspection. It is also important to recognize the combination of exposure hazards that may confront service and plant maintenance engineers, who are frequently required to work in normally inaccessible and poorly ventilated areas of the plant and who may thereby be exposed to high concentrations of both dust and fume.

Since the different processes (see Section III) may be associated with different exposure hazards, it is important to recognize the occupational health implications that may arise:

(<u>a</u>) variations in production and control technology,

(<u>b</u>) variations in process requirements for different products, and

(<u>c</u>) variations in work practice.

4. Difficulties in determining the relation between exposure and disease

When, in 1949, 2-naphthylamine was shown to be a significant impurity in some of the rubber antioxidants then in general use, it was possible to establish with reasonable certainty a direct causal link between that usage and the excess of bladder cancer cases observed by Case and Hosker (1954) in the British rubber industry. Although it now appears that the removal of those suspect chemical compounds from the industrial process has effectively eliminated that particular occupational cancer hazard, it has since become evident — from epidemiological studies carried out in several countries — that other and hitherto unsuspected cancer risks may be confronting the rubber process worker. More specifically, excesses of mortality from lung and stomach cancer among some groups of rubber workers have been reported in both the American and British rubber industries.

Only in recent years has there been any general recognition of the need for systematic monitoring of the industrial environment; and today there is a need to standardize monitoring techniques, to define acceptable hygiene standards and codes of practice, and for a greater dissemination of information on industrial hygiene. The search for carcinogenic agents that could account for the observed excesses of lung and stomach cancer is a much more difficult and complex task than the search for the causative agent for bladder cancer. Since lung and stomach tumours are frequent in the general population and the excesses observed are small, it would be difficult to determine the specific exposure(s) responsible unless detailed <u>ad hoc</u> epidemiological studies were carried out. Although some occupations and processes appear to be incriminated more than others, the contribution that any one of the many chemicals used in the industry may make to the cancer expeience of workers in those occupations is not known.

The main reasons that it is difficult to assess exposure are that:

(a) An individual experiences a multiplicity of exposures, arising both from the variety and change in chemicals used in a given job, and cross-contamination between jobs in large plants.

(b) Several hundred chemicals are used in the rubber industry (see Appendix 1); when, as frequently happens, they are referred to only by trade names, it is difficult for occupational health workers to ascertain when changes occur in their composition, or what significance such changes may have.

(c) Few workers in the industry remain in the same job during the whole period of their employment. A worker may be moved from job to job within a single department, even during the course of a single working shift, and may be transferred from one department to another in an entirely different location. The industry has not developed a system to record adequately all individual exposures through detailed documentation of work histories.

(d) Cancer excesses currently observed in the industry almost certainly result from chemical exposures that occurred many years ago. There is, however, inadequate information about the nature and extent of those exposures, and there is little available documentation of individual work histories.

(e) An industrial process may result in the formation of new materials, as by-products, or in interactions of known chemicals to produce other entities (e.g., N-nitrosamines and carbon disulphide).

Another reason behind the poor understanding of exposure-effect relationships in these industries is the missing link between occupational titles and exposures. The epidemiologist usually relies on occupational descriptions (job title or title of industry), of varying degrees of specificity, for an indirect, qualitative assessment of possible exposures. In contrast, the industrial hygienist focuses on the actual exposures that occur in the workplace. What is missing is a historical and up-to-date data source that cross-references job titles within specific industries and specific exposures. For example, 'tyre assembly' might appear to be a simple, well-defined job title on the surface;   but two individuals whose occupation can be described in that way may work in two entirely different exposure milieux.

Finally, industrial hygienists find practical difficulties in 'keeping up' with continually changing work environments. Data gathered at one point in time may not be representative of the industry over the twenty- or thirty-year time span covered by an epidemiological study. It is essential, therefore, that a system be established that would effectively provide for continuous collection and coherent organization of such information.

5. References

Case, R.A.M. & Hosker, M.E. (1954) Tumour of the urinary bladder as an occupational disease in the rubber industry in England and Wales. Br. J. prev. soc. Med., 8, 39-50

IARC (1979) IARC Monographs on the Evaluation of the Carcinogenic Risk of Chemicals to Humans, Vol. 19, Some Monomers, Plastics and Synthetic Elastomers, and Acrolein, Lyon

The International Rubber Study Group (1981) Rubber Statistical Bulletin, Vol. 35, No. 8, London, pp. 13, 35

Scabell, D. (1978) Changing rubber industry trends in western Europe. Elastomerics, 110, 17-20, 35

United Nations (1977) Yearbook of Industrial Statistics, 1975 ed., Vol. 1, General Industrial Statistics, New York, Department of Economic and Social Affairs, Statistical Office of the United Nations

1.   The origins of the rubber industry
      (for a review, see Schidrowitz & Dawson, 1952)

1.1   The discovery of rubber

      Rubber was among the first of many new discoveries to
impress the early European explorers of the New World. Columbus,
during his second voyage of discovery (1493–1496) noticed that
the natives of Hispaniola (now known as Haiti) played games with
solid balls. These balls were astonishingly resilient and
elastic, and able to bounce much higher than the hollow, inflated
leather balls used in Europe at that time. They were made from a
dried milky liquid which could be obtained by cutting into the
bark of certain trees. The South American Indians called these
trees 'haeve' or 'cauchuc' which meant 'weeping wood'; and it is
from these two Indian words that the genus name 'Hevea' for the
rubber tree, and the French and English term for rubber
'caoutchouc' originated.

      Excavations have shown that rubber was used in religious
ceremonies by the Aztecs as early as the sixth century AD. Copies
of an ancient fresco found at Teotihuacán in Mexico depict a
squatting priest making offerings that include two balls of
rubber. Early writers also stress that rubber was a magical
substance of great ritual significance for both the Aztecs and
the Mayas, and it was thought sometimes to be associated with
human sacrifice. Rubber effigies, over 500 years old, have been
found in the Well of Sacrifice in the ruined Maya city of Chichén
Itzá in Mexico. Such figures were used as offerings to the rain
gods with whose worship the Well was associated.

      In a contemporary drawing dated about 1529, Aztec players
brought back to Spain by Cortes are shown tossing a solid rubber
ball to each other using only their buttocks in the game, while
their hands remain touching the ground. They wore leather trunks
and gloves in order to lessen the impact of the hard ball on
their skin. It is also interesting that the then King of Spain
sent a physician called Francisco Hernandez to explore the
natural resources of the New Spain. Hernandez, in his book Rerum
Medicarum Novae Hispaniae Thesaurus, published in Rome in 1649,
described the gum that flowed out of the trees when the bark was

cut. This gum was shaped into balls by the natives, but he also made special reference to the numerous medical uses to which 'holli' (the Indian name for the gum) was put — to cure all manner of diseases by internal and external application.

The ancient Mexicans used these solid rubber balls for games, and a popular variety described in 1535, called 'Tlachtli', was a mixture of basketball, football and hockey. It called for a considerable degree of skill since the ball, about 9–12 cm in diameter, had to be propelled through a stone ring not much greater in size. A play-ball of this description, thought to be over 350 years old, has been found in the grave of a Peruvian child.

Man's first attempts to fashion something useful from rubber probably originated among the Amazonian natives, who dipped their feet into a container of rubber latex, thereby fashioning for themselves a pair of rubber shoes. The next step for the Amazonian shoemaker was to use a former, corresponding to the shape of his foot, which he made from clay. In order to improve on his manufacturing technique, he soon learned to dry successive latex dippings faster by using heat from a fire. This, in turn, led to the observation that a smoky fire preserved the pair of shoes longer and gave them strength and durability, not apparent in the naturally coagulated product. Present-day methods still rely on the antiseptic function of smoking to preserve natural rubber from its usual tendency to ferment and become mouldy.

The natives of Haiti made shoes, bottles, waterproof cloth, syringes and other useful objects from the elastic gum; but although the early Spanish and Portuguese explorers took samples of the gum home with them, their discovery had little impact on the civilization of the time.

1.2 The birth of an industry

Several centuries were to elapse before the new material was to be brought into commercial use in Europe. The eighteenth century expeditions of the Frenchman, Charles de la Condamine, in the equatorial regions of South America, and his subsequent writings, did much to stimulate interest in rubber in the laboratories of Europe. It was La Condamine and his engineering colleague, François Fresneau, who first described the Hevea rubber tree, as well as the methods used by the natives for extracting the latex (the Latin word for milk), and how they made useful articles from it.

Another Frenchman, Foucroy, discovered in 1791 that latex could be preserved by small amounts of ammonia, but this important discovery lay dormant for some 125 years, when it was reintroduced for use in stabilizing natural latex during transport.

By the end of the eighteenth century, the general properties of rubber were beginning to be recognized, although it was first marketed, not for its elastic properties, but to rub out pencil marks – hence the English name 'rubber', suggested by Joseph Priestley in 1770.

At the start of the nineteenth century, the use of coal-gas for illumination led to the establishment of gas companies throughout the British Isles, and in 1819 Charles Macintosh, a manufacturer of dyes, contracted to purchase the by-products of the Glasgow Gas Works. He discovered that one of those by-products, coal-tar naphtha, was an excellent solvent for rubber, for which hitherto no satisfactory solvent had been found. Macintosh used the rubber and solvent to make a solution which he spread onto one side of a fabric. Two plies of the fabric were then pressed together (rubber sides adjacent) to form the first 'Macintosh' waterproof cloth. In 1823 Macintosh patented his discovery, thus adding a new word to the English language. So successful was his business for this waterproof fabric that a new works was built as the first rubber factory in Manchester. Unhappily, the rubber that coated these 'Macintosh' garments was subject to temperature changes, becoming sticky when hot, and stiff and brittle to the point of cracking when cold and on ageing.

Public demand for rubber footwear in the US is said to have started in 1823 when a Boston merchant, T.C. Wales, began marketing rubber footwear imported from Brazil. The first rubber footwear factory, the Roxbury India Rubber Company, was started in Boston in 1833; but the products were subject to the same problems encountered by Macintosh. It was those problems which prompted Charles Goodyear into the work which finally led to his discovery of vulcanization in 1839, heralding the start of an important industry (Goodyear, 1855).

Charles Goodyear lived and worked in Naugatuck, Connecticut. His plant, also located in Naugatuck, later became a part of the US Rubber Company, now Uniroyal, Inc. Goodyear found that rubber mixed with sulphur, and then heated, resulted in a dough-like product that was unaffected by hot or cold weather. He did not patent his discovery until 1844; however, Thomas Hancock, a London coachbuilder, obtained a British patent for the vulcanization process in 1843, admitting quite openly that he had seen samples of sulphur-vulcanized rubber probably made by Goodyear himself. 'Metallic Gum-Elastic' was the term given by Goodyear to his 'cured' rubber, but the process was soon to be given the name of 'vulcanization' which derives from mythology: Vulcan, the mythical Roman god of fire, had his workshops in volcanic mountains, an abundant source of both heat and sulphur (the essential requirements for the vulcanization process). Thus, between 1835 and 1845, the work of Goodyear, Hancock and others led to the successful development on a commercial scale of the vulcanization process, by which an unsatisfactory material was converted into one with outstandingly valuable elastic properties suitable for a wide variety of industrial uses. At about the same time, it was discovered that the addition of inorganic basic oxides or hydroxides such as litharge, zinc oxide and lime, increased the vulcanization rate and improved the properties of the product.

An alternative vulcanization technique (discovered by Alexander Parkes in the UK) (British Patent No. 11147/1846) in the same period was the so-called 'cold-cure' process and was used extensively for upwards of 100 years. It involved exposing thin sheets or films of rubber to the action of sulphur chloride in a solvent at room temperature. Some time later, modifications were introduced in which sulphur chloride in vapour form or in carbon disulphide was used. With the further development of organic accelerators the cold curing process became obsolete.

Raw rubber can be much more readily shaped hot than cold, with less energy demand. Thomas Hancock in 1820 developed a machine, called the 'Pickle', which enabled him both to soften and then join together small pieces of rubber into a larger piece. This was the forerunner of the modern internal mixer. As he wrote, '... the discovery of this process was unquestionably the origin and commencement of the india-rubber manufacture properly so-called. Nothing that had been done before amounted to a manufacture of this substance, but consisted mainly in experimental attempts to dissolve it.[1] Later on, Hancock developed more powerful masticating machines which were the precursors of the modern two-roll mills (Hancock, 1857).

After the discovery of vulcanization by Goodyear, the demand for crude rubber increased considerably, and it soon became apparent that the manufacturing industry could no longer rely on the supply of rubber obtained from trees growing wild in inaccessible tropical jungles. In 1876, Henry Wickham, acting as an agent for the British India Office, was commissioned to obtain seeds of the rubber tree, <u>Hevea brasiliensis.</u> With the help of local natives, Wickham gathered over 70 000 seeds of the <u>Hevea</u> tree, in Brazil on the banks of the Tapajós River; and then, after an exciting race against time and the authorities, brought the highly perishable seeds back to Kew Gardens in London. Approximately 2500 seeds of the original total eventually germinated. From these comparatively few seedlings, distributed to Ceylon, India and Malaya, and from there throughout the east, the whole plantation industry has developed. The achievement earned Sir Henry Wickham (1841-1928) the title of 'the father of plantation rubber'. Plantation rubber was first marketed about 1900 and production has since increased steadily; wild rubber is now of little commercial importance. The rubber tree flourished in Malaysia, where large areas of jungle were cut down and planted. Henry Nicholas Ridley, who was appointed Director of the Singapore Botanic Gardens in 1888, did perhaps more than anybody to encourage planting of this new crop. By the end of the nineteenth century there were 5000 acres of rubber in Asia. Today, the major producing countries include Malaysia, Indonesia, Thailand, India and Sri Lanka; Liberia and Nigeria; and The People's Republic of China.

By 1910, stimulated by the development of Henry Ford's famous motor car and the consequently burgeoning demand for rubber, the rubber planters in Asia achieved one million acres of plantation. With the spread of motoring in every part of the world and the development of the general rubber goods section of the industry, even today's vast acreage (about 15 million acres in all) and greatly increased yields brought about by plant breeding and fertilization are insufficient to meet world demand. The industrial applications of rubber also multiplied. Many of the early articles, manufactured by Thomas Hancock (1786-1865),

are described in his book (Hancock, 1857; see Fig. 2). Some of
the equipment (not very different from that still used today) is
also depicted.

1.3 The invention of the pneumatic tyre

The first rubber tyres were used on horse-drawn vehicles and
bicycles; they were solid and grew rapidly in popularity. In
1845, R.W. Thomson was granted a patent for a tyre embodying an
air-inflated tube and a non-stretching outer cover. Although
these 'ariel wheels' were successfully used on horse-drawn
carriages, the comparatively slow speed did not establish the
advantage of the pneumatic principle, and Thomson's work was
overlooked for many years.

In 1888, J.B. Dunlop, who was unaware of the earlier patent
(and so, apparently, was the Patent Office), developed a similar
type of tyre which was tried out on a bicycle. The superiority of
this tyre over its solid counterpart was quickly realized, and
the opportunity to develop a substantial business in pneumatic
cycle tyres led to the establishment of the Dunlop Tyre Company
in Dublin in 1889. Almost at once the existence of Thomson's
patent was re-discovered. It had expired, but because of it,
Dunlop's patent was invalidated. The field was, therefore, left
wide open to competitors, and development of this new invention
was pursued with intense activity. The logic of driving on a
cushion of air instead of on a solid circular block of rubber is
simple, but the effects of the change were to have a tremendous
impact on transportation. A major problem was how to fix the tyre
onto the rim of the wheel. The idea of applying a rigid bead
containing a wire was patented by Charles K. Welch in 1890
(British Patent No. 145631); and in the same year W.E. Bartlett
invented the 'clincher' (clamp) method of attaching the tyre to
the wheel (British Patent No. 11900). In 1891, the French firm of
Michelin developed the first detachable pneumatic cycle tyre. The
tyre was capable of being changed in minutes, and its use by the
victor in the cycle race Paris-Brest-Paris ensured its success.

A few years later, in 1895, the first pneumatic tyre was
developed for motor vehicles by the same firm. L'Eclair, the
first car to be fitted with Michelin pneumatic tyres, completed

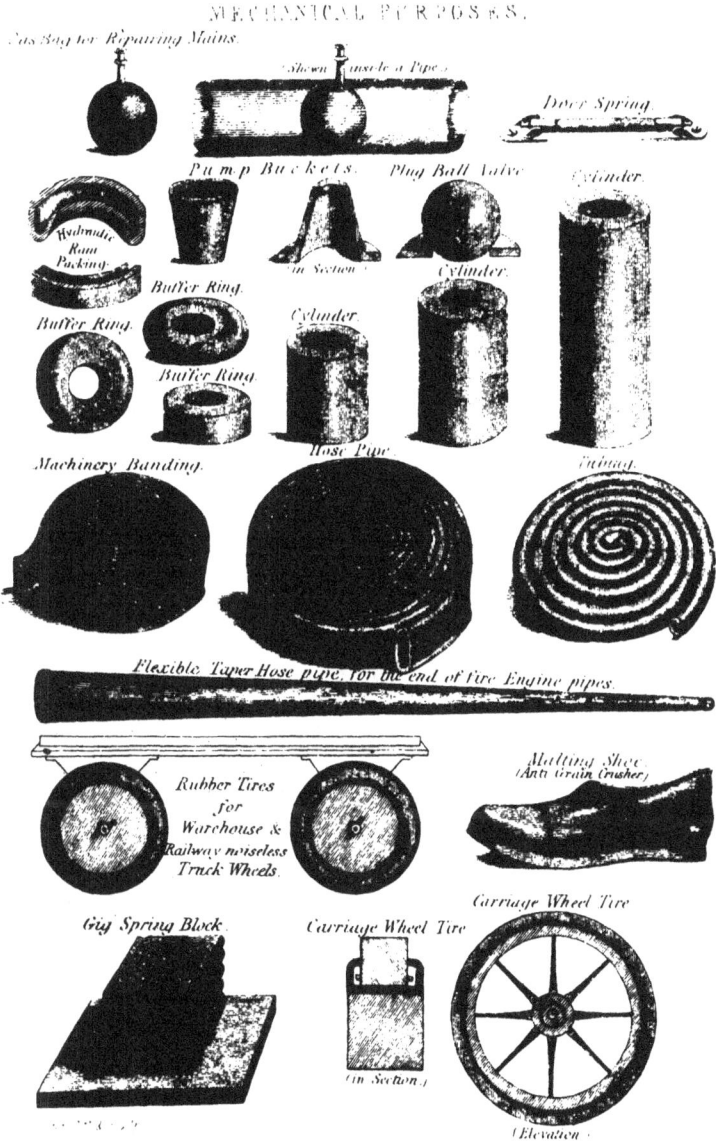

FIG. 2. ARTICLES MADE FROM OR INCORPORATING NATURAL RUBBER IN PRODUCTION BY 1857 (From Hancock, 1857)

the 1200-km course of the Paris-Bordeaux-Paris race. Despite this feat, car manufacturers were still doubtful of the absolute acceptability of the pneumatic tyre; but the motor car was at a stage of rapid development, and soon much lighter and faster models, using the new tyres, broke the 100-km/h barrier. By 1899, the tyre's life expectancy had increased from 100 miles to over 3000 miles.

Thus, at the beginning of the twentieth century, when the coming of the motor car required a phenomenal increase in the amount of crude rubber, the production of plantation rubber was also stimulated. The same stimulus prompted the development of the synthetic-rubber industry in the West after the outbreak of the Second World War in 1939. Further expansion of the motor car industry at that time would not have been possible without an adequate supply of both natural and synthetic rubber, accompanied by corresponding developments and growth in the production of petroleum products. The latter, apart from being sources of fuel, now also play an important part in all rubber manufacturing operations, and they are the most important raw materials required for the manufacture of modern synthetic rubbers.

1.4   Development of chemical compounding

The vulcanization, or curing, process, which is based on the reaction of unsaturated rubber hydrocarbon molecules with sulphur in the presence of zinc oxide and other inorganic bases, continued to be used during the latter half of the nineteenth and the early years of the twentieth century, with steady but limited improvements. The process suffered from several disadvantages, including the requirements of a high temperature and a long reaction time of several hours, the difficulty of control, and the applicability of the process only to solid raw natural rubber and not to latex. However, in 1906, Oenslåger in the US found that incorporation of the organic base aniline markedly speeded up and improved the process; and although aniline itself was found to be too toxic for commercial application, it was replaced by the non-toxic derivative thiocarbanilide, with even better results. This discovery marked the beginning of intensive research activity to identify synthetic organic chemicals that would improve both the process and the product; this scientific approach has formed the basis of the rubber chemical compounding industry as it is now constituted.

Following the First World War, research laboratories were set up by several rubber companies to improve rubber. At first, the emphasis was simply on improving performance and/or on lowering the cost of production. As time went on, more thought was given to overcoming obvious odour and health problems (dermatitis, etc.) as well as to reducing fire hazards.

2.   The developing rubber industry and its occupational health hazards

2.1   The factory environment

Today, the rubber industries that have been established in many different parts of the world produce a very wide range of manufactured goods; and, although they are founded on the use of traditional materials and processes, they also use a technology of ever-increasing complexity. The industry is heavily dependent on the use of chemical engineering skills, and in its compounding processes it now requires the use of some hundreds of different chemical compounds. Those who work in it may, therefore, be exposed to the potential hazards involved in the handling and use of those chemicals, in addition to the mechanical hazards that are common to all engineering and production work. The identification, control and elimination of those hazards is now recognized to be a matter of urgent and substantial concern.

Among the earliest references to occupational health hazards in the rubber industry, it is interesting to note especially the observations made by Dr J.T. Arlidge in his book The Hygiene Diseases and Mortality of Occupations, published in 1892 (Arlidge, 1892). He wrote then that:

'India-rubber manufactories exemplify a fact heretofore insisted on; viz., the great variety of operations carried on within a factory. Here the operatives themselves are popularly spoken of as india-rubber workers, although they have little in common beyond working on the same premises. Thus we have strong mechanical labour in connection with the powerful engines which flatten out the crude rubber submitted to them; in other departments, dust; in others, steam and the vapours of sulphur and bi-sulphide of carbon, and in the finishing rooms, nothing else save a pervading vapour of naphtha, along with sedentary employment.'

Thus, he accurately identified a number of hazards which might then have been encountered and some which were later to be brought under control by the India Rubber Regulations. In a later and more detailed report that Arlidge submitted to the Chief Inspector of Factories in 1894 (Arlidge, 1894), he noted with satisfaction evidence of a reduction in the use of carbon di-sulphide (resulting from the abandonment of many 'cold' cure processes), and he discussed at length the potential problems arising out of the extensive use of naphtha in the industry. In that context, he reported on his own observation of workers affected by headaches, giddiness, nausea and mental confusion and he noted also that the affects of such exposure were greatly augmented by 'the taking of intoxicating drink'. He considered the use of lead compounds in some of the industrial processes, but was evidently reassured by his finding that such use was diminishing and that reports of lead poisoning were infrequent. Indeed, it is apparent that the greater part of his report on the health of rubber workers was firmly reassuring. He found no evidence of anaemia and few, if any, occurrences of 'cutaneous affections'; and he stated on the evidence of his own examinations that:

'... the health of the people employed in rubber factories, coupled with verbal questioning of many hands, male and female, and likewise of foremen and others connected with such works for months and years, in several instances 20 years and upwards, has led me to the conclusion that the occupation is productive of no definite disease, nor of lasting inconveniences. This is the concurrent testimony of all the employed, as well as of the employers.'

In 1914, Dr Alice Hamilton undertook an investigation of the US rubber industry: she reported a few cases of carbon disulphide poisoning, associated with the 'cold-curing' process, but pointed out that use of this process in the US was limited and declining (Hamilton, 1943). Exposure to litharge, however, was a problem among rubber compounders, and some of the most serious cases of

lead poisoning documented in the US had occurred among these
workers (Hamilton & Hardy, 1974). Hamilton (1943) also noted
exposure to benzene, especially among those using solvent-based
rubber adhesives and sealers.

When, in 1922, the Indiarubber Regulations (HM Government,
1922) eventually came into force in the UK, it became clear that
they were intended primarily to deal with the handling of lead
compounds and with fume processes involving the use of carbon
disulphide, sulphur chloride, benzene and chlorinated hydrocarbons. It was the obvious intention of the regulations to deal
in the main with those problems that had been identified by
Arlidge so many years before.

Although the UK Registrar General had noted an excess of
mortality from cancers at specific sites among rubber workers in
data for 1920-1922 and again in data for 1929-1931 (see Mancuso
et al., 1968), it was not until the middle of the present century
that attention was once again focused upon the occupational
health hazards to which workers in the rubber industry might be
exposed. It was, of course, recognized that dermatitis was a
troublesome, recurrent, and prevalent problem; and it was
beginning also to be appreciated that environmental conditions in
the factories, where substantial exposure to solvents and to airborne chemical dusts were a commonplace, could no longer reasonably be tolerated. In some factories, mass radiographic chest
examinations had led to the identification of talc pneumoconiosis
as a disease affecting rubber workers and there was also some
concern about the possible long-term effects of exposure to
solvents on the skin and on the haemopoietic system. Unfortunate-
ly, there is available today little in the way of contemporary
and documentary evidence to establish the full extent or severity
of worker exposure to potential hazardous dust and fume associated with the manufacturing process during the first half of this
century. There are numerous anecdotal accounts of impenetrable
dust clouds arising from mixing and milling operations carried
out in the industry, and there is also some early photographic
evidence of unacceptably large amounts of fume being given off by
heated rubber compound in the milling and curing areas. It
appears to have been largely accepted that such conditions were
an inevitable accompaniment to rubber manufacturing operations,
and such improvements as were from time to time made in the
environmental conditions were the result of little more than a
simple subjective assessment of those conditions. Only in recent

years has a more systematic and scientific approach been adopted by the performance of industrial hygiene surveys, capable of providing accurate documentary evidence of exposure as the basis for the installation and implementation of environmental control.

2.2   The identification of bladder cancer as an occupational disease in the rubber industry and the development of epidemiological studies

The association between occupational exposures to chemicals and malignant tumours of the lower urinary tract was first suspected in the dyestuffs industry in 1895, when the German surgeon Rehn described three cases of papillary bladder tumour arising in workers engaged on the manufacture of fuchsine (Rehn, 1895). Although it was subsequently noted (International Labour Office, 1921) that men engaged in the manufacture of some aromatic amines – among which benzidine and 2-naphthylamine were particularly mentioned – developed bladder tumours, it was not then suspected that the products would extend the area of hazard beyond the manufacturing process in the dyestuffs industry; and until the late 1940s no suspicion existed that bladder tumours could result from exposure to rubber chemicals. It was not until Case and Hosker (1954), in the course of detailed epidemiological studies on the British dyestuffs industry, unexpectedly identified an excess of bladder tumours affecting rubber workers that this came to light. They discovered that 41 cases of bladder cancer reported between 1921 and 1950 within the county borough of Birmingham had occurred in people who either were working or had worked in the rubber industry and noted that this figure was substantially in excess of the expectation for the whole of the county borough during the observation period. On the evidence of these preliminary studies, the compounding chemicals chiefly indicted in the rubber industry were withdrawn from use in the UK in 1949.

Although this action was taken, the full implications of Case's work were not well-understood, and little further action was taken, until, in 1957, the British rubber manufacturers, recognizing the continued appearance of new cases of bladder cancer attributable to previous exposure, established a cyto-diagnostic screening unit. This unit was later to develop into the British Rubber Manufacturers' Association occupational health research unit. During the late 1950s, fears continued to be expressed that unidentified and hitherto unsuspected bladder carcinogens might still be in use in the industry. It was this fear, coupled with the impact of several widely reported inquests on rubber and cable industry workers (Anon., 1965a,b,c,d,e, 1966), correspondence in the medical journals (Anon., 1964; Boyland & Haddow, 1964; Case, 1964; Parkes, 1964a,b; Wallace, 1964) and a report by Case and Davies (1965), which indicated the need for further action; and in June 1966 a papilloma committee for the rubber industry with representatives from management, trade unions and government, was established to promote and coordinate research and epidemiological studies. Although these studies were initially designed to explore whether or not there was evidence of a continuing bladder cancer hazard, they were later extended and developed to examine the overall mortality experience of British rubber workers.

In 1970, an important common law action was started in the British High Court in which the Trades Unions, acting on behalf of two workers affected by bladder cancer, claimed damages from Imperial Chemical Industries and from Dunlop (Anon, 1971; Cassidy & Wright versus Dunlop & ICI, 1971). Judgement was given for the plaintiffs, and the case, which went to and was upheld on appeal, established the principle of an employer's liability for the safety of his products, not only during the manufacturing process but also in the circumstances in which he may reasonably expect that product to be used.

It was not in Britain alone that epidemiological studies in the rubber industry were undertaken. In the US, Mancuso followed the development of epidemiological studies in the industry; and, reporting on his own observations, starting in 1949 (Mancuso, 1963; Mancuso et al., 1968; Mancuso & Brennan, 1970; Mancuso, 1975, 1976, 1982), he indicated the need for a systematic inquiry into the health of the US rubber worker.

In 1970, following negotiations between the United Rubber Workers and six major rubber companies, agreement was reached to establish joint occupational health programmes (Wolf, 1970, 1971). Under joint contract to management and labour, the Schools of Public Health at the University of North Carolina and Harvard University undertook to conduct a wide-ranging epidemiological study, with major emphasis on cancer incidence, mortality and distribution. These programmes continued until 1979 and 1980, respectively.

3. <u>References</u>

Anon. (1964) Annotations: Cancer Research. <u>Lancet</u>, <u>ii</u>, 25-26

Anon. (1965a) Leading article: Bladder cancer in the rubber industry. <u>Br. med. J.</u>, <u>i</u>, 329-330

Anon. (1965b) Leading article: Occupational bladder tumours and the control of carcinogens. <u>Lancet</u>, <u>i</u>, 306-307

Anon. (1965c) Medicine and the Law: Industrial cancer of the bladder. <u>Lancet</u>, <u>i</u>, 328

Anon. (1965d) Leading article: Bladder tumours in industry. <u>Lancet</u>, <u>ii</u>, 627-628

Anon. (1965e) Medicine and the Law: Death of a rubber worker. <u>Lancet</u>, <u>ii</u>, 635

Anon. (1966) Medicine and the Law: Inquest on a former rubber worker. <u>Lancet</u>, <u>ii</u>, 1259

Anon. (1971) Medicolegal: Damages for rubber workers. <u>Br. med. J.</u>, <u>ii</u>, 412-413

Arlidge, J.T. (1892) <u>The Hygiene Diseases and Mortality of Occupations</u>, London, Percival & Co., pp. 483, 487

Arlidge, J.T. (1894) In: <u>Annual Report of HM Chief Inspector of Factories and Workshops</u>, London

Boyland, E. & Haddow, A. (1964) Letters to the Editor: Cancer Research. <u>Lancet</u>, <u>ii</u>, 527

Case, R.A.M. (1964) Letter to the Editor: Cancer Research. <u>Lancet</u>, <u>ii</u>, 309-310

Case, R.A.M. & Davies, J. (1965) Occupational bladder cancer: some recent observations. <u>Br. J. prev. soc. Med.</u>, <u>19</u>, 51

Case, R.A.M. & Hosker, M.E. (1954) Tumour of the urinary bladder as an occupational disease in the rubber industry in England and Wales. <u>Br. J. prev. soc. Med.</u>, <u>8</u>, 39-50

Cassidy & Wright versus Dunlop & ICI (1971) London, High Court of Justice; 1968 C. No. 3455; 1969 C. No. 4678; 1969 W. No. 2443; 1969 W. No. 2750

Goodyear, C. (1855) Gum Elastic and its Varieties, with a Detailed Account of its Applications and Uses and of the Discovery of Vulcanisation, New Haven, CT, published for the Author

Hamilton, A. (1943) Exploring the Dangerous Trades, The Autobiography of Alice Hamilton, Boston, Little, Brown & Co., pp. 294–296, 388

Hamilton, A. & Hardy, H.L. (1974) Industrial Toxicology, 3rd ed., Acton, MA, Publishing Sciences Group, Inc., p. 90

Hancock, T. (1857) Personal Narrative of the Origin and Progress of the Caoutchouc or India-Rubber Manufacture in England, London, Longman, Brown, Green, Longmans & Roberts

HM Government (1922) The Indiarubber Regulations, 1922, dated March 31, 1922, made by the Secretary of State under section 79 of the Factory and Workshop Act, 1901 (1 Edw. 7, c.22), for Certain Processes Incidental to the Manufacture of Indiarubber and of Articles and Goods made wholly or partially of Indiarubber (Statutory Rules and Orders, 1922, No. 329), London, His Majesty's Stationery Office

International Labour Office (1921) Cancer of the Bladder among Workers in Aniline Factories (Studies and Reports, Series F., No. 1), Geneva

Mancuso, T.F. (1963) Tumors of the central nervous system. Industrial considerations. Acta unio int. contra cancrum, 19, 488–489

Mancuso, T.F. (1975) Epidemiological investigation of occupational cancers in the rubber industry. In: Levinson, C., ed., The New Multinational Health Hazards, Geneva, International Chemical Federation, pp. 3–59

Mancuso, T.F. (1976) Problems and perspectives in epidemiological study of occupational health hazards in the rubber industry. Environ. Health Perspect., 17, 21–30

Mancuso, T.F. (1982) Epidemiological study of tumors of the central nervous system. Ann. N.Y. Acad. Sci. (in press)

Mancuso, T.F. & Brennan, M.J. (1970) Epidemiological considerations of cancer of the gallbladder, bile ducts and salivary glands in the rubber industry. J. occup. Med., 12, 333-341

Mancuso, T.F., Ciocco, A. & El-Attar, A.A. (1968) An epidemiological approach to the rubber industry. A study based on departmental experience. J. occup. Med., 10, 213-232

Parkes, G. (1964a) Letters to the Editor: Cancer Research. Lancet, ii, 254-255

Parkes, G. (1964b) Letters to the Editor: Cancer Research. Lancet, ii, 414

Rehn, L. (1895) Bladder tumours in Fuchsine workers (Ger.). Arch. Klin. Chir., 50, 588-600

Schidrowitz, P. & Dawson, T.R., eds (1952) History of the Rubber Industry, Cambridge, W. Heffer & Sons, Ltd

Wallace, D. (1964) Letters to the Editor: Cancer Research. Lancet, ii, 365

Wolf, R.F. (1970) American letter. Peace reigns in Akron for another three years... we hope. Rubber Journal, July, p. 22

Wolf, R.F. (1971) American letter. Rubber health studies start. Rubber Journal, August, p. 27

Reviews of various rubber manufacturing processes are available in Stern (1967) and Blow (1978). Much of the information in this section was obtained from publications of the US Environmental Protection Agency (1980; Foster D. Snell, Inc., 1976).

1. Introduction

The basic manufacturing operations to be found in any rubber factory can be identified and distinguished as follows:

- raw materials handling, weighing and mixing;
- milling;
- extruding and calendering;
- component assembly and building;
- 'curing' or vulcanizing;
- inspection and finishing;
- storage and dispatch.

A typical flow diagram for the manufacture of rubber goods is shown in Figure 3.

(a) Raw materials handling, weighing and mixing

All the materials required for the manufacture of the finished product are assembled. The raw polymer, either natural or synthetic is brought together at this stage with a variety of compounding chemical additives before being introduced into a mixer. The extensive range of chemicals required and the volume of raw material which has to be handled can give rise to substantial quantities of airborne dust.

(b) Milling

From the mixer, the uncured rubber compound usually passes to one or more milling machines, where it is thoroughly blended to ensure an even dispersion of its chemical constituents. At this stage, considerable heat is generated, and, although many improvements have been introduced in recent years, the job of mill operator still involves a considerable degree of physical exertion and exposure to fume arising from the heated compound.

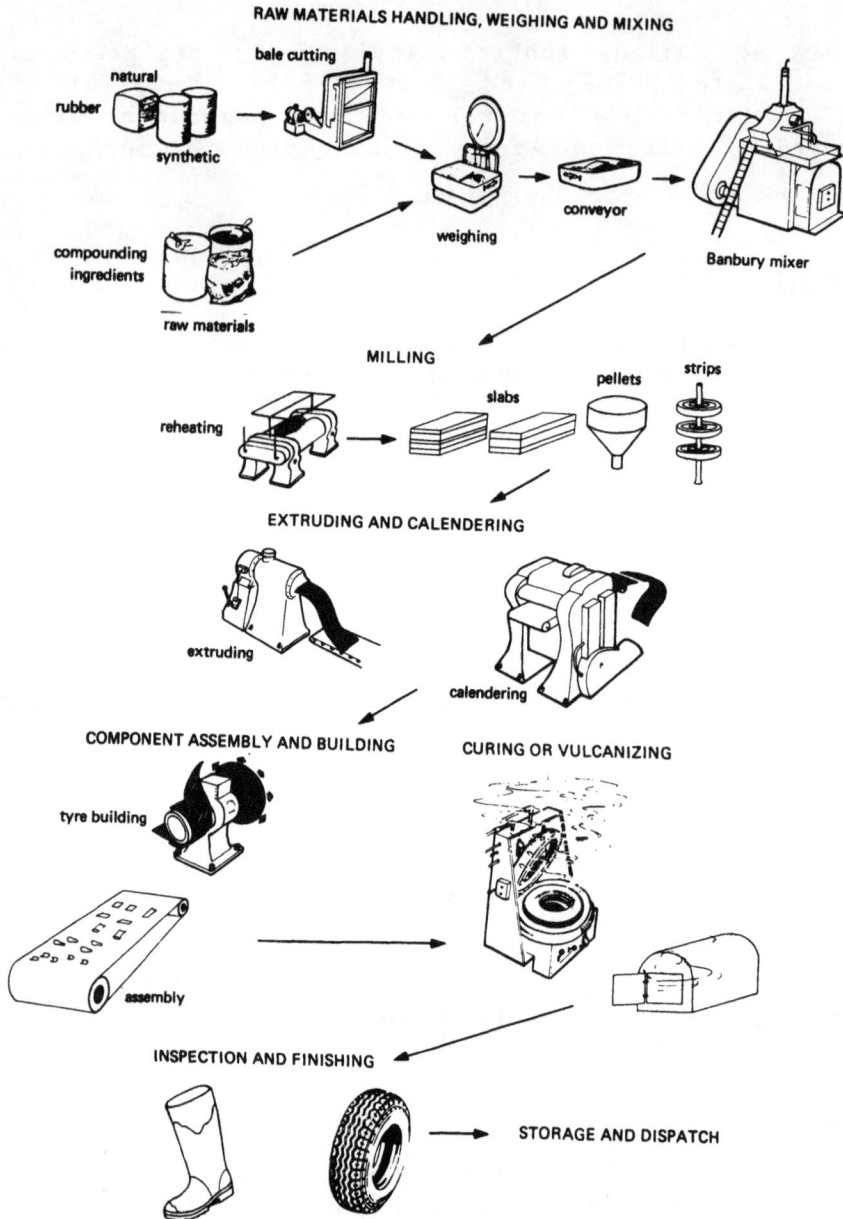

FIG. 3. TYPICAL FLOW DIAGRAM FOR RUBBER GOODS' MANUFACTURE

(c) Extruding and calendering

These processes depend upon the use of machinery and ancillary equipment that largely relieve the operator of heavy physical effort. The extruders force rubber compound through a die into various forms, which are then cut by a guillotine into appropriate lengths suitable for making up. Calenders, multiple-roll milling machines, fed with strips of softened rubber compound, are used to form rubber sheeting or to apply rubber directly onto a woven textile fabric which can then be wound off on to a roll. During such manufacturing operations fumes are often generated.

(d) Component assembly and building

According to the requirements of the finished product, a varying amount of skilled manual work is required in fabrication prior to vulcanization. At this stage, rubber solvents are frequently used, with the possibility of inhalation of solvent vapours or of direct solvent action on the skin of the operator.

(e) 'Curing' or vulcanizing

After fabrication the process of curing or vulcanizing takes place. Heat, usually in the form of steam, is applied to the product in a curing mould, press, autoclave, etc; operators working in the area are exposed both to heat from the presses and to fumes given off from the heated rubber products. Chemical reactions which take place throughout the manufacturing process may give rise to new, more volatile, and possibly more toxic chemicals.

(f) Inspection and finishing

This involves the handling, frequently while still hot, of cured rubber products. It usually requires direct and extensive skin contact with the surface of the finished article (during inspection) and may also involve exposure to vulcanizing fume. Grinding, trimming, repair, painting and cleaning may also involve exposure to rubber dust, fume and solvents.

(g) Storage and dispatch

Large quantities of stored rubber goods may release toxic substances, either as vapours or as constituents of the 'bloom' on the surface of finished goods. In tyre and tube warehouses, N-nitrosamines have been measured in the $\mu g/m^3$ range (see Section V, 2.6).

It will be appreciated that the precise nature of the finished product necessitates some variation in the basic manufacturing operations. Although the stages described above are applicable to the majority of goods manufactured from solid polymer, it should be recognized that a substantial area of production involves the use of liquid latex. This applies to the manufacture of dipped rubber goods (such as rubber gloves and some footwear), foam latex products (such as mattresses, cushions, etc), and extruded thread products (such as elasticated fabrics and surgical hose). These processes are not considered further here, but their relevant features are discussed later, in the appropriate section of the Monograph.

2.   Tyres, tubes, remoulds and retreads

2.1   Tyres

More rubber is used in the production of tyres than in any other segment of the industry. Natural rubber and styrene-butadiene synthetic rubber are much the most frequently used polymers in tyre manufacture. Polybutadiene is, however, now used in some quantity for treads and sidewalls; and halobutyl polymers for inner liners. Since most industrial processes that take place elsewhere in the rubber industry are found in some variant in tyre manufacture, that process is described in some detail, emphasizing those aspects which are of significance to industrial hygiene. The description of a particular manufacturing process generally adequately describes the occupations involved.

(a) Raw materials handling, weighing and mixing

(i) <u>Handling of raw materials</u>: Rubber arrives at a factory in wrapped bales on pallets. The bales may be dusted with an anti-tackifying powder. Although many factories do their own compounding, others may receive partially compounded rubber.

Solid additives may be in the form of powders, flakes or pellets, mostly supplied in bags, drums or other small units. Some are incorporated in rubber, either sheets (masterbatch), which the worker cuts to obtain the desired quantity of additive, or as pelletized predispersions. Carbon black and, occasionally, zinc oxide, arrive in bulk, either loose in tankers or in rigid metal, transportable containers (tote bins), for transfer to a storage and mixer feeding system, or, increasingly, in returnable containers consisting of collapsible rubber bags, which hold up to 4500 kg of material and can be connected directly to the feeding system.

Antioxidant oils are usually received in 55-gallon (208-l) drums. Extender oils may be received in drums, but are more commonly handled in bulk systems, whereby they are transferred from tank cars to heated storage tanks in the mixing area and are pumped directly into the mixers. Solvents may be used to make doughs, solutions and adhesives, and in fabrication and assembly. They are supplied in drums or in tank cars for transfer to storage tanks.

Exposure to dust or fume during the handling of raw materials may result from over-dusted rubber, damage to containers by handling equipment, leaks in conveyor or piping systems used for transferring bulk materials, or spillage from rail cars, tankers and trailers during bulk transport operations.

(ii) <u>Weighing</u>: Carbon black, extender oils and some other bulk materials are commonly measured directly into the mixer by an automatic feed. Dry materials in drums or bags may be loaded by a precompounder into a 'semi-bulk' system for direct weighing into the mixer or for delivery to compounding stations, and exposures may occur at this stage. Since the conveying and control equipment requires frequent servicing, maintenance personnel may also be exposed.

At the compounding stations, materials are hand-weighed into paper or plastic bags on scales, which sometimes have provision for dust control. New automatic weighing stations are being made available, incorporating carousel-type dispensing equipment with an integrated exhaust/extraction system. As materials are often stored in the compounding area in open drums, and bagged materials transferred from bags to drums for weighing, this operation, and the disposal of empty bags, are often quite dusty. Antioxidant oils may be transferred from drums to small plastic bags for weighing, and spillage can occur.

The amount of rubber required for a batch is cut by guillotine. Often, the guillotine, scales and mixer-loading conveyor are combined to form a continuous mixer-feeding line. Preweighed materials from the compounding department may be dumped onto the conveyor or directly into the mixer; or materials may be added in sealed plastic bags.

(iii) Mixing: The Banbury mixer, first introduced in 1916 and used throughout the rubber industry, is an internal, batch-type mixer. Rubber and additives are fed by conveyor or by hand into a hopper and fall into the mixing chamber, where two lobed rotors mix them between the rotors and against the walls of the chamber while pressure is applied from above by a plunger or ram. The chamber is usually water-cooled to reduce heat (although in some operations, the chamber may be steam-heated to reduce the viscosity of the mixture). Mixer capacity ranges from less than 0.5 kg (for laboratory use) to over 400 kg; the most popular production size is 370 pounds (170 kg). With larger mixers, the operation is usually arranged on three levels: bulk materials are stored on the top level so that bulk loading of the mixer is gravity-assisted. The mixer hopper is located on the second level. The mixing-chamber rotor-drive motor and discharge door mechanism are located on a mezzanine between the first and second levels. A typical mixing cycle takes less than half an hour, at the end of which the discharge doors open to drop the batch onto a two-roll mill.

Two types of mixing operations are performed. In first-stage mixing, retarders, antidegradants, processing aids, reinforcing agents and fillers are added to the raw rubber stock; vulcanizing agents and accelerators are omitted, so that the resulting stock can be stored. In the second mixing operation, these materials are added to the first-stage mix along with additional small quantities of other materials. This stock is for immediate use. Mixing temperatures range from 90-180°C, the lower temperature being used for final mixing to prevent premature curing.

Loading of the mixer is liable to be a dusty operation, and almost all Banbury mixers are provided with some means of exhaust ventilation at the hopper. Inadequate maintenance of the ventilation system, leaks from faulty seals, from the bulk charging system and materials spilled during transportation to and from the compounding department contribute to airborne dust exposures, Since no production work is done on the mezzanine, heavy accumulations of dust can lead to exposure of maintenance personnel, unless routine cleaning is carried out.

(b) Milling

The mixer discharges its batch directly onto the rolls of a two-roll mill. (In some operations, an extruder known as a 'transfer mixer' may be used between the Banbury mixer and the mill.) Further mixing takes place on the mill and the stock is cooled to approximately 65-80°C. Since milled stock must be removed, usually by conveyor, this 'open' mixing operation does not lend itself to enclosure for ventilation. Overhead canopy hoods are used instead, with the idea that the hot fumes will rise. However, since mill operators often work directly at the hot mill rolls, cooling fans sometimes are used, which may create cross-drafts which defeat the ventilation system. The mill operator is thus exposed to vapours and aerosols from the hot rubber and may be exposed to dust from the Banbury mixer overhead. In some plants, mill and Banbury mixer operators rotate jobs midway through the shift, or on a daily or weekly basis.

Rubber stock normally comes off the mill in a continuous sheet which is fed by conveyor through an antitackifying dip. Mineral dust slurries and soap solutions are common antitackifying agents, and spillage of the liquid may result in exposure to dust. The dipped rubber sheet is dried, folded and placed on pallets. First-stage rubber is stored; second-stage rubber is ready for fabrication into the components from which the tyre is built: tread and sidewall beads and plies, belts and inner liners.

(c) Extruding and calendering

(i) Extrusion: The tread and sidewall are produced by an extrusion process. Cold final-batch rubber is fed into a two-roll mill, where it is warmed; it is then carried by conveyor to a feed mill and fed into the tread or side-wall extruder.

The tread and sidewall may be manufactured separately or in the same operation. The tread/sidewall extruder laminates the two types of strip to form a tyre tread and two sidewalls. The strips are bonded by heat and pressure generated by a rotating extruder screw. The tread and sidewall may also be formed separately, in similar types of production lines, and the components bonded only when the 'green' (uncured) tyre is constructed.

Extrusion temperatures are generally in the range of 80°C and may result in volatilization of stock constituents. The extruder operator may also be exposed to volatile organic compounds used in nearby operations.

Component parts are assembled with the use of solvent or s-olvent-based adhesives. After extrusion, a cushioning layer (undertread or tread base) is added to the underside of the tread or tread/sidewall combination, and this is tackified, usually by the application of an adhesive, with a felt roller. Solvents typically used include naphtha, heptane, hexane, some isopropanol and toluene. The tread strip is then cooled by air drying on a conveyor and/or by passing through a water bath.

Vapours of solvent evaporating from the container, the application assembly and the tread component as it passes along the conveyor contribute to workers' exposure to organic vapours.

The continuous rubber tread is then cut to the specified length for each tyre series. The tread ends may be tackified by one of two methods: they can be sprayed automatically with an adhesive prior to stacking in trays for transport to the tyre-building area; alternatively, the adhesive can be applied manual-ly, prior to stacking or as the tread is wrapped around the tyre-building drum. Naphtha, hexane and heptane are the solvents typically used; isopropanol and toluene are used less frequently.

Roller and spray adhesive operations may be equipped with local exhaust ventilation; manual adhesive operations usually rely on ambient airflow or general ventilation to reduce concentrations of solvent vapours. Exposure to organic vapours might result from use of excess adhesive, from the container itself and from the tread ends.

Tyre beads are rubber-covered wires which ensure a seal between the tyre and the rim of the wheel on which it is mounted. In general, beads are formed by extruding rubber onto several strands of braided copper or brass-plated steel wire which are then shaped into rings. They may be tackified to ensure proper adhesion to the sidewall when the tyre is built, by dipping, spraying, rolling or swabbing the bead assembly with a solvent-based adhesive. Thus, bead packages or bundles may be immersed into an adhesive vat, then raised and allowed to drip; the beads are then racked by hand for drying. Individual beads may be placed on conveyorized hooks, which dip the beads, allow excess adhesive to run off and carry the beads to a drying area. Solvent may also be applied manually to the assembled bead. In an alternative method, the rubber-coated wire is passed through a trough of adhesive, and a bead is formed from the bonded material. Finally a layer of rubber-coated fabric is often wrapped around the bead and either natural tackiness is relied on for adhesion or the tackifying agent is incorporated into the rubberized fabric wrap. The solvents used are the same as those for tackifying treads, and the same potential exposure exists.

Adhesives for bead dipping, tread and sidewall bonding, and those used in tyre building, spraying, repairing, etc, may be prepared in a separate building (cement or solution house). Solvents are usually stored indoors, in tanks or drums, and are prepared in mixing tanks ranging in size from 200-500 litres. Local exhaust ventilation may be provided at the mixing tanks, the storage tanks, or both, but this is not invariable. Dilution ventilation is employed primarily for fire control: air is exhausted from the floor level, where heavier organic vapours tend to collect, and clean air may be provided near mixing areas. The highest exposures occur during measuring or mixing of solvents at open tanks. Spills, the accumulation of solvent-soaked rags and other poor housekeeping practices may contribute to ambient exposure levels, which may exceed acceptable industrial hygiene standards for mixtures of organic solvents.

(ii) <u>Calendering</u>: Plies and belts are the body of the tyre; they give it strength and stability, and are composed of rubber reinforced with synthetic fabric, steel wire or glass fibre. The inner liner is an unsupported rubber sheet which makes the finished tyre airtight. Plies, belts and liners are made on a calender, a multiple-roll mill which produces stock of carefully controlled thickness.

First, a roll of fabric (normally, rayon or other synthetic fiber) is spliced, either by adhesive or by a high-speed sewing machine, onto the end of a previously processed roll. This continuous sheet of fabric is then dipped under controlled tension into a tank containing latex. Solutions of formaldehyde, caustic soda and resorcinol, or other synthetic adhesive combinations may be added to the latex to improve bonding characteristics. After dipping, the fabric travels past either rotating beater bars or vacuum suction lines and then through a drying oven to remove excess solvent. Many tyre manufacturers purchase fabric that has been latex-dipped.

The latex-dipped fabric is then passed through a calendering machine, which impregnates it with rubber. With four-roll calenders, both sides of the fabric can be coated simultaneously, and these are the most commonly used type of calender. The plasticity of the fabric is maintained by steam-heating the calender rolls, typically to temperatures of 70-80°C. Emissions from calendering are therefore similar in character and magnitude to those from milling or extrusion.

The rubberized fabric is now cooled and cut to the proper angle and length. These strips are wound on a roll, separated by a reusable cloth liner, and conveyed to the tyre-building work stations.

(<u>d</u>) <u>Component assembly and building</u>

Passenger car and lorry tyres are built as cylinders on a collapsible, rotating drum. First, the inner liner is wrapped around the drum, followed by a variable number of rubber-impregnated fabric plies. Next, the edges of the fabric and inner liner are wrapped around the bead assemblies. Then, pressure is applied, manually or automatically, from the tread centre out to the beads in order to expel air trapped between the assembled components. Then belts, made of fabric, steel or glass fibre, are laid onto the cord. Finally, the tread and sidewall components are wrapped around the assembled components and are bonded. In the construction of large, cross-country tyres for use in agriculture, mining and construction, the tread may be built up by continuous wrapping of a narrow, extruded strip of rubber. Application of an adhesive to the tread end at the extruder is thereby eliminated, but extensive 'swabbing' of solvent onto the components is common. These operations produce an uncured or 'green' tyre.

There are three variations to the method of assembling tyres. In one-stage tyre building, all of the components are assembled on one machine. In the two-stage operation the carcass is constructed at one site, and at a second site, the subassembly is rechecked and the belts, tread and sidewall are applied and bonded. In three-stage tyre building, carcass assembly, belt/-tread construction and final tyre assembly are each carried out at a different station. Cross-ply tyres are usually made in single-stage construction, and radial tyres by two- and three-stage building methods; however, exposures are reported to be similar in the two types of operation.

Organic solvents, such as naphtha, heptane, hexane, isopropanol, methanol and toluene, are normally used during building to tackify the rubberized tyre components, either because they have lost natural tack or because a solvent is required for a particular tyre type. The purpose is to keep the tyre components together prior to curing.

Local exhaust ventilation is rarely found at tyre building operations. Potential sources of exposure at such stations are the solvent container and applicator and tackified tyre components. Exposure may vary, however, since the quantity of solvent used for component assembly can be altered by the machine operator, and solvent use varies with the type of tyre produced by a particular process, with the type of operation (one-, two- or three-stage) and with the machine used for each step of two- or three-stage tyre assembly processes.

(e) Curing or vulcanizing

Prior to curing, the assembled, unvulcanized tyre is inspected and repaired if necessary. It is then placed in a ventilated booth where it is sprayed on the inside with band-ply lubricants and on the outside with mould-release agents. Band-ply lubricants allow air to be removed from the inside of the tyre as the moulding/curing bladder expands. Mould-release agents prevent the outside of the tyre from sticking to the mould after curing. Either organic solvent-based lubricants or water-based suspensions of silicone solids may be used for outside sprays. Solvent-based lubricants are much more common than water-based lubricants for the inside sprays. The solvents used include naphtha, hexane, heptane, isopropanol and toluene. The ventilation system in the spray booth may be defeated by poor spraying technique or by improper location of cooling fans. Evaporation of solvents from coated tyres and poor housekeeping may contribute to exposure.

The tyre is then moulded and vulcanized in a curing press (Fig. 4). In this process, the tyre is shaped, the tread design created and the chemical cross-linking of the rubber is triggered, allowing the tyre to hold its shape. In a manual press, the tyre is loaded and unloaded from the mould by hand; however, mechanically assisted loading and unloading with automatic presses is far more common in tyre factories today.

The tyre is positioned in the mould, and a rubber bladder is inflated inside it so that it takes the characteristic doughnut shape. As the bladder inflates, the mould is closed. Steam is applied to the outside of the tyre, through the mould and to the inside. Excess rubber and trapped air are forced out through 'weepholes' in the mould. The time, pressure and temperatures of the cure are controlled; then, the press is cooled, the bladder is deflated, and the tyre, complete with grooved tread and raised lettering, is removed from the mould. Curing usually takes 20-60 min at a temperature of 100-200°C. After removal from the mould, some cured tyres (mostly those of cross-ply construction) are sometimes placed on a former, inflated and allowed to cool under controlled conditions (post-cure inflation, PCI).

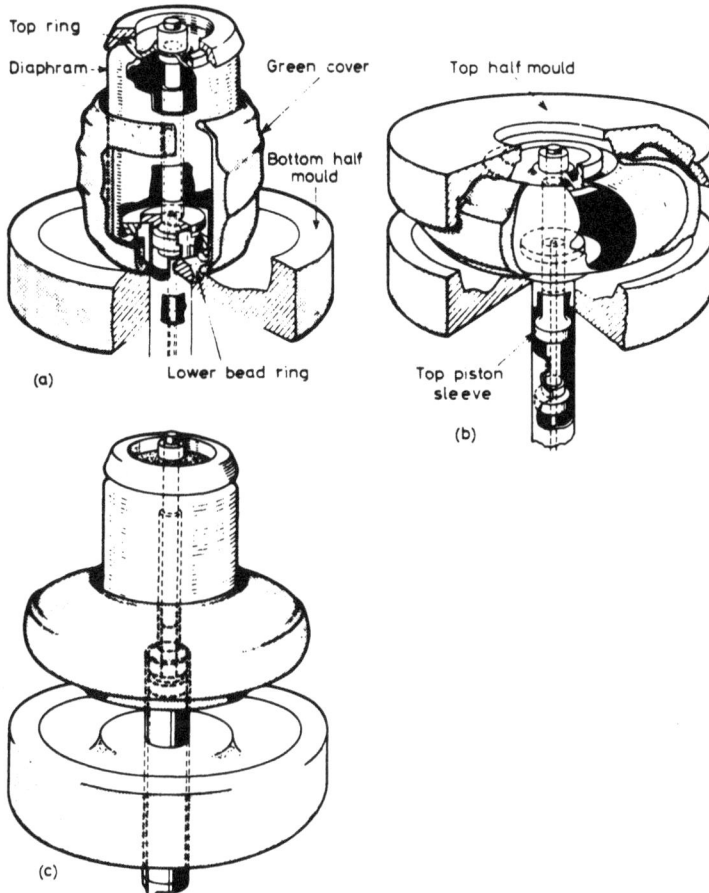

FIG. 4.   AN AUTOMATIC (BAGOMATIC) PRESS
           (From Morton & Quinton, 1978)

(a) diaphragm bladder assembly at tyre–loading stage;
(b) final tyre–shaping during mould closure;
(c) diaphragm bladder stripped from tyre prior to removal of tyre
     from press

The major problem in most curing areas is that all freshly moulded tyres, as they are ejected from the presses discharge substantial volumes of fume into the atmosphere and continue to do so as they are transported to the finishing area. Another source of exposure is the heated, contaminated air emitted through the curing mould weepholes. Curing presses are rarely provided with local exhaust ventilation. In some curing rooms, contaminated air is exhausted above the presses and conveyors, and fresh air is supplied where the curing operators work. Short-circuiting of the supply and exhaust air is prevented by dropping a curtain from the ceiling to the top of the press line, enclosing the area above the presses and the conveyor. When combined with automatic presses, this system can be quite effect-ive in reducing exposures of curing operators. It is still common, however, to find curing rooms in which no attempt has been made to reduce exposures through proper design of dilution ventilation. The positioning and density of the curing presses and the building in which they are installed are factors of major importance in controlling environmental exposure.

(f)   Inspection and finishing

After curing, the tyres are inspected for faults. Inspectors are frequently exposed to substantial quantities of curing fume from freshly moulded tyres, which may be delivered and stacked up near them while still giving off fume.

Rubber whiskers or 'flash', formed from excess rubber that was cured in the weepholes of the mould, are removed by a grind-ing machine or manually with a knife. Blemishes are ground out, cleaned with solvent and refilled with a cold-curing compound. Most tyre treads are then buffed and ground to ensure proper balance. Some tyres may receive decals or other manufacturer markings, with the use of organic solvent-based inks, paints or sprays. Finishing operations thus result in exposure to rubber dust and solvents. Buffing and grinding, in particular, involve risks due to exposure to fume, dust and rubber particles.

(g)   Storage and dispatch

For storing of tyres, powered tractors, forklifts and mechanical conveying systems aid the warehouse workers, but there is some manual handling of the tyres. A recent, surprising observation was the discovery of levels of several $\mu g/m^3$ N-nitrosamines in the air of tyre warehouses (see Section V, 2.6).

2.2   Tubes

Tube manufacture is similar to tyre manufacture, and the health aspects of the process are essentially the same. One distinction of inner tube compounding is the use of large quantities of butyl rubber; also different accelerators are used.

Mixing and milling are carried out as described above. The compounded rubber is then fed into an extruder via a warm-up mill and strip-feed mill and formed into a continuous cylinder. To keep the inner walls from sticking together, a mineral powder (traditionally, talc) is sprayed inside the tube as it is formed. Very heavy exposure to talcs of unknown fibre content undoubtedly occurred in the past; today, talc has been partially replaced with calcium carbonate, and exposures have been much reduced by the use of liquid slurries. The tube is then passed through a water cooling tank, the water is blown off, and a lubricating agent is sprayed onto the outside.

Once extruded, the tube is cut to length. The ends are then spliced together, and a valve is attached.

The curing cycle is very much shorter than that required for a tyre, and a line of curing presses making tubes opens and closes much more frequently than with tyres. Substantial amounts of fume may thus be released into the atmosphere as the tubes are extracted from the moulds and carried away on a conveyor system.

2.3   Remoulds and retreads

Remoulding and retreading are processes for replacing the worn tread on sound tyre carcasses. Whether independent or owned by rubber manufacturers, most remould and retread shops are fairly small, employing 10-30 workers. Some shops operate in conjunction with new-tyre warehouses.

Used tyres are inspected, and damaged carcasses rejected; the sound tyres are then buffed to remove the old tread. Buffing produces substantial quantities of both fume and dust; ventilation more easily controls dust than fume. Minor defects are ground out by hand, cleaned with solvent and patched with a compound rich in natural rubber.

In the remoulding process, unvulcanized tread rubber is applied to a prepared carcass, and the tyre is heated to cure and mould the tread design and to adhere it to the carcass. In the retreading process, a prevulcanized tread is applied to a prepared carcass over an uncured cushion of gum. The tread is bonded to the carcass by heating the tyre and curing the gum. Rubber for either process is normally produced at tyre factories, and the exposures are as described above. Application of an adhesive to the undertread and application of the uncured gum may be done either by a supplier or by a retread shop.

When an adhesive is applied to the tyre carcass and allowed to dry, application is generally done in a ventilated spray booth. In some operations, the process is automated and completely enclosed during the actual spraying. In poorly designed or maintained bonding operations, solvent exposure may occur during the spraying itself or during handling of freshly sprayed tyres. In retreading, the prevulcanized tread is then cut to length, an adhesive is applied to the tread ends, and the tread is applied to the carcass.

In the remoulding process, the tyre is moulded and vulcanized in a curing press similar to those used in new-tyre curing. In retreading, the tyre is heated to cure the gum cushion; because only the gum cushion and the splice are cured, less curing fume is released than in remoulding. In one, older method, the tread was pressed onto the tyre with a metal band, and curing was done in an ambient-pressure, hot-air chamber. In another method, the tyre was encased in a flexible rubber envelope and immersed in hot water under pressure. With both methods, several tyres were cured at a time. In current methods, a curing tube is generally used to apply pressure from the inside of the tyre, and steam is circulated through an unpatterned mould, flexible rubber bladders, or against an envelope applied to the tyre itself. Each tyre is cured in an individual chamber, although several chambers may be mounted on a single machine.

3. General rubber goods

3.1 Introduction

The basic principles of the manufacture of miscellaneous rubber goods are similar to those involved in tyre manufacture, although factories producing miscellaneous rubber goods are more likely to use non-automated methods for handling raw materials. Variations that occur at the beginning of the process – handling of raw materials, mixing and milling – are generally due to the fact that smaller and much more varied batches are prepared than in the tyre industry. Thus, the use of open mills for mixing (rather than internal mixers) is still retained for smaller batch sizes and is considered necessary for closer quality control of certain special materials. When open mills are used, operators are exposed to large amounts of dust containing the various rubber compounding substances. Many manufacturers purchase rubber which has already been masterbatched (partially mixed), and some buy the final-mix rubber, dispensing with mixing altogether.

Fabrication processes vary widely, but they can be broadly divided into building and moulding methods. As in tyre manufacture, building involves the assembly of previously extruded and calendered components. The level of machine assistance varies, but many building operations require extensive manual labour involving direct contact with rubber components and adhesives. Building is followed by a separate curing operation. Moulding methods, by contrast, combine forming and curing into a single operation. There are three variations of this technique: compression, transfer and injection moulding. Compression and transfer moulding involve use of hydraulic presses with steam- or electrically-heated platens. In compression moulding, the rubber is compressed between the two faces of the mould. In transfer moulding, it is forced out of a main cavity, the 'pot', to flow into the cavities of the moulding section. In injection moulding, the stock is extruded directly into the mould. Transfer moulding is used when the rubber is to be bonded to a metal support or is to enclose a metallic insert. In this type of moulding, there may be a greater amount of waste rubber than in other types of forming operations because it is not possible to empty the 'pot' completely. This gives rise to a cured slab of waste rubber, which may increase the operator's exposure to curing fume. Injection moulding, a more recent technique, obviates the problem of excess cured rubber, because only the material in the mould cavity becomes cured. In this type of operation, extreme care has to be used in the formulation, mixing and compounding of the stock; and, generally, it requires the use of more expensive ingredients. Exposure to curing fume commonly occurs during the stripping of hot components from the mould.

Variations in building and moulding techniques, curing and finishing generally reflect the form and use of the final product.

3.2 Wire and cable (largely derived from Rowley, 1978)

Elastomers are used both to insulate electrical wire and to jacket (or sheathe) and protect the insulation. Those used include natural rubber, styrene–butadiene rubber, butyl and ethylene propylene rubbers of both copolymer and terpolymer types. Polyethylene and ethylene–vinyl acetate, originally used only in communications wire and cable, are now also cross–linked and used in other wire and cable applications. Chlorosulphonated polyethylene, neoprene, fluoroelastomers and silicone elastomers are also used in specialized applications. Neoprene, because of its good weathering properties, oil resistance, flame resistance, and mechanical strength, is currently the most widely used jacketing material. Lead compounds have been commonly used as compounding ingredients for all of these materials, especially the vinyls, and significant exposures may occur during weighing and mixing.

Rubber coverings are applied to wire or cable by one of two basic methods – conventional extrusion and continuous vulcanization. Conventional extrusion is that in which extrusion and vulcanization are separate operations. Usually, dual extruders are used, permitting the simultaneous application of insulation compound and sheath compound (see Fig. 5). To prevent distortion prior to vulcanization, the uncured wire or cable may be extruded into a pen containing a supporting bed of soapstone or similar material or cooled in a water bath or trough containing a slurry or emulsion of antistick agent. Larger size cables may be taped before cure to prevent flattening, and lead covers are frequently applied to serve as the mould during vulcanization. (See also 'hose manufacture', below.) Curing is done in an open steam vulcanizer, with direct contact between the steam and the cable.

FIG. 5. PRINCIPLE OF SYNCHRONIZED DUAL EXTRUSION MACHINE (From Pollard, 1971)

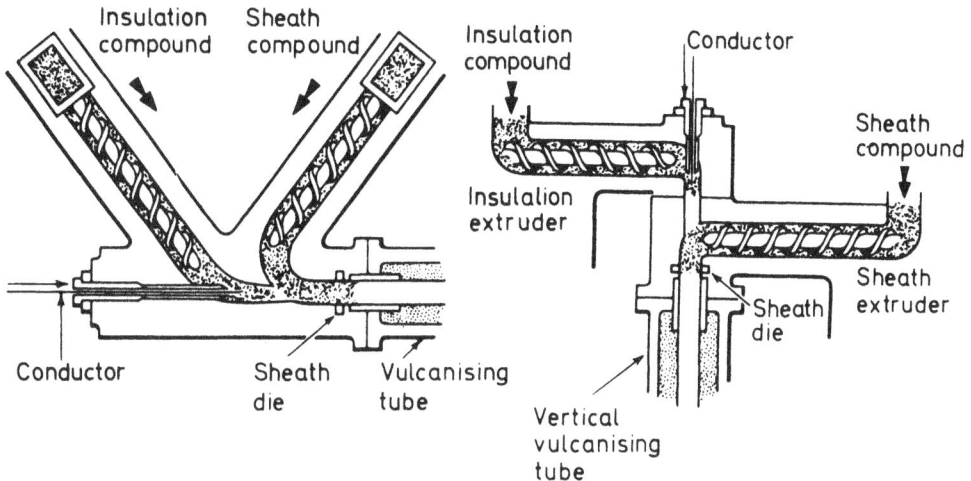

In continuous vulcanization operations (Fig. 6), the wire or cable goes through an extruder, where it is covered with insulation, as above, and then directly into a curing tube in which high-pressure steam is confined. The vulcanized product may be discharged into the atmosphere through mechanical seals or through a water seal in which pressure is maintained just below the steam pressure in the adjacent curing tube.

After curing, the cable is labelled, and samples are tested for the conducting properties of the wire and the insulating properties of the rubber. The cable is then coiled, packaged and prepared for shipment.

3.3 Belting

Natural and styrene-butadiene rubber are among the most common elastomers used in the manufacture of belts; neoprene (polychloroprene) may be used where oil resistance is required; and other elastomers are used to provide wear-resistant surfaces

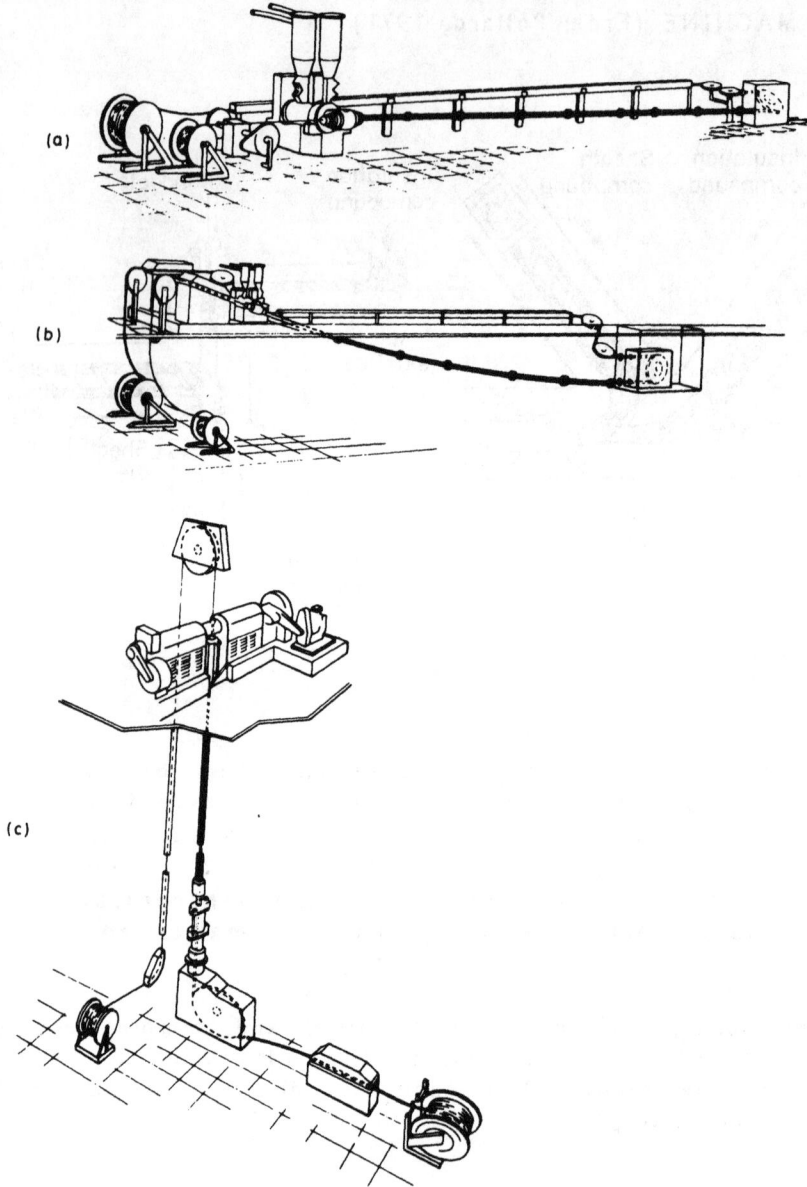

FIG. 6. CONTINUOUS VULCANIZATION OF
         CABLES (From Pollard, 1971)

(a) horizontal continuous vulcanization;
(b) catenary continuous vulcanization;
(c) vertical continuous vulcanization, showing tower

for conveyor belts. Use of ethylene-propylene terpolymer and epi-chlorohydrin in belt covers increases the temperature range and extends the service life of conveyor belts used with high temper-atures. Natural rubber, isoprene, nitrile and butyl rubbers continue to be used generally in conveyor belting for a wide range of services, while silicone and fluoroelastomers are used in special cases where extreme heat or solvent conditions warrant the use of these premium materials (Wade, 1978).

Milling and calendering operations are essentially similar to those used to produce calendered stock in the tyre industry. Cotton and synthetic textiles dominate, but for special purposes, such as heat resistance, asbestos, glass and aromatic polyamide fibres have been used. Sophisticated, heavily loaded belts for long haulage often include steel cable.

The flat belt components – calendered gum and coated fabric – are assembled in the proper sequence and bonded together with a pressurized roller. As in tyre building, significant exposure to solvent can occur. 'Cut-edge' transmission belting, the main type manufactured, is then slit by machine to the required widths and lengths; 'folded-edge' belts are made in narrow widths, with the outer plies folded around a central core to form a jacket. End-less belts are built on a two-pulley building machine, similar to an extended tyre-building machine. Spliceable belting is assem-bled on a building table; its length is limited only by the prac-tical size of the wind-up spool (Neller, 1978).

Vulcanization of flat belting is carried out either in a press or in a continuous-drum curing machine (Fig. 7). Flat-platen presses, up to 18 m in length, are used; several lengths may run side by side on the same platen, and the use of stacked platens can further increase the capacity of the press. These presses are rarely ventilated by a local exhaust system, and substantial exposure to fume can occur. Two continuous drum curing machines in common use are the Beistoff and the Rotocure, in which the belt is fed between a large, heated curing drum and a tension belt which holds the belt around the circumference of the drum. This system lends itself more easily than the flat press to the control of fume. Curing may also be used to splice belting stock to increase its length or to produce an endless belt (Wade, 1978).

FIG. 7. DRUM MACHINE FOR CONTINUOUS VULCANIZATION
(From Crowther & Edmondson, 1971)

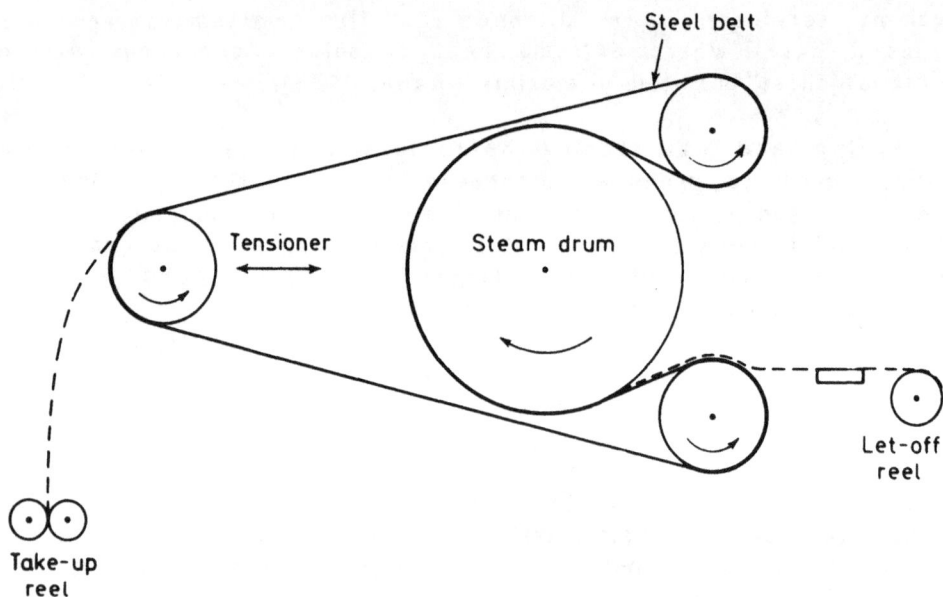

Steel belt

Tensioner

Steam drum

Let-off reel

Take-up reel

The V-belt building operation is quite similar to tyre building but much less complicated. Layers of calendered rubber stock are wrapped around a metal bar; a reinforcing cord is spiralled around the wrapped calendered stock, and additional rubber sheeting is applied to cover the reinforcing cord. This assembly may then be cured in an autoclave and the completed tube lathe cut and skived to form the completed belts. Alternatively, when a cover is required over the total belt surface, the uncured tube may be cut and skived to uncured belts, which are wrapped in special machinery with a thin layer of rubberized, friction-calendered textile. Such uncured belts are then consolidated and cured by autoclave or press moulding on specially designed moulds or in unique, small Rotocure-type machines.

3.4 Hose

The elastomers and compounding ingredients used in the manufacture of rubber hose are similar to those used in belt-making. The compounding, mixing and calendering steps are identical, and it is common for these processes to be carried out on the same pieces of equipment in facilities designed for the manuacture of both belt and hose.

Hose generally consists of an extruded liner tube, a re-inforcing carcass, generally of calendered fabric or individually wound cords, and a cover to protect and identify the hose. Several different processes may be used to assemble these components: machine wrapping, hand wrapping, the lead-sheath process and minor variants of each of these processes.

(a) Machine-wrapped ply hose

In this type of construction, bias cut rubber-coated fabric is produced exactly as in the manufacture of cross-ply tyres.

The hose is built by wrapping the required number of plies generated by calendering and bias cutting around an extruded rubber tube, which is mounted on a mandrel for internal support. Finally, the plies are covered with a calendered rubber sheet. The assembled hose is then wrapped in a reusable cotton or nylon wrap, which provides pressure during curing.

(b) Hand-built hose

For this type of hose, a chuck-driven steel mandrel is used for support. For sizes up to 100 mm, the inner tube is produced by extrusion and slipped over the mandrel. Larger diameters of tube are constructed by wrapping layers of unsupported calendered rubber sheets by hand around the hose by rotating the mandrel. Hoses made by this process may also be reinforced with wire. The position of the wire in relation to the plies is dictated by the service to which it is to be put. Afterwards, a rubber cover is applied. Before the hose is cured, several criss-crossed reusable nylon or cotton wraps are applied under tension to provide pressure during curing.

(c) Lead-sheathed or moulded hose

In the manufacture of moulded hose, strands of reinforcing wire or fibre are braided or spiralled around a firm, unsupported inner tube. The hose is then passed through an extruder which applies a seamless outer cover. It is then encased in lead, which is extruded in semi-molten condition around the hose.

Hoses are cured in direct-steam autoclaves. The cotton or nylon wrap is then removed from machine-wrapped or hand-built hose and rolled up for further use; with lead-sheathed hose, the lead is stripped and remelted for subsequent reuse. Significant exposures to lead dust can occur as the lead is scored and stripped from the hose. Workers who clean the oxide from the surface of molten lead in pots may be exposed to high levels of lead oxides. Workers who handle lead in any of these operations may have slightly elevated blood lead levels.

As batch vulcanization of rubber hose is energy- and time-consuming, several methods of continuous vulcanization have been developed. The oldest method is continuous steam tube vulcanization, a technique borrowed from the wire and cable industry. Hose, built on a flexible mandrel is passed through a long small-diameter tube into which high-pressure steam is introduced.

A second technique for continuous vulcanization is the fluid-bed continuous vulcanization system (FBCV), wherein hose is passed through a long, narrow bed of small glass spheres, which are transformed into a pseudo-liquid by the passage of hot air or steam up through the bed. The hose thus receives the heat energy necessary to effect vulcanization. The FBCV method has evolved so that consolidation is effected by variations in compounding, including the use of different cure activators, different process aids and the addition of dessicants to absorb moisture present in the compounds. A natural outgrowth of this technique is the pressurized unit, which is essentially a compromise between steam vulcanization and basic FBCV methods (Williams, 1978).

Some supplies of glass beads used in the FBCV process bear labels warning of the presence of free silica. Dust is generated by abrasion during the fluidization process, and workers may be exposed.

Several methods have been developed for the continuous vulcanization of lead-sheathed moulded hose: air, low-pressure steam, hot liquid and molten heat-transfer salts (usually mixtures of sodium or potassium nitrate and nitrite) have been used as the heating medium. Currently, microwave heating and irradiation vulcanization techniques are being developed, both of which will require adjustment to the formulations of the compounds used (Williams, 1978).

3.5 Ebonite

Ebonite (vulcanite, or hard rubber, as it is known in the US) is a rubber containing large amounts of sulphur and generally heavily reinforced with anthracite coal dust, limestone (calcium carbonate) and/or reclaimed hard-rubber dust. Styrene-butadiene rubber is the most commonly used elastomer, although natural, nitrile or neoprene rubber may be used.

Batches are typically prepared in an internal mixer and conveyed to a warm-feed extruder, where the screw-action of the extruder mixes the batch further. A thick ribbon of rubber is extruded and cut into slugs for moulding. When compounded from latices, hard rubber can be sprayed or dipped to provide a protective coating or lining for chemical tanks, etc; for most applications however, hard rubber is moulded. It is used in the manufacture of battery cases, bowling balls, caster wheels, steering wheels, electrical equipment (Cooper, 1978) and as an interlayer in bonding rubber to metal (Heinisch, 1974).

Curing times and temperatures vary widely (from 5 min to 15 h; from 100 to 200°C) depending on the compound and the form of the final product. Certain precautions are necessary when vulcanizing thick articles because of the evolution of hydrogen sulphide gas.

After moulding and curing, parts are trimmed to remove flash and inspected.

3.6 Rubber footwear

Rubber footwear includes rubber-soled canvas shoes and waterproof boots and shoes.

The primary elastomer is natural rubber, but lower-cost synthetics such as isoprenes, styrene-butadienes and polybutadienes may also be used. Conventional compounding and mixing methods are used, but in the production of white canvas goods, oxides of zinc, titanium and magnesium replace carbon black, and much greater care is taken to prevent contamination and discolouration of the stock. Extruded strip, calendered gum and rubber-coated fabrics are produced for construction of the upper part of the shoe and are often shipped to a separate facility for cutting and assembly.

The components of the uppers are assembled on a foot-shaped 'last'. Rubber stock, specially compounded with sodium bicarbonate or azodicarbon amide blowing agents, is extruded to produce the foamed inner sole, and scrap from reprocessed rubberized fabric is used to make the insole 'rag'. These are adhered to the uppers with hot-melt glues, latex adhesives or solvent-based bonding agents. Where rubber is joined to rubber or to rubberized fabric, a curing-type adhesive is used, which is usually manufactured at the plant from compounded rubber dissolved in naphtha, hexane, toluene, etc, mixed with sulphur or sulphur compounds.

The soles for hand-built footwear are formed by calendering or moulding. They are deflashed and buffed, treated with a bonding agent, and adhered to the upper by a bottom press. In the case of machine-built footwear, the sole is moulded directly to the upper.

Shoes are cured on racks in a hot-air tunnel vulcanizer or autoclave. The process takes 1 to 1 1/2 h at about 130°C under a pressure of 1.4–2.1 kg/cm². Large amounts of fume are released into the atmosphere during removal of racks of shoes from the autoclave. Anhydrous ammonia may be injected into the oven or autoclave to complete the cure: this produces surface gloss and eliminates the residual tackiness associated with rubber that is cured conventionally. About 5–10 kg of ammonia are used for every thousand pairs of shoes cured. At the end of the curing cycle, the ammonia/air mixture is vented to the atmosphere. Some shoes are cured without ammonia, when the tackiness of the product is not important or when the compounding recipe can be modified to eliminate the tackiness. Steam is not used for curing because, in many cases, the steam would stain the canvas parts of the shoe.

3.7   Food-processing equipment

The manufacturing techniques used in the production of rubber items intended for contact with food are not unique. Tubing is extruded, proofed fabric containers are calendered or dipped into latex and assembled, gaskets are die-cut and moulded, etc. Common polymers are used for these products. The compounding of these materials, however, must be carefully controlled for health reasons, and the selection of both elastomers and additives is often regulated by law. US Food and Drug Administration regulations governing 'Rubber articles intended for repeated use', 'Closures with sealing gaskets for food containers', and 'Antioxidants and/or stabilizers for polymers' are given in the US Code of Federal Regulations (US Food & Drug Administration, 1980). In the Federal Republic of Germany, recommendation XXI of the Federal Health Authority (B.G.A.) controls the composition of rubber articles intended for contact with foodstuffs.

3.8   Aircraft deicing equipment

Deicers remove or prevent the buildup of ice on critical surfaces of airplanes, helicopters, etc. Pneumatic deicers have been produced for some 50 years. They form part of the leading edge of wings, stabilizers, etc., and consist of parallel tubes of rubber-coated fabric (generally nylon) covered with sheet rubber. The tubes are inflated with air; when they are deflated, they flex and break free any ice that has formed. Electric deicers are used on propellers, helicopter rotors and around air intakes, and consist of electrical heating elements sandwiched between double layers of sheet rubber. Heating the deicer prevents the formation of ice or melts any ice that has formed.

The deicer assembly plant receives sheet rubber, coated fabric and bonding agents which have been prepared at other locations. Natural and neoprene rubber are the major elastomers used in producing these components, although small amounts of chlorobutyl rubber may occasionally be used; and standard internal mill mixing methods are used. Coated fabrics are prepared either by dipping into resorcinol-formaldehyde latex or by calender frictioning. Sheet gum is calendered to the required thickness. The bonding agent is prepared by dissolving rubber in a solvent (naphtha); it may be further diluted at the deicer assembly plant.

The deicer is assembled on a flat metal form, which is coated with a bonding agent, generally applied by roller. Sheeted gum, cut to the required size, is applied to the metal to form the outer surface of the deicer. Sewn or folded tubes are assembled and bonded on top of the sheeted gum. Considerably more manual work is required to assemble the individual folded tubes than the multiple sewn tubes; the change to sewn tubes has therefore reduced workers' exposure to solvents. The parallel tubes are connected by a manifold tube, held in place by a bonding agent or by Velcro. More bonding agent may be applied to the top surface of the tubes, and a final sheet of gum is placed on top of the assembly. The top surface of the sheet becomes the inside surface of the deicer, which is attached to the wing, stabilizer, etc. An impression fabric is placed on this surface, and during curing the pattern of the fabric is transferred to the gum, creating a rough surface to improve adherence to the metal of the aircraft. Several deicers of simple design can be assembled per shift, while more complex designs may require two or more shifts for assembly.

The assembled deicer is placed in a curing blanket which is evacuated to compress the components during the cure. The units are then placed on racks, which are rolled into a steam vulcanizer where heat and pressure are applied for 1-2 h. After curing, the blanket and impression fabric are removed, and the deicer is stripped from the metal; valves are installed and cured in place with small plate heaters.

The steps in assembling electric deicers are generally similar. The heating element consists of copper resistance wire arranged in a zig-zag pattern on sheeted gum stock; this unit is assembled on a wire-winding jig. In the early 1970s, an etched metal resistance element was introduced. The element is sandwiched between the bottom gum stock and a second sheet of rubber. The unit, approximately 30-cm square, is then ready for assembly.

As with the pneumatic deicer, sheeted gum stock is cemented to a flat metal form. As many as thirty deicers are then laid out on the gum stock, and these are covered with another sheet of rubber. Very little bonding agent is used in the building of electrical deicers. The assembled deicers are placed in a curing blanket and cured in a steam vulcanizer. After curing, the blanket is removed, the deicers are stripped from the metal, and the individual deicers are separated in a die-cutter. Each unit is examined by fluoroscopy for broken wires; assembly of the lead wires is completed; and electrical resistance is checked. Complete assembly of a unit (not including curing time) takes 1-2 h.

3.9   Automobile parts (seals, mountings, bushings)   (largely derived from Walter, 1976)

Other rubber components of automobiles are hoses, body seals, bearings and mountings, bellows joints, sleeves, and engine and transmission seals. These parts may be exposed to high temperature, continual vibration, petrol, lubricating or transmission oils, antifreeze and brake fluids. The elastomers are chosen accordingly: styrene-butadiene and natural rubbers are used for body seals; chloroprene rubber and ethylene-propylene terpolymer are replacing the former types for manufacture of seals exposed to the atmosphere. Natural rubber is used in the manufacture of bearings and mountings, but where oil resistance is required, significant amounts of nitrile, styrene-butadiene and polyurethane materials are preferred. Natural, styrene-butadiene and chloroprene rubbers are used in making sleeves over the drive shaft tunnel or on the steering column, in dust seal sleeves on electrical components, on brake and clutch cylinders and on other hydraulic components, where there is little, if any, contact with oil-based lubricants, or where contact is with hydraulic fluid based on polyglycol. Chloroprene and soft poly-vinylchloride can be used for grease-filled sleeves on steering rods and gear levers and on axle joints. Nitrile rubber is the most common material used for engine and transmission seals, although polyacrylate, silicone and fluoroelastomers are chosen for some sealing applications.

The shape of the final product determines the forming and curing method used: flat gaskets are die-cut from flat calendered stock; long strip seals may be either press-moulded or extruded. O-rings may be produced by cutting a tube of rubber, which is made by extrusion or building on a mandrel and curing in an autoclave. With some compounds the cutting process is lubricated with water; when dry cutting is done, a considerable amount of fine rubber dust and smoke may be generated. O-rings may also be press-moulded.

Bearings and mountings are generally moulded parts and often include metal components. To ensure a good rubber-to-metal bond, the metal parts must be thoroughly cleaned, usually with tri-chloroethane or a similar degreasing solvent, and may subsequent-ly be sandblasted. The metal parts are then sprayed or brush-painted with a bonding agent and allowed to dry. The prepared metal part and a rubber blank are placed into the mould cavity and mated, shaped and cured in the moulding operation.

Deflashing may be done by cutting or grinding; die-cutting can be used to remove flash from some parts. Alternatively, most rubber compounds can be frozen to a brittle state with liquid carbon dioxide, dry ice or liquid nitrogen in a tumbling barrel; the tumbling action then breaks thin, frozen flash from the piece before thicker sections are frozen. In a variation of this process, a grit blast is used to break off the flash while the parts are being tumbled (Anderson, 1978).

4. Proofed rubber fabrics, adhesives and sealants

4.1 Proofed rubber fabrics (largely derived from West, 1978)

A number of elastomers and polymers are used in the manu-facture of proofed rubber fabrics, e.g., natural rubber, styrene-butadiene rubber, nitrile, neoprene, chlorosulphonated polyethylene, polysulphide, butyl, silicone and polyacrylic types. Other polymers such as polytetrafluoroethene (Teflon), vinyls, urethanes and phenolics are also used.

In the past, substrates were generally limited to various types of cotton; however now, nylon, polyester, fibre-glass, asbestos and blends of those fabrics are also used. Non-woven substrates have been introduced in the last 10-15 years. Woven fabrics used in the coating industry are generally treated before use to remove finishes that may have been applied to the fibres during spinning and weaving, and to stabilize the fibres and minimize shrinking at the processing temperatures used by coated fabric manufacturers.

Special fabrics may be supplied by textile finishers and weavers for various product applications. Some such fabrics are treated with special finishes to give better adhesion, weather resistance or mildew resistance. Many coating manufacturers have their own adhesive systems, consisting of isocyanates or special resins.

Two methods are used to apply rubber compound to a textile fabric: a dry method, which involves calendering; and spreading, in which the rubber compound is dissolved in a solvent, such as toluene or methyl ethyl ketone, and then spread on a textile substrate. Generally, the thickness of the coat of rubber required dictates the method of manufacture: thin coatings are applied by the solution method, and heavier coatings by the dry method.

The rubber used in the dry method is compounded in the conventional manner. A three- or four-roll calender is then used to form the rubber into the correct thickness and to combine it to the textile fabric. This method is also used extensively for making rubber sheet material (calendered gum) that is not attached to fabric.

For preparation of spreading solution, the compounded rubber is mixed in a mill or Banbury mixer, cut into small pieces and dissolved in a churn at a concentration of 10–35% solids. The rubber can be applied to the textile material by impregnation, reverse-roll coating or conventional spreading. In a 'spread', or direct-coating machine, fabric is pulled through the gap between a knife and a rubber roller. The solvents from the coatings are expelled from the solution by passage through hot ovens and may then be recovered for recycling. The temperatures of the ovens on the spreaders vary depending on the type of solvent and the rubber compounds that are being applied. Ovens have three, two or one zone(s) at increasing temperatures, from 65–120°C.

Within the last 20 years, a new method for solution coating has been introduced, called 'cast' or 'transfer' coating, which involves application of the solution onto a base such as coated paper or a steel belt. An adhesive base is then applied to the first cast coating, laminating the fabric substrate to the total composite. The material is then stripped from the paper carrier or metal belt. This method was originally used for vinyl casting, but more recently it has been used widely for polyurethane coatings to simulate leather goods, and for very thin, lightweight, air-holding products.

Vulcanizing is generally done by festooning in a dry-heat chamber under specific conditions of time and temperature, which vary with the rubber compound and with the specific requirements of the finished goods. Coated fabrics are also vulcanized in roll form: the material is dusted with mica or talc and wrapped around metal drums; water-resistant covers are put over the metal drums; and the total assembly is rolled into a closed-chamber steam vulcanizer. The material is then cured for long periods, 3-4 h, at 150-165°C, because of the time required for heat to penetrate the entire roll. Sometimes, special paper is used to interline the roll and give better surface appearance or to prevent sticking. Coated material may also be vulcanized by processing over heated drums, with pressure applied by a metal sheet.

4.2 Adhesives and sealants

(a) Adhesives (largely derived from Goken, 1979)

Elastomeric adhesives consist of compounded polymer dissolved or suspended in an appropriate liquid vehicle. In solvent adhesives, an organic solvent is used; in latex adhesives, the vehicle is water. The rubber is compounded and mixed by conventional methods, pelletized or otherwise divided, and weighed into appropriate batches. The solvent is metered into a churn of a capacity of up 1000 litres, and the rubber and other dry compounding ingredients are added. After an appropriate mixing time, the churn is tapped, and shipping containers are filled, sealed and labelled. Adhesives used as backings for sheet or ribbon materials may be applied by the methods described above.

Both natural and synthetic rubbers are used in adhesives and sealants. New or reclaimed materials may be used; reclaims are used widely in the manufacture of sealants that are not required to have strength and elasticity.

Solvent-based rubbery adhesives can be applied in solution or dispersion or as preformed films. Natural rubber is widely used, due mainly to its unique surface adhesion. Chemically modified natural rubber and reclaims are used primarily for bonding to flexible substrates, and other elastomers may be chosen depending upon the surfaces to be joined and on other conditions.

Most 'contact adhesives' are based on polychloroprene. Such adhesives do not depend on curing to develop bond strength but rely instead on crystallization. Oxides added to combat the hydrogen chloride formed during decomposition can crosslink the polymer in time. Many elastomeric adhesive formulations are vulcanizable and can be co-cured with rubber parts in a bonding process to other rubbers or metal.

Pressure-sensitive adhesives are a special class of elastomeric adhesive, and are generally less defined than other types. The bulk of such adhesives are based on natural rubber, although some synthetics are used. Most adhesives are preapplied to film, foil or fibrous backings, slit into narrow widths and used as tapes. The tapes are used for masking, insulating, bundling, sealing, protecting, identifying, holding, etc.

(b) Sealants

Production of sealants is similar to that of adhesives, but because sealants are generally of higher viscosity, special mixing and packaging equipment may be necessary.

Unvulcanized sealants are usually referred to as 'mastics' and are formulated from bituminous materials or caulks. They require 'skinning' agents to form a dry protective surface. Asphalt dispersions and various fillers (including asbestos fibre) may be added to sealants, depending on the intended use.

Masticated rubbers of various types, polybutenes and butyls are the most common elastomers used in caulks. They are formed into tapes with some degree of pressure-sensitive adhesion and curing possibilities and are used extensively in automotive applications where the sealant is also the primary adhesive holding glass in place.

The principal exposure hazards associated with the production of adhesives and sealants arise from the inhalation of solvent vapours and from skin contact with solvents and rubber chemicals in solution, especially resins. Many rubber chemicals have dermatitic properties, which are enhanced by the action of industrial solvents and can give rise to skin irritation and sensitization.

5.   **Dipped latex products and foams** (largely derived from Hoogheem et al., 1977)

5.1 **Latex-based, dipped goods**

The most widely produced latex-based, dipped goods are household gloves, surgical gloves, contraceptives, baby-bottle teats and balloons. The very thin-walled goods are produced by straight-dipping; thicker walled items are made by coagulation dipping. Latices are also used in the carpet industry, as backings, foam backings and underlays, in binders for non-woven fabrics, papers and woven textiles, in a multitude of water-based adhesives, in so-called emulsion paints, in dipping processes, in moulded latex foam rubber, and in latex thread and rubberized hair. Medical applications usually involve natural rubber latex, and one of the dipping processes is used. For example, straight dipping is employed for the manufacture of condoms; coagulant dipping is used to make surgical gloves; and heat-sensitized dipping is used for teats, catheters, etc. In all cases, the dipped product is thoroughly leached to remove water-soluble impurities.

(**a**) Compounding

The rubber latex and compounding ingredients must first be brought into solution or dispersion form. Solution is used when all of the ingredients are water-soluble; dispersion is used when it is necessary to emulsify the liquid ingredients and to disperse the solid materials in water.

Dispersions are prepared from coarse slurries of powder and water containing small quantities of dispersing agents and stabilizers. Typical dispersing agents are sodium 2-naphthalene sulphonate reacted with formaldehyde and an alkyl metal salt of sulphonated lignin; such materials are usually employed in concentrations of less than 1% by weight. Physically, the dispersions are prepared with grinding equipment such as colloid mills, ball and pebble mills, ultrasonic mills and attrition mills. Colloid mills, which break aggregates but do not change particle size, are used for clay, precipitated whiting, zinc oxide and other such materials. The other types of mills are used to prepare dispersions of sulphur, antioxidants and accelerators that require both aggregate and particle-size reduction.

Emulsions are prepared by exposing a coarse, aqueous suspension of ingredients to intense shearing in a colloid mill, an ultrasonic mill or a homogenizer.

In itself, the preparation of the latex compound is a very simple operation, consisting of weighing and mixing the proper amounts of various solutions, emulsions and dispersions, including stabilizers, sulphur, vulcanization accelerators, antioxidants and sensitizers. This is done in a large tank with a mechanical agitator. A flow diagram for the production of dipped latex-based goods is shown in Figure 8.

FIG. 8.   FLOW DIAGRAM FOR THE PRODUCTION OF TYPICAL
LATEX-BASED DIPPED ITEMS
(From Hoogheem et al., 1977)

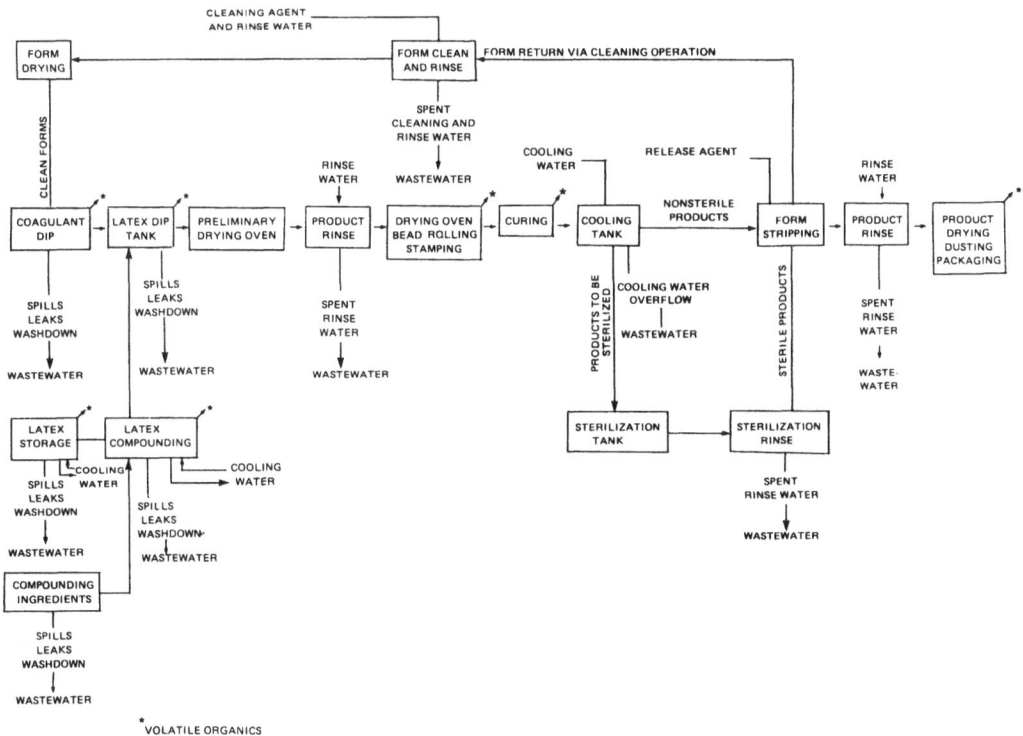

Prevulcanized latex can also be obtained.

(b) Coagulation dipping

The coagulation solution is usually a mixture of coagulants and organic solvents, such as ethanol and acetone. Typical coagulants are calcium nitrate, calcium chloride and zinc nitrate. A surfactant is sometimes added to the mixture to ensure good 'wetting' of the forms; and release agents are added when the form has a complicated shape and removal of the dipped goods would be difficult. Talc, clay and diatomaceous earth are commonly used release agents.

The dipping operation is carried out by transporting glazed porcelain or polished metal forms through the various processing units on a closed-loop conveyor. After being coated with coagulants, the forms are dipped into the rubber latex compound. The coagulant film on the surface of the form causes the rubber emulsion to 'break', and the latex solids coalesce to produce a film of rubber that covers and adheres to the form. These coated forms are passed through a preliminary drying oven (with subsequent emission of volatiles) so that the film does not disintegrate and wash away during the next washing step.

In the washing operation, the soluble constituents of the rubber film are leached out and rinsed away in a water-bath maintained at 60-71°C. Emulsifiers used in the original production of the latex and metal ions from the coagulant mixture appear in the leachate. The washed forms are sent through a drying oven and heated to 100-120°C (with subsequent emission of volatiles) in a conditioning oven prior to reuse.

In some applications, such as rubber-glove manufacture, the goods are not only dried but they are heated sufficiently to roll the rubber coating downward on itself to form a reinforced cuff bead. Usually, the rubber goods are stamped with proprietary brands and other information, such as size, in a stamping unit after drying.

The rubber products are cured in an oven at temperatures ranging from 65-95°C. After curing, the items are cooled in water and mechanically stripped from the forms, usually with the aid of a lubricating detergent. The detergent is subsequently washed from the goods in a rinse tank. The final manufacturing operation consists of drying the goods, dusting them inside and outside with talc to prevent sticking, and packaging.

For the manufacture of sterilized products, such as surgical gloves, the goods are immersed in a chlorine dip-tank, typically containing 1000 mg/l free chlorine. After disinfection, the goods are dipped into a water-bath at 75–80°C to remove residual chlorine. These two operations generally occur between the post-cure cooling and the final drying and packaging.

About once a week, it is necessary to wash the forms in a bath containing a cleaning agent. If porcelain forms are used, the cleaning agent is usually chromic acid (a mixture of potassium dichromate, sulphuric acid and water). Once cleaned, the forms are passed through a rinse tank fed with fresh water, from which the accumulation of cleaning agent overflows.

(c) Straight dipping

The straight-dip method is the simplest of the latex dipping operations. Warm forms are dipped directly in the latex and removed slowly. After dipping, the forms are slowly rotated while the film is drying to ensure uniform thickness. The films are dried at room temperature or in warm air at 50–60°C. Thicker articles can be made by multiple dipping with intermittent drying. Latex deposits vary from 0.13–2.5 mm per dip, depending on the viscosity of the latex compound used.

(d) Rubber goods from porous moulds

Dolls, squeeze toys and other rubber sundries may be produced by the porous mould technique. The moulds used in this process are made from plaster of Paris or unglazed porcelain with pore sizes smaller than the smallest rubber particles. Latex, compounded in the manner described above, is poured through a funnel-shaped opening into the mould where it is allowed to rest until a deposit of the desired thickness has developed on the mould wall. The mould is then emptied of excess compound and placed in an oven to dry at 60°C. The interior surfaces of the rubber article are dusted with talc to prevent sticking when it is removed from the mould. Once it is removed, the article may be returned to the oven for 30 min.

(e) Latex thread

Latex thread is produced by extruding the latex compound through fine orifices into a coagulant bath, where it is gelled. The thread is then toughened, washed, dried and cured. Dilute acetic acid is commonly used as the coagulant.

All the dip and extrusion processes described above may involve exposure to volatile material, such as formaldehyde, ammonia, hydrogen chloride, chlorine, in addition to curing fume.

5.2 Latex foam

The latex used in foam manufacture may consist of natural rubber, styrene-butadiene rubber or a combination of the two, and is compounded with a variety of ingredients. The foams are generally produced in slab or moulded form at a density range of 64-128 kg/m³. They are used to manufacture automotive seating, mattresses, pillows, carpeting, mats, upholstery and many other products.

(a) Dunlop process

In the Dunlop process, foam is produced by mechanically whipping latex to a froth. This can be done on a batch basis, but the Cakes continuous mixer is the standard piece of equipment used. Once frothed, the latex must be coagulated, or gelled, to give a stable foam, by adding sodium silicofluoride and zinc oxide to the mix, which remains dormant long enough to allow the froth to be poured into moulds. When stable latices are used, secondary gelling agents, such as cationic soaps, other salts and amines may be required to induce coagulation.

As soon as the gelling agents are added, the foam is poured into steam-heated moulds and cured, with subsequent emission of volatiles. The product is removed when the curing cycle is completed, and washed with water to remove those ingredients in the compounded latex that are not permanently held in the foam matrix. The foam is then dried in a hot-air dryer and inspected, prior to storage and shipment.

(b) Talalay process

In this process, the froth is produced by chemical rather than mechanical means. Hydrogen peroxide and enzymatic catalysts are mixed with the latex, and the mixture is placed into a mould. The enzyme decomposes the peroxide, thus liberating oxygen, which causes the latex mix to foam up and fill the mould. This foam is rapidly chilled, and carbon dioxide is introduced to effect gelation. The gelled foam is handled in a manner similar to that used in the Dunlop process. A flow diagram is shown in Figure 9.

FIG. 9. FLOW DIAGRAM FOR THE PRODUCTION OF TYPICAL
         LATEX FOAM ITEMS
         (From Hoogheem et al., 1977)

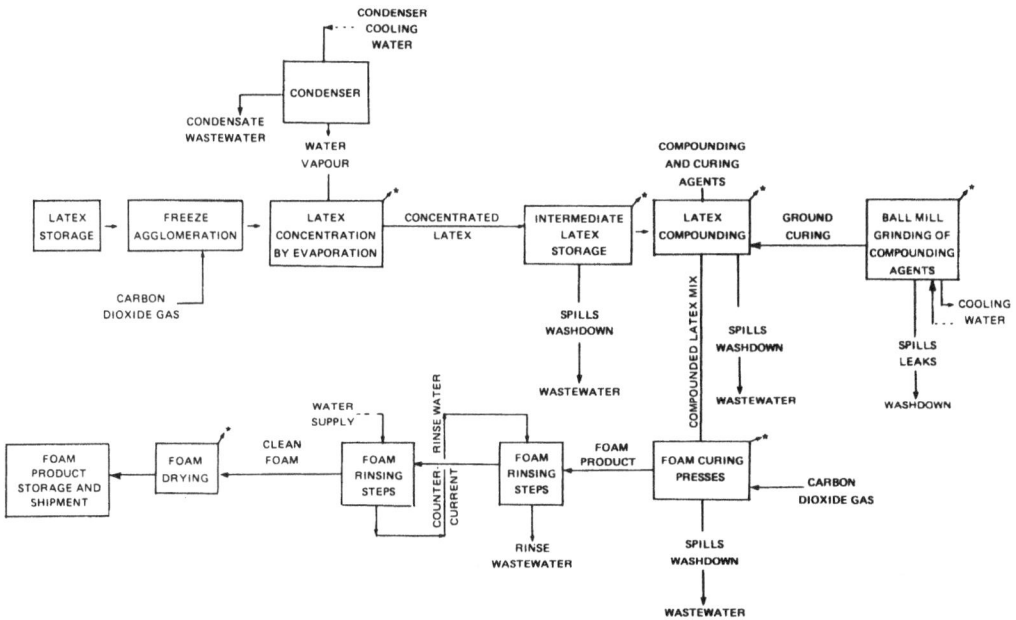

*VOLATILE ORGANICS

The major emission given off during the curing of latex foam articles is ammonia.

(c) Foam backing

For supported, flat foam, either ammonium acetate or ammonium sulphate is employed in combination with zinc oxide as the gelation agent. The froth is prepared in a Cakes mixer; the gelling agent is added, and the foam is applied to the fabric by direct spreading. In some cases, the foam is spread on a belt which transfers it to the fabric. The gelling is carried out at elevated temperatures, usually with the aid of infra-red lamps. To prevent uneven shrinkage, the fabric is carried through a high-temperature zone and drying ovens on tenters.

6. <u>References</u>

Anderson, H.H. (1978) <u>Molded goods.</u> In: Babbit, R.O., ed., <u>The Vanderbilt Rubber Handbook</u>, Norwalk, CT, R.T. Vanderbilt Co., p. 697

Blow, C.M., ed. (1978) <u>Rubber Technology and Manufacture,</u> London, Newnes–Butterworths

Cooper, D.L. (1978) <u>Hard rubber.</u> In: Babbit, R.O., ed., <u>The Vanderbilt Rubber Handbook,</u> Norwalk, CT, R.T. Vanderbilt Co., pp. 810–812

Crowther, B.G. & Edmondson, H.M. (1978) <u>Processing technology.</u> In: Blow, C.M., ed., <u>Rubber Technology and Manufacture</u>, London, Newnes–Butterworths, p. 304

Foster D. Snell, Inc. (1976) <u>Assessment of Industrial Hazardous Waste Practices, Rubber and Plastics Industry, Draft Final Report.</u> Prepared for the US Environmental Protection Agency, Office of Solid Waste Management Programs, Washington DC, pp. 111–30, 35, 71, 74–76, 118–120, 122–123, 154

Goken, G.L. (1979) Elastomers' role in adhesives. <u>Elastomerics,</u> June, pp. 24–27, 37

Heinisch, K.F. (1974) <u>Dictionary of Rubber,</u> New York, John Wiley & Sons, p. 225

Hoogheem, T.J., Chi, C.T., Rinaldi, G.M., McCormick, R.J. & Hughes, T.W. (1977) <u>Identification and Control of Hydrocarbon Emissions from Rubber Processing Operations.</u> Draft Report. Prepared for the US Environmental Protection Agency, Office of Air and Waste Management, Washington DC, p. 217

Morton, G.F. & Quinton, G.B. (1978) <u>Manufacturing techniques.</u> In: Blow, C.M., ed., <u>Rubber Technology and Manufacture</u>, London, Newnes–Butterworths, p. 367

Neller, W.C. (1978) <u>Belting.</u> In: Blow, C.M., ed., <u>Rubber Technology and Manufacture,</u> London, Newnes–Butterworths, pp. 378–379

Pollard, D. (1978) Cables. In: Blow, C.M., ed., Rubber Technology, London, Newnes-Butterworths, pp. 431, 434

Rowley, A.C. (1978) Wire and cable compounding and processing. In: Babbit, R.O., ed., The Vanderbilt Rubber Handbook, Norwalk, CT, R.T. Vanderbilt Co., pp. 751, 757-758

Stern, H.J. (1967) Rubber: Natural and Synthetic, 2nd ed., London, MacLaren & Sons

US Environmental Protection Agency (1980) Rubber Tire Manufacturing Industry - Background Information for Proposed Standards, Preliminary Draft, Research Triangle Park, NC, Office of Air Quality Planning and Standards, pp. 3-15 - 3-28

US Food & Drug Administration (1980) Food and drugs. US Code fed., Regul., Title 21, parts 177.1210, 177.2600, 178.2010, pp. 191-195, 249-253, 259-266

Wade, W.E. (1978) Flat belting. In: Babbit, R.O., ed., The Vanderbilt Rubber Handbook, Norwalk, CT, R.T. Vanderbilt Co., pp. 702-703

Walter, G. (1976) Elastomers in the automotive industry. Rubber Chem. Technol., 49, 813, 816

West, G. (1978) Coated fabrics. In: Babbit, R.O., ed., The Vanderbilt Rubber Handbook, Norwalk, CT, R.T. Vanderbilt Co., pp. 797-800

Williams, A.E. (1978) Hose. In: Babbit, R.O., ed., The Vanderbilt Rubber Handbook, Norwalk, CT, R.T. Vanderbilt Co., pp. 711-712

This subject has been reviewed by Stern (1967) and by Blow (1978).

1. Components required and historical changes in the substances used

The basic materials used in rubber compounding consist of:

- elastomers (natural or synthetic rubber)
- fillers (e.g., China clay)
- antidegradants (antiozonants, antioxidants)
- vulcanizing agents (e.g., sulphur or sulphur donors, organic peroxides, phenol resins, metal oxides)
- accelerators (e.g., benzothiazoles, guanidines, dithiocarbamates)
- retarders (e.g., organic acids, N-nitrosodiphenylamine)
- pigments (inorganic pigments and organic dyes and lacquers)
- reinforcing agents (e.g., carbon black)
- processing aids (e.g., mineral oils, solvents, talc)
- activators (e.g., zinc oxide)

The use of these raw materials and the changes in compounding that have taken place in recent years can be illustrated by a comparison of a pre-war tyre formulation with its modern counterpart. A typical formulation described by Russell in 1937 consisted of:

- smoked sheet (natural rubber)   100 parts
- pine tar   3 parts
- stearic acid   4 parts
- antioxidant   1 part
- zinc oxide   5 parts
- carbon black (channel process)   50 parts
- sulphur   3 parts
- mercaptobenzothiazole   1 part

Today, the equivalent product might be made up as follows:

- oil–extended styrene–butadiene rubber (SBR) (37.5% highly aromatic oil)   137.5 parts
- aromatic process oil   10.0 parts
- stearic acid   1.0 part
- N–isopropyl–N'–phenyl–para– phenylenediamine (antiozonant)   2.5 parts
- zinc oxide   5.0 parts
- improved (high–abrasion furnace) carbon black   75.0 parts
- sulphur   1.8 parts
- paraffin wax   2.0 parts
- N–cyclohexyl–2–benzothiazole– sulphenamide (accelerator)   1.5 parts

Although it is true that increased complexity and substantial advances in rubber technology were already in evidence before the start of the Second World War, the outbreak of war, bringing with it the urgent problem of a shortage of raw materials, was a stimulus for intensive research activity into the development of new materials and alternative formulations. Among such can be identified three fundamental and highly important changes in the pattern of raw material supply and usage which have been taking place over the past 35 years, involving changes in the rubber polymer, carbon blacks and process oils. The changes involved not only the physical and chemical composition but also the volume of usage. Table 2 indicates the general nature and direction of these changes.

(a) Changes in the production, composition and use of elastomers

During the first quarter of this century, the bulk of all rubber polymer used in manufacturing processes consisted of natural rubber, produced for the most part in Malayan plantations. Although patents for synthetic polymers were first taken out in 1912, it was not until 1930 that in Germany and in Russia work on the development of synthetic rubber polymer was intensified. By 1939, a number of synthetic rubbers, some of which had additional – and eminently desirable – oil-resisting properties, were in commercial production in Europe. In the US, production was negligible prior to the Second World War; but, when supplies

Table 2. Changes in raw materials used in rubber compounding over time

Dates	Rubber[a]	Blacks	Oils	Approx. % of oil in tyres
Before 1943	NR	Channel	Pine-tar	2 – 3
1944–1946	NR/SBR (25/75)	Channel & furnace	Mineral oil	5 – 7
1946–1950	NR	Channel	Mostly pine-tar	2 – 3
1951–1955	NR	Channel/ furnace	Mostly pine-tar	2 – 3
1956–1960	NR/SBR (75/25)	Furnace/ channel	Pine-tar/ mineral oil	4 – 7
1961–1965	NR/(SBR+BR) (50/50)	Mostly furnace	Mostly mineral oil	20 – 23

[a] NR: Natural rubber; SBR: styrene–butadiene rubber; BR: polybutadiene rubber

of natural rubber were cut off, existing plans to start a synthetic rubber industry were expedited and expanded, so that by 1944 87 factories had been completed (Stern, 1978). Thus, in the US, in 1939, a total of 1750 long tons of synthetic rubber were produced; between 1940 and 1944, a total of 1 028 989 long tons were made, of which 856 475 were SBR; and between 1945 and 1949, a total of 2 951 113 long tons were produced, of which 2 429 627 were SBR (Dunbrook, 1954). In the UK, commercial use of synthetic rubber was limited until the mid-1950s, due to a restriction on imports and a limited capacity for production.

In the mid-1950s, there were only four main types of synthetic rubber – SBR, butyl, nitrile and polychloroprene; at that time, oil-extended SBR also began to be used. It had been found that by polymerizing SBR to a higher viscosity, a large amount of cheap extender oil could be added, resulting in an excellent rubber for tyres. Initially, the types and amounts of oil used in these rubbers varied from naphthenic to highly aromatic, and up to 37 1/2 parts of oil added to 100 parts of SBR during the coagulation process; by 1956, SBR 1712, containing this amount of highly aromatic oil, became the standard oil-extended polymer for use in tyre manufacture. In the US, production of latex-masterbatched, oil-extended, high-Mooney, cold SBR was started in April 1951. During the 1960s, advances in the synthesis of elastomers produced polyisoprene (a synthetic rubber more like natural rubber), polybutadiene and the ethylene propylene rubbers.

The market share of synthetic rubbers has grown rapidly. In 1955, the US and Canada manufactured most of the synthetic rubber in the western world; small amounts were manufactured in the Federal Republic of Germany, the USSR and the German Democratic Republic. Worldwide production at that time was only 1 542 000 tonnes. By 1978, worldwide production had risen to 8 720 000 tonnes, a growth rate of 7.8% per year. Use of natural rubber during the same period grew from 1 928 000 to 3 725 000 tonnes, a growth rate of 2.9% per year (Davis, 1980).

However, synthetic rubber production is firmly linked to the petrochemical industry. Present concern about the future avail-ability and cost of petrochemicals, and the increasing use of natural rubber in radial tyres has again stimulated interest in natural rubber. In 1980, world consumption of synthetic rubber declined by 5%; however, that was not a typical year: the average rate of growth over 1975-1980 was 4.1% per annum, and the rate of growth of natural rubber use was 2.7% (The International Rubber Study Group, 1946-1981).

The development and usage of synthetic polymers is perhaps the most important of all the process changes that have taken place in recent years, and its possible relevance to recent epidemiological findings must be considered carefully.

(b) Changes in the production and use of carbon black

The major compounding ingredient in tyre compounds, apart from the polymer, is carbon black; and until 1951 the majority of the carbon black supplied to the rubber industry was manufactured by the 'channel' process (see p. 105 of this section). Today, furnace blacks (see p. 105) have virtually displaced the channel variety (see Table 2). The relevance and the possible significance of this change in practice have been considered by industrial physicians and by hygienists in the light of the fact that whereas channel blacks have a negligible content of polycyclic aromatic hydrocarbons, they are undoubtedly present at a higher level in furnace blacks (see Section V).

(c) Changes in the composition and use of process oils

The traditional process oil used in rubber compounds — and especially in tyre formulations — until 1943 was pine-tar oil. Today, the majority of tyres produced by the industry probably have 20% or more of aromatic oil in their composition. The potential hazard of the continued and increasing use of extender oils by the rubber manufacturing industries must be considered in the light of the presence of carcinogenic polycyclic hydrocarbons in these oils. Occupational exposure to extender oils may occur at any stage of the manufacturing process: and, although mechanical handling and automatic feed of oil to the Banbury mixers significantly reduces the risk of skin contact at the 'front' end of the process, exposure to curing fume during and immediately following vulcanization may involve an element of risk for those concerned.

Although the principal changes in compounding of identifiable significance are referred to above, many other changes have also taken place. Some, at least, have served to reduce the probability of exposure to risk: the use of carbon disulphide has been virtually abandoned and exposure to benzene greatly reduced.

2.   Chemical compounds used in rubber compounding (see also Appendix 1, Tables 1, 3, 4)

Elastomers are the basic polymers used in rubber manufacture. Natural and various types of synthetic rubbers are employed, which usually contain some unsaturation on which to build a cross-linking system (Fig. 10).

FIG. 10. NATURAL AND SOME SYNTHETIC RUBBERS, SHOWING THE UNSATURATION WHICH PERMITS CROSS-LINKING ON VULCANIZATION

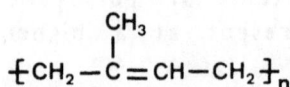

$$\underset{\substack{| \\ CH_3}}{+CH_2-C=CH-CH_2+_n}$$

cis-1,4-polyisoprene
(natural rubber)

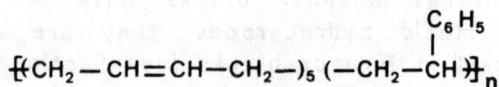

$$+CH_2-CH=CH-CH_2-)_5 \ (-CH_2-\underset{\substack{| \\ C_6H_5}}{CH}+_n$$

polybutadiene-co-styrene (styrene-butadiene rubber)

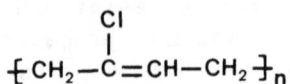

$$+CH_2-\underset{\substack{| \\ Cl}}{C}=CH-CH_2+_n$$

polychloroprene (Neoprene)

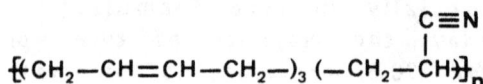

$$+CH_2-CH=CH-CH_2-)_3 \ (-CH_2-\underset{\substack{| \\ C\equiv N}}{CH}+_n$$

polybutadiene-co-acrylonitrile (nitrile rubber)

Latex is the sap of rubber-yielding plants or a colloidal dispersion of rubber particles in an aqueous medium. The rubber particles are approximately one-thousandth of a millimetre in diameter and constitute 40-70% of the mass of the latex.

There are many types of rubber latex, which contain one of the following rubbers:

> Natural rubber (cis-polyisoprene)
> Styrene-butadiene rubber
> Acrylonitrile-butadiene rubber
> Chloroprene rubber

Natural rubber latex was originally preserved with ammonia alone, but in recent years small amounts (< 0.1%) of the combination of tetramethylthiuram disulphide and zinc oxide have been used in addition to improve the quality. Synthetic rubber latices contain small amounts (usually <0.1%) of residual monomers (styrene, acrylonitrile, etc), and these may be released during processing (Rappaport & Fraser, 1977). In addition, the raw elastomers supplied to an industry may contain aromatic extender oils (oil-extended polymer) or may be masterbatches containing carbon black.

Elastomers can be divided into the following classes:

(i) General purpose

American Society for Testing Materials (ASTM) designation

natural	N R
polyisoprene	I R
styrene-butadiene	SB R
butyl	II R
ethylene-propylene	EPM, EPDM
polybutadiene	B R

(ii) Solvent-resistant

polysulphides	T
nitrile	NB R
polychloroprene	C R
polyurethanes	A U, E U
epichlorohydrin	CO

(iii) Heat-resistant

silicone	MQ
chlorosulphonated polyethylene	CSM
polyacrylates	ACM
fluoroelastomers	CFM

- SBR is now the major synthetic rubber produced, comprising about 40% of world production (Davis, 1980). (See Appendix 1, Table 4). In comparison with natural rubber, SBR is weaker and less resistant to fatigue, but it has the merit of ageing more slowly.

- Butyl rubbers have a low permeability for air and gases and have thus been used for inner tubes. Polybutadiene is difficult to process, and so it is usually unsuited for use on its own; its value lies in its capacity to blend with SBR or natural rubber. In tyre treads, however, it lowers the build-up of heat and improves wearing quality (abrasion resistance). It has the disadvantage of reducing skid resistance.

- Nitrile rubbers generally have excellent abrasion resistance, but their oil-, water- and chemical-resistance are the major factors dictating their use.

- Synthetic polyisoprene contains a high percentage of cis-isoprene but differs from its natural counterpart, and its main function is as a blending component with other types of rubber.

- Polychloroprene rubber, originally known as Neoprene, has most of the advantages of SBR and of natural rubber, but in addition it is flame-resistant and wears longer. It also possesses oil-, heat- and solvent-resistance, but despite these undoubted attributes its high price limits its production. The polychloroprene rubbers are used mainly in the transport industry, and for rubber boats, cables, sealants, coatings and adhesives.

- The ethylene-propylene rubbers possess improved resistance to sunlight, ozone, aging and weathering. In particular, they can accept large loadings of extender oils and fillers without serious loss of their physical properties.

The following specialized synthetic rubbers are made, with particular properties; but they are expensive to produce and their market is limited. They comprise about 2% of synthetic rubber production (Davis, 1980):

- Silicone rubbers are effective in extremes of temperature and are used in the aerospace industry. They also seem to be well tolerated by human tissues, which makes them of value in surgery.

- Solid polyurethane rubbers are used in the soles and heels of-shoes, in solid tyres and in automotive applications.

- Polysulphide rubbers, being very resistant to solvents, are used mainly as sealant putties in the construction and building industries.

- Chlorosulphonated polyethylene rubber is used for cable coverings.

- Polyacrylic rubbers are plastic rubbers that resist oil and aging. They are used in seals and gaskets for vehicles.

- Fluoroelastomers, the most costly of all the special purpose synthetic rubbers, have been used in the aerospace programme, because of their high thermal stability.

- The thermoplastic elastomers melt at higher temperatures (unlike conventional rubbers, which would tend to crosslink under the same conditions) and then resolidify on cooling, without significant loss of their elastic properties. They are usually extruded without further curing.

The aim of the rubber compounder is to formulate a composition which will be: easy to put through such processes as calendering and extrusion with the minimum of energy input; stable at the temperatures encountered in those processes, but which will cure rapidly and controllably at vulcanization temperatures; and capable of giving a product with the desired physical characteristics and which is resistant to oxidation, heat, aging and attack by light, ozone and other chemicals. Hundreds of different rubber additives may be used in different blends; in a particular rubber product, however, around a dozen different components may be used (Holmberg & Sjöström, 1977; Hybart et al., 1968). Rubber additives are classified according to their function during or after rubber processing. The main groups of chemicals used for these purposes are as follows:

(a) Vulcanizing agents

These materials are necessary for the cross-linking that takes place during vulcanization, which changes the rubber from a soft thermoplastic mixture to a final product with the desired properties.

The most common vulcanizing agent, used in most general-purpose natural and SBR systems, is sulphur; both cross-links and cyclic structures are formed (Fig. 11a). Sulphur donors, such as tetraalkylthiuram disulphides, morpholine disulphide, dithiocarbamates and, more recently, dithiophosphates, are sometimes used instead of or in addition to elemental sulphur. The closely related elements, selenium and tellurium, and their compounds, have also been used as vulcanizing agents.

FIG. 11. STRUCTURAL FEATURES OF A VULCANISATE NETWORK

(a) Chemical groups present in a sulphur-vulcanized natural rubber network: (1) polysulphide cross-links, n = 1-6; (2) intrachain cyclic sulphides, m = 1-2 (From Brydson, 1978).
(b) Peroxide vulcanization, in which free radicals are formed on the polymer chains, which then combine to form carbon-to-carbon cross-links (From Stephens, 1973)

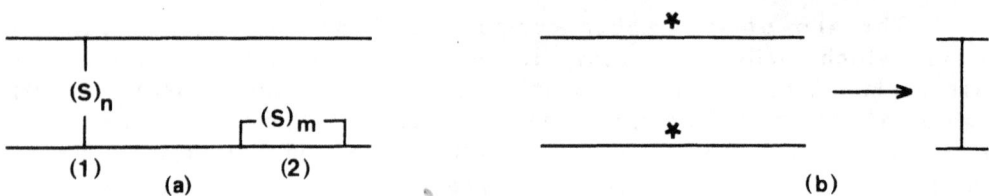

Fully-saturated elastomers, such as the silicones, cannot be vulcanized with sulphur and require the use of peroxides. In consequence of the decomposition of peroxides, free radicals are formed on the polymer chains, which can then combine to form cross-links (Stephens, 1973) (Fig. 11b).

(b) Accelerators

The reaction between sulphur and rubber is slow, and in order to obtain shorter cure times and better final properties accelerators are used. They function at normal curing temperatures (140-200°C) and (except in latex) not at lower temperatures. Often a primary accelerator is used together with a smaller amount of a secondary accelerator, to produce a synergistic effect giving better final properties than can either accelerator separately. Accelerators can be classified in various ways:

(i) Classification by sulphur demand: Accelerators can be classified by the amount of sulphur they require; less active accelerators require a relatively large amount while more active ones require a smaller quantity.

(ii)   **Classification by rate of vulcanization:**   A more commonly used classification is based on the rate of vulcanization achievable. There are slow accelerators (amines, thiourea derivatives); semi-ultra accelerators (moderately fast) (sulphenamides, 1,3-diphenylguanidine, mercaptobenzothiazole); and ultra accelerators (very fast) (thiurams, dithiocarbamates, xanthates, thiophosphates). This type of classification is inevitably a simplification, however, since accelerators often behave differently in different polymer systems.

(iii) _ **Classification by chemical composition:** The main structural groups are shown in Figure 12.

FIG. 12. ACCELERATOR TYPES CLASSIFIED BY CHEMICAL STRUCTURE

Aldehyde-amine condensates

$R_1-N=CHR_2$

Dithiocarbamates

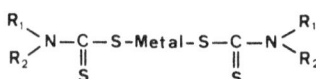

Benzothiazoles

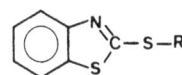

Amines

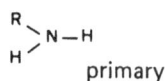
primary

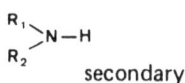
secondary

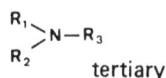
tertiary

Thiophosphates

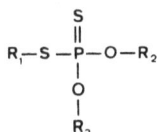

Guanidines

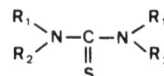

Thioureas

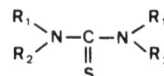

Xanthates

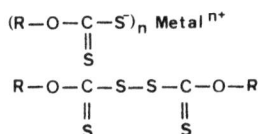

Sulphenamides

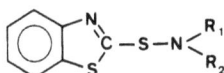

Thiuram sulphides

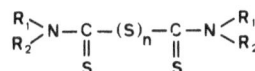

The chemistry of rubber acceleration is complex, although some simple trends can be discerned. For instance, the activity of simple amines increases with their basicity in the following order: triarylamines < diarylamines < monoarylamines and alkylarylamines < mono-, di- and trialkylamines. Compounds that contain nitrogen but no sulphur, such as the amines, fall into the class of slow accelerators; those containing sulphur but no nitrogen are in the class of semi-ultra accelerators; while the more active compounds contain both nitrogen and sulphur.

Accelerated sulphur vulcanization is thought to proceed by the following steps (Coran, 1978):

(1) The accelerator reacts with sulphur to give monomeric polysulphides of the type $Ac-(S)_n-Ac$, where Ac is an organic group derived from the accelerator. Certain initiating species may be necessary to start the reaction.

(2) The polysulphides can interact with rubber to give polymeric polysulphides of the type rubber-$(S)_n-Ac$. When mercaptobenzothiazole is used as the accelerator, the quantity present first decreases to low levels, then increases as the rubber polysulphides form.

(3) The rubber polysulphides then react, either directly or through a reactive intermediate, to give cross-links or rubber polysulphides of the type rubber-$(S)_n$-rubber.

For sulphenamide accelerators, these steps can be written as shown in Figure 13.

Vulcanization may also take place _via_ free-radical mechanisms in the presence of accelerators. There are often strong synergistic effects among different groups: thus, guanidines have strong synergistic secondary accelerating effects with dithiocarbamates and benzothiazoles, so that 1,3-diphenylguanidine is in fact most often used in combination with mercaptobenzothiazole or mercaptobenzothiazole disulphide.

For a more detailed account of the various classifications and interactions of accelerators, see Kempermann (1978, 1979).

FIG. 13. ACCELERATED SULPHUR VULCANIZATION
          (From Coran, 1978)
          (See text for explanation)

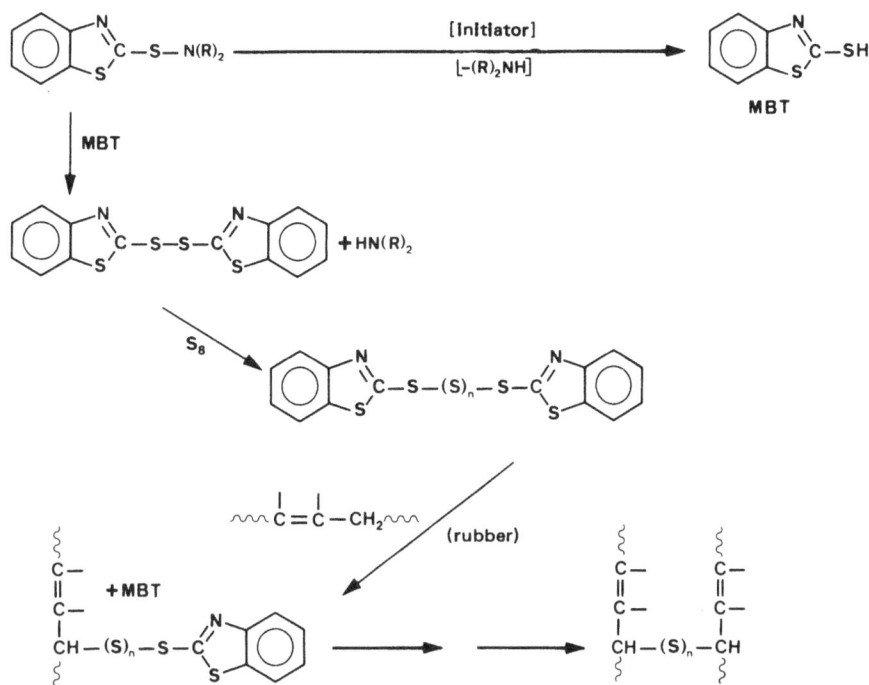

(c) Activators

These materials are used to make accelerators more effective, probably by forming intermediate complexes; for instance,
zinc ions may react with an accelerator to produce a chelated
form that is more active than the free accelerator (Coran, 1978)
(Fig. 14).

The main types of activator in use are inorganic compounds,
which are mainly metal oxides, such as zinc oxide, litharge
(PbO), red lead (Pb_3O_4), magnesium oxide and sodium carbonate.
Organic acids such as stearic acid or lauric acid, are used to
increase the solubility of the metal in the rubber formulation.
The most common activation system is thus zinc oxide in

FIG. 14.   AN ACTIVATED SYSTEM, IN WHICH ZINC ION REACTS
          WITH THE ACCELERATOR, GIVING A CHELATED FORM
          THAT IS MORE ACTIVE THAN THE FREE ACCELERATOR
          (From Coran, 1978)

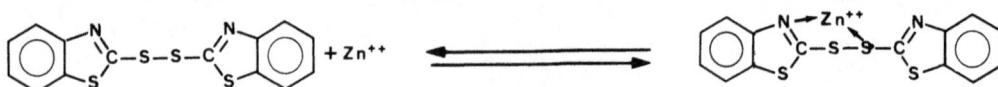

combination with a fatty acid, which produce a rubber-soluble
soap (zinc stearate) in the rubber matrix.

(d)   Retarders

Highly accelerated rubber compounds may tend to cure prema-
turely during intermediate processing operations or during
storage: such compounds are said to be 'scorchy'. To delay the
action of an accelerator, retarders are sometimes used. The ideal
retarder has no effect on the final rate of cure or on the properties of the vulcanisate. Organic acids (e.g., salicylic acid),
N-nitrosodiphenylamine, cyclohexylthiophthalimide, and a sulphon-
amide derivative (Vulcalent E) are the retarders commonly used.

Cyclohexylthiophthalimide is converted to phthalimide during
vulcanization (Fig. 15) (Leib et al., 1970).

FIG. 15.   DECOMPOSITION OF THE RETARDER N-CYCLOHEXYL-
          THIOPHTHALIMIDE DURING VULCANIZATION

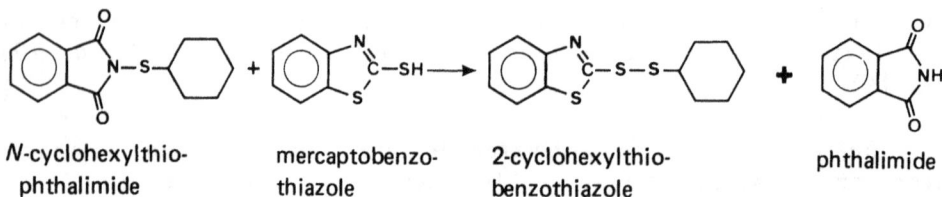

N-cyclohexylthio-   mercaptobenzo-   2-cyclohexylthio-   phthalimide
phthalimide   thiazole   benzothiazole

(e)   Antidegradants

Rubbers deteriorate with aging, particularly at elevated temperatures. To arrest or retard this deterioration, which is usually a greater problem in unsaturated than saturated rubbers, antidegradants are added to the rubber formulation.

Deterioration of rubber may be due to chain breakdown, cross-link breakdown, cross-link formation, development of polar groups, or development of chromophoric (colour-forming) groups in the polymer (Brydson, 1978). Not only the polymer chain but also the sulphide links may undergo oxidative attack, usually resulting in decreased cross-link density.

Many of these processes are caused by oxidation. The unsaturated polymer itself may be oxidized via free-radical mechanisms in a chain reaction mediated by a hydroperoxide produced during the process; this reaction is autocatalytic, i.e., the products of the process catalyse its continuation, which thus proceeds with increasing speed. Antioxidants effective against these processes act either by interrupting chain reactions or by preventing free-radical formation. Amines and phenols are the most widely used antioxidants that act by the former mechanism; those that interfere by the latter mechanism include peroxide-decomposing agents, chelating agents, ultra-violet screens, absorbers and quenchers. Of recent interest, for their association with cancer, are the aldehyde-naphthylamine-condensate antioxidants, such as Nonox S, which have now been withdrawn from use (see p. 160).

Ozone, normally present in traces in the atmosphere, is also important in rubber deterioration. In unprotected rubbers under tension, ozone causes deep cracks perpendicular to the direction of stress. This reaction is initiated by addition of ozone to the double bond of the unsaturated rubber, followed by rearrangement and hydrolysis (Fig. 16).

In general, the antioxidants mentioned above do not give protection against ozone cracking. The original agents used were waxes, insoluble in rubber, which act by diffusing slowly to the surface and forming a protective film (bloom) that protects the rubber surface physically from ozone attack. Waxes are still used, especially in static applications; in dynamic applications, however, the film tends to be broken, exposing the surface to

FIG. 16. PROPOSED MECHANISM FOR OZONE ATTACK
ON RUBBER

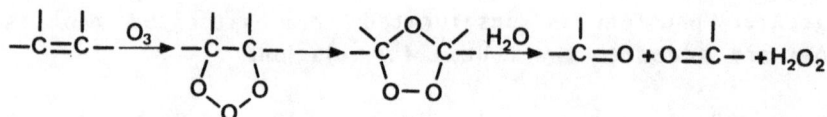

$$-\overset{|}{C}=\overset{|}{C}-\xrightarrow{O_3}-\overset{|}{\underset{O-O}{C}}\overset{|}{\underset{O}{C}}-\longrightarrow-\overset{O}{\underset{O-O}{C}}\overset{}{C}-\xrightarrow{H_2O}-\overset{|}{C}=O+O=\overset{|}{C}-+H_2O_2$$

further attack. para-Phenylenediamine derivatives, particularly
the branched alkylaryl diamines, are widely used for protection
against ozone, but the mechanism by which they act is not
completely clear.

(f) Processing aids

The largest group of processing aids are used to make
uncured rubber softer and more easily mixed, extruded or calendered. Historically, pine tars were used, but these have now been
almost completely replaced by mineral oils. Paraffinic,
naphthenic and aromatic mineral oils are in use – and of these
types, the aromatic grades have become particularly widespread.
They give good properties to the finished rubber, and are cheap;
many rubber formulations contain 20% or more of mineral oil. The
aromatic oils are obtained from the residues remaining from
solvent-refining, lubricating and cutting oils, and contain relatively large quantities of polycyclic aromatic hydrocarbons.
Typical figures reported by oil companies show that 4-6-ring
polycyclic hydrocarbons are present at a concentration of about
20% in these oils, and a typical aromatic processing oil may
contain 50 ppm of benzo[a]pyrene (Nutt, 1979). Other materials
used include vegetable oils, coal-tar pitch, phthalates, organic
phosphates and various types of factice (polymerisates of
unsaturated vegetable or animal oils with sulphur or sulphur
chloride).

Peptizing agents are sometimes used to soften the rubber by
chemical interaction. Most such materials contain –SH groups
which function as chain terminating agents for the radicals
formed by rupture of the polymer chains during mastication.
Examples are mercaptan derivatives, benzimidazoles, thiophenols
and mercaptobenzothiazole.

Tackifying agents are used to increase adhesion among un-cured rubber parts, useful when building up rubber components. The most widely used materials are the resins based on petroleum hydrocarbons and the phenolic resins.

(g)   Reinforcing agents

Certain fillers are crucially important in rubber techno-logy in that they have dramatic effects on the tensile strength and abrasion resistance of the vulcanized rubber. This effect is known as 'reinforcement'. The most important reinforcing agents are carbon black and amorphous silicas.

The original form of carbon black was lamp black, but this was largely superseded in the period 1910-1942 by 'channel' black. Channel black was made from natural gas by burning in small sooty flames impinging on a cool surface, such as channel iron. Since the 1940s, the channel blacks have been almost completely replaced by furnace blacks. Although originally made from natural gas by the furnace process, furnace blacks are now manufactured from oil: a fuel, either gas or oil, is burned with an excess of air to generate high temperatures. The heavy aroma-tic tar oil is injected into this hot air and decomposes to fine-ly divided carbon within milliseconds. The hot smoke stream is then quenched with water. Furnace blacks contain a higher level of polycyclic aromatic hydrocarbons than channel blacks (see Section V). As a consequence, the US Food & Drug Administration (1980) restricts the carbon black content of packing materials used in contact with foodstuffs.

Physical and chemical properties of the two types of carbon black are given in Table 3.

The silicas used as rubber reinforcement agents are synthetically produced. Two types are in use: precipitated silica, made by direct precipitation from sodium silicate solu-tion, and pyrogenic silica, made by reacting silicon tetra-chloride with water vapour in a hydrogen-oxygen flame.

(h)   Fillers and diluents

For non-critical applications a significant proportion of filler can be added to the rubber formulation without detracting from the properties of the vulcanisate. Calcium carbonate

Table 3. Physical and chemical properties of of carbon blacks[a]

Property	Furnace black		Channel black
	Oil	Gas	
Composition			
Carbon (%)	98	99.2	88.4-95.2 (avg, 91.2)
Oxygen (%)	0.8	0.4	3.6-11.2 (avg, 7.8)
Hydrogen (%)	0.3	0.3	0.4-0.8 (avg. 0.6)
Ash-Ca, Mg, Na (%)	0.1-1.0	0.1-1.0	0.01
Volatile matter (%)	1-2	1-2	5-18
Average particle diameter (μm)	0.018-0.06	0.04-0.08	0.01-0.03
Specific surface (m^2/g)	25-200	25-50	100-1000
pH	8-9	8-9	3-5
Benzene extractables (%)	0.05-0.1	0.05-0.15	-

[a] From National Institute for Occupational Safety & Health (1978)

(whiting), clays, barytes, magnesium carbonate and other inorganic solids are in common use. The clays used may contain crystalline silica; 'China' clays may contain up to 1% and 'ball' clays up to 20% silica. Some fillers have weakly reinforcing effects.

(i)   Miscellaneous additives

(i) Blowing agents are used to produce foam rubbers by decomposing at cure temperature to produce gases. The main blowing agents and routes of decomposition are shown in Figure 17.

(ii) Promoters are materials added in small quantities to uncompounded rubber (usually butyl rubber) before the other compounding ingredients, to increase the resilience and tensile strength of the cured rubber, and to lower the build-up of heat in products such as tyres.

(iii) Mould-release agents are usually sprayed onto moulds to aid removal of the cured rubber items. Soaps, synthetic detergents, silicones, fluorinated hydrocarbons and polyethylene glycols are all in use.

(iv) Both inorganic pigments (e.g., titanium dioxide, cadmium sulphide, chromium oxide) and organic dyestuffs are used to produce coloured rubbers.

(v) Bonding agents are used to bond rubber to the textile or steel used in the construction of tyres or rubber/-metal articles. Many of the systems in use are proprietary mixtures, often of undisclosed composition, which may contain isocyanates and/or para-dinitrosobenzene. Resorcinol-hexa-methylenetetramine bonding systems are also used.

(vi) Antitack agents include stearates of metals (e.g., zinc stearate), mica and talc.

(vii) A variety of organic solvents are used in compounding and processing, including aliphatic hydrocarbons, acetone, 1,1,1-trichloroethane, methyl ethyl ketone, methylene chloride, perchloroethylene, trichloroethylene, toluene, xylene, tetrahydrofuran and dimethylformamide.

FIG. 17.   SOME BLOWING AGENTS AND THEIR ROUTES OF DECOMPOSITION

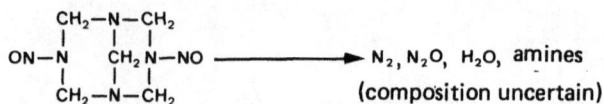

CH$_2$—N—CH$_2$
ON—N   CH$_2$ N—NO ⟶ N$_2$, N$_2$O, H$_2$O, amines
CH$_2$—N—CH$_2$
                                              (composition uncertain)

dinitrosopentamethylene-
   tetramine

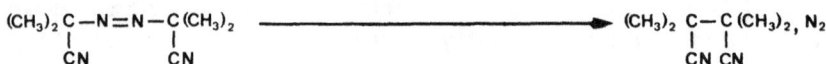

(CH$_3$)$_2$ C—N≡N—C (CH$_3$)$_2$ ⟶ (CH$_3$)$_2$ C—C (CH$_3$)$_2$, N$_2$
         CN   CN   CN CN

azobisisobutyronitrile   tetramethylsuccino-
                                              dinitrile

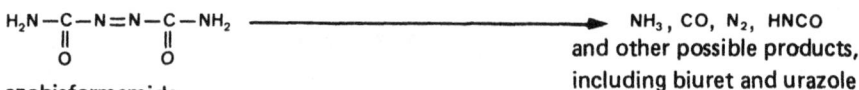

H$_2$N—C—N≡N—C—NH$_2$ ⟶ NH$_3$, CO, N$_2$, HNCO
         O   O   and other possible products,
                                          including biuret and urazole
azobisformamide

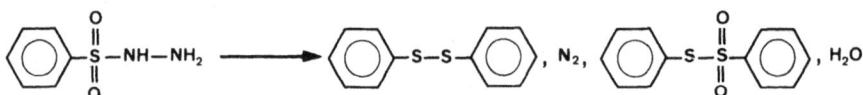

benzenesulphonyl   diphenyldisulphide   phenyl benzene-
   hydrazide   thiosulphonate

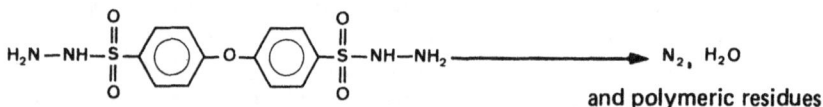

⟶ N$_2$, H$_2$O
and polymeric residues

para, para'-oxybis(benzenesulphonyl
   hydrazide)

(viii) Other rubber additives are <u>flame-proofing agents</u>, such as antimony trioxide, aluminium hydrates and halogenated aliphatic hydrocarbons; <u>odorants</u>, blends of perfumes and oils; and <u>coupling agents</u>, mostly silanes.

(ix) Materials unique to latex processing are dis-persing agents, stabilizers, emulsifiers, wetting agents, thick-eners, preservatives, coagulants, foaming agents and antifoaming agents.

Stabilizers, such as casein and a sodium alkylsulphate, are used. Dispersing agents are usually polyalkylarylsulphonates. As wetting agents, alkyl sulphonates, organic phosphates or a nonyl-phenol-ethylene oxide adduct may be used. Thickeners used are, for example, polyacrylates, cellulose derivatives or other high molecular-weight carbohydrate derivatives. Preservatives include formaldehyde and pentachlorophenates. Coagulants include sodium silicofluoride.

3. Chemical by-products (see also Appendix 1, Table 2)

Very few data are available on chemical species generated during rubber processing (with the exception of N-nitrosamines). Because the maximum temperature of vulcanization is approximately 240°C, pyrolysis reactions do not normally occur.

During vulcanization, the mould contains a reducing atmo-sphere because air is excluded. Products that could be formed during vulcanization and be released from the surface include amines and organic sulphides derived from the accelerators. For example, cure systems containing tetramethylthiuram disulphide may produce carbon disulphide and dimethylamine during cure (Willoughby & Lawson, 1981). The accelerator N-tert-butyl-2-benzothiazole sulphenamide has been reported to break down to tert-butylisothiocyanate at curing temperatures (Rappaport & Fraser, 1976).

Sulphenamide accelerators yield mercaptobenzothiazole and characteristic amines (Brock & Louth, 1955; Kleeman & Erben, 1964; Manik & Banerjee, 1970; Potts et al., 1972). Thiourea accelerators may decompose to give isothiocyanates (e.g., diethylthiourea produces ethyl isothiocyanate) (Groves & Smail, 1969). The retarder cyclohexylthiophthalimide is converted to phthalimide (Leib et al., 1970). (See Fig. 18.)

Upon removal from the mould, oxidizing reactions can occur, in which peroxy-substituted amines and acids may be formed (Tsurugi et al., 1971).

In a simulated vulcanization process, Rappaport and Fraser (1976) identified the following volatile compounds in the stock effluent (Table 4).

Table 4. Volatiles released from a rubber stock during simulated vulcanization, as identified in the stock effluent[a]

Compound	Probable source
Methylbenzene	cis-Polybutadiene rubber
4-Vinylcyclohexene	cis-Polybutadiene rubber
Ethylbenzene	Aromatic oil
Dimethylbenzene(1,3- and 1,4-)	Aromatic oil
Styrene	Styrene-butadiene rubber
tert-Butylisothiocyanate	N-tert-Butyl-2-benzo-thiazole-sulphenamide
1,5-Cyclooctadiene	cis-Polybutadiene rubber
Benzothiazole	N-tert-Butyl-2-benzo-thiazole-sulphenamide
N-sec-Butylaniline	N-Phenyl-N-sec-butyl-para-phenylenediamine
1,5,9-Cyclododecatriene	cis-Polybutadiene rubber
Methylnaphthalene	Aromatic oil
1,3-Butadiene trimer	cis-Polybutadiene rubber
Ethylnaphthalene	Aromatic oil
Dimethylnaphthalene	Aromatic oil

[a] From Rappaport & Fraser (1976)

Nitroso compounds

The occurrence of volatile N-nitrosamines in the rubber and tyre industry has been described by Fajen et al. (1979) Preussmann et al. (1980), Yeager et al. (1980), McGlothlin et al. (1981) and Spiegelhalder & Preussman (1982). The following N-nitrosamines have been detected: N-nitrosodimethylamine, N-nitrosodiethylamine, N-nitrosodibutylamine, N-nitrosopiperidine, N-nitrosopyrrolidine and N-nitrosomorpholine. [The Working Group noted that the corresponding nitrosatable precursor of each of these compounds, with the exception of N-nitrosopyrrolidine, is used in rubber compounding.]

The analytical methods used to determine these nitrosamines are based on wet-sampling techniques, such as impinger traps; on adsorption of organic material on solid samplers, for air sampling; or on extraction and distillation methods, for chemicals and rubber products. For qualitative and quantitative determination of N-nitrosamines in extracts, nitrosamine-specific chemoluminescence detection was used after separation by gas chromatography. Usually, identity was confirmed by combined gas chromatography/high-resolution mass spectrometry. The possibility of artefact formation during clean-up was excluded by the addition of nitrosation inhibitors such as alkali or sulphamic acid.

The formation of N-nitrosamines from precursors has been described in a previous IARC Monograph (IARC, 1978). The general reaction can be described as follows:

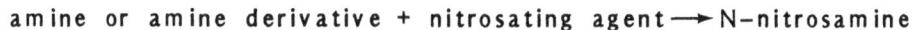

amine or amine derivative + nitrosating agent ⟶ N-nitrosamine

In addition to the familiar nitrosation of secondary amines, reactions involving tertiary amines or amine derivatives such as dialkyl dithiocarbamates, dialkyl thiuram sulphides and sulphenamides are possible in the rubber industry, where these types of chemicals are used as vulcanization accelerators and stabilizers (Fig. 18). Some nitrosatable accelerators which yield nonvolatile nitrosamines after nitrosation are shown in Figure 19.

Nitrosation can occur in aqueous systems, in solid systems as well as in the gas phase. The following two nitrosation reactions are possible:

(1) Nitrosatable compounds dissolved or dispersed in latex solution may be nitrosated during the production of latex articles. Nitrogen oxides from air have been proposed as the nitrosating agents.

(2) Chemicals that contain nitro or nitroso groups are potential nitrosating agents. As some of these chemicals may decompose thermally during processing to form nitrogen oxides, direct nitrosation of nitrosatable compounds contained in solid

FIG. 18. GROUPS OF CHEMICALS THAT CAN BE CONVERTED TO $\underline{N}$-NITROSAMINES

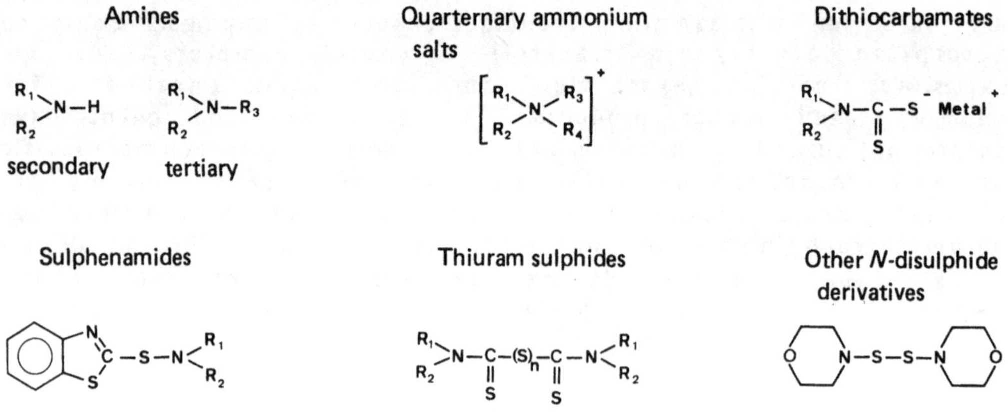

rubber is possible (Rappe & Rydström, 1980). Figure 20 shows potential nitrogen oxide-releasing chemicals used in the rubber industry.

Replacement of $\underline{N}$-nitrosodiphenylamine by other retarders results in a decreased level of detectable nitrosamines in rubber factories (Preussmann **et al.**, 1980; McGlothlin **et al.**, 1981; Spiegelhalder & Preussmann, 1982).

In western Europe, and to a lesser extent in the US, some rubber products are cured in a bath consisting of a mixture of molten nitrate and nitrite salts (salt-bath curing). In continuous vulcanization, the extruded rubber material is transferred continuously through the molten heat-transfer salt. Nitrosatable chemicals present at the surface of solid rubber can react directly with nitrite to form nitrosamines.

Nitrosamines are not only formed during the manufacture of rubber but may be present in rubber chemicals as contaminants (Table 5). The origin of these nitrosamines is probably nitrosation by ambient nitrogen oxides during production or storage.

ACCELERATOR   NITROSAMINE

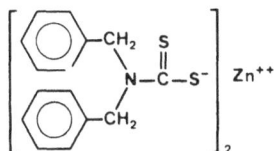

zinc dibenzyldithiocarbamate   nitrosodibenzylamine

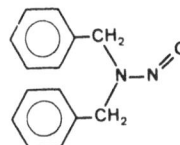

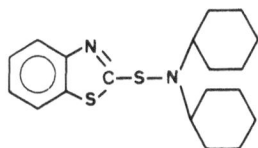

N,N-dicyclohexyl-2-benzo·
thiazolesulphenamide   nitrosodicyclohexylamine

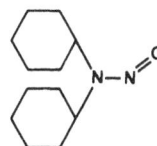

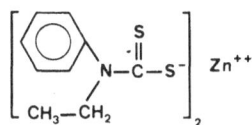

zinc ethylphenyldithiocarbamate   nitrosoethylphenylamine

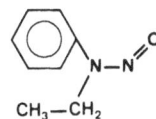

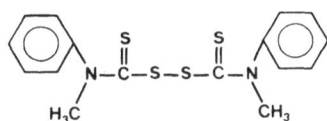

dimethyldiphenylthiuram disulphide   nitrosomethylphenylamine

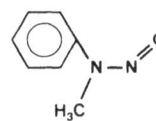

FIG. 19. ACCELERATORS AND CORRESPONDING NON–VOLATILE
NITROSAMINES
(From Spiegelhalder & Preussmann, 1982)

RETARDERS

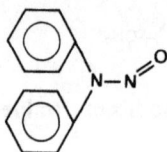

N-nitrosodiphenylamine

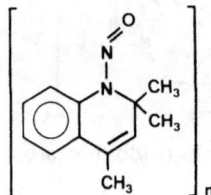

poly-N-nitroso-2,2,4-trimethyl-
1,2-dihydroquinoline

ACCELERATORS

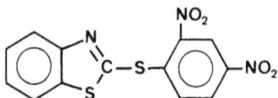

2-(2,4-dinitrophenylthio)-
benzothiazole

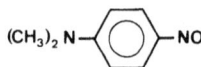

N,N-dimethyl-para-nitrosoaniline

PROMOTOR

BLOWING AGENT

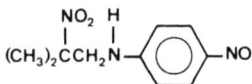

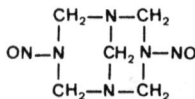

N-(2-methyl-2-nitropropyl)-
4-nitrosoaniline

dinitrosopenta-
methylenetetramine

FIG. 20.   NITRO AND NITROSO COMPOUNDS USED IN THE RUBBER
           INDUSTRY THAT CAN ACT AS PRECURSORS OF
           NITROGEN OXIDES

Natural atmospheric levels of 30–70 ppb nitrogen oxides may be complemented by combustion processes such as open flames, industrial pollution and exhausts from gas- and diesel-powered fork-lift trucks and other transport vehicles. Propane-powered vehicles for indoor use, which emit low levels of carbon monoxide, have been shown to increase the level of nitrogen oxides up to 1000 ppb. Nitrosamine levels in such areas are elevated (Spiegelhalder & Preussmann, 1982).

Table 5. Examples of nitrosamine contamination in commercial samples of rubber chemicals[a]

Accelerator	Nitrosamine present	Concentration (μg/kg)
N-Pentamethylene dithiocarbamate, piperidine salt	N-nitrosopiperidine	200
Tetramethylthiuram disulphide	N-nitrosodimethylamine	4– 800
Tetraethylthiuram disulphide	N-nitrosodiethylamine	25 – 80
Zinc-pentamethylene dithiocarbamate	N-nitrosopiperidine	60 – 450
Zinc-dibutyldithiocarbamate	N-nitrosodibutylamine	65 – 2500
Zinc-diethyldithiocarbamate	N-nitrosodiethylamine	10 – 100
Morpholine derivatives	N-nitrosomorpholine	60 – 3500

[a] From Spiegelhalder & Preussmann (1982)

4. Summary

In the industry as a whole, several hundred different chemicals are or have been involved in the manufacture of various rubber products. The choice of chemicals employed at different stages of processing varies from company to company and in different factories within the same company. During the development of the industry, there has been increasing use of synthetic elastomers (after the Second World War); changes in the materials used for compounding, such as the types of carbon black used in the late 1940s and the withdrawal of certain aromatic amines around 1950; and the introduction of the use of highly aromatic extender oils during the late 1950s. Other compounds are formed during rubber processing, including amines, sulphides and volatile compounds produced during vulcanization. The occurrence of nitrosation, resulting in the formation of volatile N-nitrosamines during rubber processing, has been studied in particular. Some nitrosamine precursors, such as morpholine derivatives and thiocarbamates, were introduced for use in the 1930s.

5. References

Blow, C.M., ed. (1978) Rubber Technology and Manufacture, London, Newnes-Butterworths

Brock, M.J. & Louth, G.D. (1955) Identification of accelerators and antioxidants in compounded rubber products. Anal. Chem., 27, 1575-1580

Brydson, J.A. (1978) Rubber Chemistry, London, Applied Science Publishers Ltd, pp. 197, 260

Coran, A.Y. (1978) Vulcanization. In: Eirich, F.R., ed., Science and Technology of Rubber, New York, Academic Press, pp. 300, 305

Davis, A.J. (1980) Developments in synthetic rubber since 1955. Rubber World, 181, 29-34

Dunbrook, R.F. (1954) Historical review. In: Whitby, G.S., Davis, C.C. & Dunbrook, R.F., eds, Synthetic Rubber, New York, John Wiley & Sons, pp. 32-55

Fajen, J.M., Carson, G.A., Rounbehler, D.P., Fan, T.Y., Vita, R., Goff, U.E., Wolf, M.H., Edwards, G.S., Fine, D.H., Reinhold, V. & Biemann, K. (1979) N-Nitrosamines in the rubber and tire industry. Science, 205, 1262-1264

Groves, J.S. & Smail, J.M. (1969) Outbreak of superficial keratitis in rubber workers. Br. J. Ophthalmol., 53, 683-687

Holmberg, B. & Sjöström, B. (1977) A Toxicological Survey of Chemicals Used in the Swedish Rubber Industry (Investigation Report 1977:19), Stockholm, National Board of Occupational Safety and Health

Hybart, F.J., Briscoe, G.B. & Daniel, T.J. (1968) Variety in compounding in the general rubber goods section of the rubber industry. J. Inst. Rubber Ind., 2, 190-193

IARC (1978) IARC Monographs on the Evaluation of the Carcinogenic Risk of Chemicals to Humans, Vol. 17, Some N-Nitroso Compounds, Lyon, pp. 35-47

The International Rubber Study Group (1946-1981) Rubber Statistical Bulletin, Vols 1-35, London. Data collated by the Rubber & Plastics Research Association of Great Britain, Shrewsbury

Kempermann, T. (1978) Concerning the relationship between the chemical compositions and effects of accelerators. Part 1. Tech. Notes Rubber Ind., 50, 29, 32, 33

Kempermann, T. (1979) Concerning the relationship between the chemical compositions and effects of accelerators. Part 2. Tech. Notes Rubber Ind., 51, 17

Kleeman, W. & Erben, G. (1964) Thermostability of sulfenamide accelerators in tire compounds. Rubber Chem. Technol., 37, 204-209

Leib, R.I., Sullivan, A.B. & Trivette, C.D., Jr (1970) Pre-vulcanization inhibitor. The chemistry of scorch delay. Rubber Chem. Technol., 43, 1188-1193

Manik, S.P. & Banerjee, S. (1970) Sulfenamide accelerated sulfur vulcanization of natural rubber in presence and absence of dicumyl peroxide. Rubber Chem. Technol., 43, 1311-1326

McGlothlin, J.D., Wilcox, T.C., Fajen, J.M. & Edwards, G.S. (1981) A health hazard evaluation of nitrosamines in a tire manufacturing plant. In: Choudhary, G., ed., Chemical Hazards in the Workplace, Measurement and Control, Washington DC, American Chemical Society, pp. 283-299

National Institute for Occupational Safety & Health (1978) Criteria for a Recommended Standard ... Occupational Exposure to Carbon Black (DHEW (NIOSH Publication No. 78-204), Cincinnati, OH

Nutt, A.R. (1979) Toxicity of rubber chemicals. Prog. Rubber Technol., 42, 141-154

Potts, K.T., Brugel, E.G., D'Amico, J.J. & Morita, E. (1972) Electron impact-induced fragmentations of 2-benzothiazole sulfenamides and related compounds. Correlation with rubber vulcanization activity. Rubber Chem. Technol., 45, 160-172

Preussmann, R., Spiegelhalder, B. & Eisenbrand, G. (1980) Reduction of human exposure to environmental N-nitroso-carcinogens. Examples of possibilities for cancer prevention. In: Pullman, B., Ts'o, P.O.P. & Gelboin, H., eds, Carcinogenesis: Fundamental Mechanisms and Environmental Effects, Dordrecht, D. Reidel, pp. 273-285

Rappaport, S.M. & Fraser, D.A. (1976) Gas chromatographic-mass spectrometric identification of volatiles released from a rubber stock during simulated vulcanization. Anal. Chem., 48, 476-481

Rappaport, S.M. & Fraser, D.A. (1977) Air sampling and analysis in a rubber vulcanization area. Am. ind. Hyg. Assoc. J., 38, 205-210

Rappe, C. & Rydström, T. (1980) Occupational exposure to N-nitroso compounds. In: Walker, E.A., Griciute, L., Castegnaro, M. & Börzsönyi, M., eds, N-Nitroso Compounds: Analysis, Formation and Occurrence (IARC Scientific Publications No. 31), Lyon,. International Agency for Research on Cancer, pp. 565-574

Russell, W.F. (1937) Practical compounding. In: Davis, C.C. & Blake, J.T., eds, The Chemistry and Technology of Rubber, New York, Reinhold

Spiegelhalder, B. & Preussmann, R. (1982) Nitrosamines and rubber. In: Bartsch, H., O'Neill, I.K., Castegnaro, M. & Okada, M., eds, N-Nitroso Compounds: Occurrence and Biological Effects (IARC Scientific Publications No. 41), Lyon, International Agency for Research on Cancer (in press)

Stephens, H.L. (1973) Compounding and vulcanization of rubber. In: Morton, M., ed., Rubber Technology, 2nd ed., New York, Van Nostrand-Reinhold, p. 28

Stern, H.J. (1967) Rubber: Natural and Synthetic, 2nd ed., London, MacLaren & Sons

Stern, H.J. (1978) History. In: Blow, C.M., ed., Rubber Techno-
    logy and Manufacture, London, Newnes–Butterworths, pp. 1–19

Tsurugi, J., Murakami, S. & Goda, K. (1971) Charge transfer
    complexing mechanism of antioxidants. Fate of aromatic
    amines during thermal oxidation of natural rubber vulcan-
    izates. Rubber Chem. Technol., 44, 857–880

US Food & Drug Administration (1980) Food and drugs. US Code Fed.
    Regul., Title 21, part 177.2600

Willoughby, B.G. & Lawson, G. (1981) Laboratory vulcanization as
    an aid to factory air analysis. Rubber Chem. Technol., 54,
    311–330

Yeager, F.W., van Gulick, N.N. & Lasoski, B.A. (1980) Dialkyl-
    nitrosamines in elastomers. Am. ind. Hyg. Assoc. J., 41,
    148–150

(A summary of environmental monitoring techniques is given as an annex to this section)

1.   Engineering controls, personal protective equipment and work practices

Engineering controls, including changes in process equipment and ventilation, can provide protection for workers in the rubber industry. Exhaust equipment should not only remove materials, thus preventing worker exposure, but should also be designed to prevent community exposure in the general environment outside the factory. Machinery design should minimize worker contact with materials, e.g., by isolating operators from the process stream or by enclosing highly toxic processes. Machinery should also be designed so that its various parts can be isolated during maintenance or repair.

The use of respirators is not recommended for protection during routine production operations. When respirators are used, a programme of proper selection, cleaning and fitting should be initiated. A medical evaluation of a worker's cardiopulmonary condition and ability to use a respirator should be evaluated. Regular monitoring of the workers' health and evaluations of the effectiveness of the programme are recommended.

Variations in work practices can substantially affect a worker's exposure. Management is responsible for supervision of these practices and for providing continuing education programmes to inform workers about hazards that exist within their workplace and about the toxic properties and guidelines for the safe handling of all materials found in their working environment.

Washroom facilities, appropriate respirators, eyewash fountains, emergency showers and other personal protective equipment should be available at locations readily accessible from all areas where hazardous materials are found. Eating areas, smoking areas and toilet facilities should be isolated from the work

areas. Workers in certain areas, such as compounding and processing, run a greater risk of prolonged skin contact with toxic
materials; they should be encouraged to take a shower after work
and to change clothes prior to returning home so as to avoid
transporting exposure to family members and prolonging their own
exposure.

2. General reviews of exposure in the rubber industry

Three general reviews of environmental contamination were
available to the Working Group. Williams et al. (1980) and Van
Ert et al. (1980) carried out comprehensive reviews of levels of
exposure to particulates and solvents in the US tyre manufacturing industry. The British Rubber Manufacturers' Association
(Parkes et al., 1975) reported an environmental monitoring study
in 10 UK tyre factories in 1974, in which high-volume area
samples were taken and in which total particulate, cyclohexane-
soluble and benzo[a]pyrene concentrations at various sites were
reported. General studies of nitrosamine exposure have been made
in the US and the Federal Republic of Germany. The surveys by the
US National Institute for Occupational Safety and Health (Fajen
et al., 1979; Ringenberg & Fajen, 1980; McGlothlin et al., 1981)
represent results obtained in five factories; Spiegelhalder and
Preussmann (1982) and Spiegelhalder (unpublished data) investigated more than 17 rubber factories in the Federal Republic of
Germany.

Abbreviations used are: NDBA – N-nitrosodibutylamine; NDEA –
N-nitrosodiethylamine; NDMA – N-nitrosodimethylamine; NDPhA –
N-nitrosodiphenylamine; NMOR – N-nitrosomorpholine; NPIP –
N-nitrosopiperidine; NPYR – N-nitrosopyrrolidine.

2.1 Raw materials handling, weighing, mixing (Table 6)

Historically and to the present day, these operations have
been among the dirtiest in the industry. In some plants, the
majority of the particulate is carbon black; when carbon black is
handled automatically, weighers may be exposed only to other
compounding materials. The separation and analysis of carbon
black and other specific compounding materials remain difficult
problems.

Table 6. Exposures during raw materials handling, weighing and mixing

Reference	Material	Level	Comments
Williams et al. (1980)	Total particulate	3.10 mg/m³ (3 plants; median) 1.27-13.0 mg/m³ (11 samples)	Personal samples; compounding
	Total particulate	1.90 mg/m³ (14 plants; median) 0.1-21 mg/m³ (19 samples)	Personal samples; mixing
Parkes et al. (1975)	Total particulate	0.25-10 mg/m³ (50 samples in 10 plants)	High-volume area samples; internal mixer loading
	Total particulate	0.4 - >10 mg/m³ (50 samples in 10 plants)	High-volume area samples; raw materials weighing
Williams et al. (1980)	Benzo[a]pyrene	0-32.3 µg/m³ (7 plants)	High-volume area samples; mixing
McGlothlin et al. (1981)	No nitrosamine detected		Personal sample; tyre
Fajen et al. (1979)	NDMA	0.1 µg/m³	Area sample; industrial rubber products
Spiegelhalder & Preussmann (1982)	NDMA	0.2-0.9 µg/m³	Area samples; tyre
	NMOR	<0.1-2 µg/m³ [a]	Area samples; tyre
Van Ert et al. (1980)	Benzene	1.5 mg/m³ (8 plants; median) 0.6-24 mg/m³ (23 samples)	Personal samples; solvent mixing
	Hexane	56 mg/m³ (8 plants; median) 2.5-808 mg/m³ (23 samples)	Personal samples; solvent mixing

[a] Process not separated from other areas

While median exposure levels as reported by Williams et al.
(1980) may give some idea of exposure throughout the industry, it
should be noted that the range of exposures is very wide. Individuals may be exposed to high levels even in plants where median
exposure levels are low. There may be cross exposures to milling
fume from drop mills.

Exposure to solvents may occur during the mixing of adhesives, used either as such or in building rubber goods. Although
hexane is not suspected of being a carcinogen, it may have
significant effects on health.

2.2 Milling, extruding and calendering (Table 7)

Mill operators may be exposed to cross contaminants from
Banbury mixers and to residual compounding material from the mill
itself. In milling, extruding and calendering, there is also
exposure to condensed volatiles, vapours and gases. Because of
the high temperatures used in these processes and the large
surface area of rubber that they generate, traces of new compounds, including nitrosamines, may be formed.

2.3 Component assembly and building (Table 8)

The solvents currently used in the building of rubber goods
are generally petroleum naphthas, although coal-tar naphthas were
used in the past. Both naphthas contained benzene, at levels of
up to several percents; current levels are generally much lower
(a fraction of a percent). There may be exposure via the skin to
mineral oils, to solvents and to fractions of rubber dissolved in
solvent during building operations; such exposures are not listed
in Table 8.

2.4 Curing or vulcanization (Table 9)

When goods are prepared for curing, they may be sprayed with
a solvent-based lubricant. The curing itself generates condensed
volatiles, vapours and gases, and the job area is subject to and

Table 7. Exposures during milling, extruding and calendering

Reference	Material	Level	Comments
Parkes et al. (1975)	Total particulate	0.02–10.0 mg/m³ (50 samples in 10 plants)	High-volume area samples; milling
	Total particulate	0.08–4.0 mg/m³ (50 samples in 10 plants)	High-volume area samples; extruding
	Cyclohexane-soluble particulate	0.02–4.0 mg/m³ (50 samples in 10 plants)	High-volume area samples; extruding
	Total particulate	0.02–1.5 mg/m³ (50 samples in 10 plants)	High-volume area samples; calendering
	Cyclohexane-soluble particulate	0.007–1.0 mg/m³ (50 samples in 10 plants)	High-volume area samples; calendering
Williams et al. (1980)	Total particulate	0.76 mg/m³ (2 plants; median) 0.16–2.18 mg/m³ (8 samples)	Personal samples; milling
	Total particulate	0.62 mg/m³ (1 plant; median) 0.28–0.89 mg/m³ (5 samples)	Personal samples; calendering
	Total particulate	18.0 mg/m³ (2 plants; median) 4.67–32.0 mg/m³ (4 samples)	Personal samples; tube extrusion
	Benzo[a]pyrene	0–15.3 µg/m³ (2 plants)	High-volume area samples; milling

Table 7 (contd)

Reference	Material	Level	Comments
Van Ert et al. (1980)	Benzene	2.4 mg/m³ (9 plants; median)	Personal samples; extruding
		0.3-40 mg/m³ (70 samples)	
Ringenburg & Fajen (1980)	NDMA NMOR	0-0.09 µg/m³ 0.9-1.4 µg/m³	Personal samples Personal samples
McGlothlin et al. (1981)	NDMA NMOR NPYR NDPhA	<0.1-0.4 µg/m³ <0.1-25 µg/m³ [a] <0.1-0.8 µg/m³ <0.1-13 µg/m³	Personal samples Personal samples Personal samples Personal samples
Fajen et al. (1979)	NMOR	1.7-27 µg/m³	Area samples; extruding
Spiegelhalder & Preussmann (1982)	NDMA NMOR	0.1-2 µg/m³ 0.1-9 µg/m³	Area samples; tyre and industry products
McGlothlin et al. (1981)	NDMA NPYR NMOR	<0.1-5.5 µg/m³ <0.1-3.9 µg/m³ <0.3-250 µg/m³	Process sample; tyre Process sample; tyre Process sample; tyre

[a] Process sample at same feed mill contained up to 250 µg/m³ NMOR

contributes to cross contamination of the work environment. The data in Table 9 demonstrate the occasional presence of benzene, benzo[a]pyrene, particulates (both total and respirable) and nitrosamines.

2.5 Inspection and finishing (Table 10)

Inspection involves the handling of hot cured rubber products, and workers are exposed to condensed volatiles, vapours and gases. The final finishing operation results in extensive skin contact with the finished product and exposure to rubber dust and solvents. These processes also contribute to cross contamination of the workplace air.

Table 8. Exposures during component assembly and building

Reference	Material	Level	Comments
Williams et al. (1980)	Total particulate	0.11 mg/m³	Single high-volume, area sample; tyre building
	Respirable particulates	0.24 mg/m³ (2 samples; median)	Personal samples; bead building
Van Ert et al. (1980)	Benzene	4.2 mg/m³ (10 plants; median) 0.3-27 mg/m³ (81 samples)	Personal samples; tyre building
		6 mg/m³ (2 plants; median) 1.2-9 mg/m³ (26 samples)	Area samples; tyre building
	Hexane	40 mg/m³ (10 plants; median) 0.4-207 mg/m³ (84 samples)	Personal samples; tyre building
		70 mg/m³ (2 plants; median) 30-850 mg/m³ (27 samples)	Area samples; tyre building
McGlothlin et al. (1981)	NDMA	0.1 μg/m³	Personal sample; tyre building
	NMOR	1.6-1.9 μg/m³	Personal samples; tyre building
Spiegelhalder & Preussmann (1982)	NDMA	0.1-1 μg/m³	Personal samples; tyre and industry products
	NMOR	0.5-3 μg/m³	

Table 9. Exposures during tyre curing or vulcanizing

Reference	Material	Level	Comments
Parkes et al. (1975)	Total particulate	0.03–2.0 mg/m³ (50 samples in 10 plants)	High-volume area samples; curing area
	Cyclohexane-soluble parti-culate	0.05–2.0 mg/m³ (50 samples in 10 plants	High-volume area samples; curing area
Williams et al. (1980)	Total particulate	1.33 mg/m³ (2 plants; median) 0.28–10.27 mg/m³ (23 samples)	Personal samples
	Respirable particulate	0.43 mg/m³ (3 plants; median) 0–1.5 mg/m³ (11 samples)	Personal samples
	Benzo[a]pyrene	0–8.8 μg/m³	High-volume area samples
Van Ert et al. (1980)	Benzene	2.4 mg/m³ (9 plants; median) <0.3–33 mg/m³ (22 samples)	Personal samples
Ringenburg & Fajen (1980)	NDMA NMOR	0.08 μg/m³ 1.5 μg/m³	Area samples; tyre curing Area samples; tyre curing
McGlothlin et al. (1981)	NDMA NMOR NDMA NMOR	0.1–0.3 μg/m³ 0.4–1.8 μg/m³ <0.1–0.2 μg/m³ <0.1–6.4 μg/m³	Personal samples; tyre curing Personal samples; tyre curing Tyre-process sample Tyre-process sample
Fajen et al. (1979)	NMOR	2.2–7.1 μg/m³	Area samples; tyre curing
Spiegelhalder & Preussmann (1982)	NDMA NDMA	0.1–2 μg/m³ 15–130 μg/m³	Personal samples; tyre curing Personal samples; tube curing (NDPhA used)
	NDMA	1–4.5 μg/m³	Personal samples; tube curing (NDPhA not used)
	NDMA	17–28 μg/m³	Personal and area samples; tube curing
	NDPA	1–2.5 μg/m³	Personal and area samples; tube curing

Table 9 (contd)

Reference	Material	Level	Comments
Spiegelhalder & Preussmann (1982)	NDBA	1 µg/m³	Personal and area sample tube curing
	NMOR	0.1-17 µg/m³	Personal samples; tyre curing
	NDMA	1-40 µg/m³	Personal samples; salt-bath curing
	NDEA	0.1-5 µg/m³	Personal samples; salt-bath curing
	NDBA	<0.1-1 µg/m³	Personal samples; salt-bath curing
	NMOR	0.1-3 µg/m³	Personal samples; salt-bath curing
	NPIP	<0.1-1.5 µg/m³	Personal samples; salt-bath curing
	NDMA	40-90 µg/m³	Personal samples; injection
	NMOR	120-380 µg/m³	moulding (TMTD,dithiomorpholine and NDPhA in use)
	NDMA	500-1060 µg/m³	Process samples; as above
	NMOR	200-4700 µg/m³	Process samples; as above
	NDMA	0.5-1 µg/m³	Personal and area samples; water hose
	NDEA	0.1-5 µg/m³	Personal and area samples; water hose
	NDBA	0.1-1 µg/m³	Personal and area samples; water hose
	NPIP	<0.1-0.3 µg/m³	Personal and area samples; water hose
	NMOR	0.1-2 µg/m³	Personal and area samples; water hose
	NDMA	1-3.5 µg/m³	Personal and area samples; window seals
	NMOR	3-9 µg/m³	Personal and area samples; window seals
	NDMA	0.2-3.5 µg/m³	Personal and area samples; injection moulding
	NDMA	1 µg/m³	Area samples; latex goods production
	NDEA	3 µg/m³	Area samples; latex goods production

Table 10. Exposures during inspection and finishing

Reference	Material	Level	Comments
Parkes et al. (1975)	Total particulate	0.08-2.0 mg/m³ (50 samples in 10 plants	High-volume area sample; inspection
	Cyclohexane-soluble particulates	0.02-2.0 mg/m³ (50 samples in 10 plants)	High-volume area sample; inspection
Williams et al. (1980)	Particulate (respirable)	0.22 (11 plants) 0-2.83 mg/m³ (55 samples; median)	Personal samples
	Benzo[a]pyrene	<1-15.3 µg/m³ (7 plants)	High-volume area samples
Van Ert et al. (1980)	Benzene	3.3 mg/m³ (3 plants) 0.3-81 mg/m³ (11 samples; median)	Personal samples
Fajen et al. (1979)	NMOR	0.6 µg/m³	Personal samples; tyres
Spiegelhalder & Preussmann (1982)	NDMA NMOR NDMA	0.1-1.5 µg/m³ 0.1-20 µg/m³ up to 10 µg/m³	Personal samples; tyres Personal samples; tyres Personal samples; tubes

2.6 Storage and dispatch (Table 11)

Storage and dispatch are carried out in the plant warehouse. The products that may be emitted are off-gases of solvents (e.g., benzene) and nitrosamines. Nitrogen oxides may occur due to the use of gasoline- and propane-driven fork-lift trucks.

3. Studies of specific exposures in the rubber industry

A number of smaller studies of the industry help to create a picture of the diversity of worker exposures. They are summarized in Table 12.

Table 11. Exposures during storage and dispatch

Reference	Material	Level	Comments
Van Ert et al. (1980)	Benzene	0.03-1.4 mg/m³ (32 samples in 2 plants)	Area samples; tyre warehouse
McGlothlin et al. (1980)	NDMA	0.04-0.1 μg/m³	Personal samples; tyres
	NMOR	<0.01-1.7 μg/m³	Personal samples; tyres
Spiegelhalder & Preussmann (1982)	NDMA	0.2-10 μg/m³ [a]	Personal samples; tyres
	NDMA	1-19 μg/m³	Personal samples; tubes
	NDMA	30-40 μg/m³	Personal and area samples; tubes
	NDPA	1.5-2.5 μg/m³	Personal and area samples; tubes
	NMOR	0.3-17 μg/m³	Personal samples; tyres
	NDMA	0.2-1 μg/m³	Industrial rubber production

[a] Higher values due to presence of tubes stored nearby

Between July 1972 and January 1977, the US Occupational Safety and Health Administration (1977) conducted 85 surveys with regard to carbon black to determine compliance with the occupational exposure limit of 3.5 mg/m³. Approximately 20% of the workplaces inspected were in violation of the standard, and levels in about 60% of these were 1-2 times above the standard.

Sands and Benitez (National Institute for Occupational Safety & Health, 1978) reported in 1961 concentrations of carbon black (measured as total dust) at three rubber factories ranging from 0.14-38.9 mg/m³: 1.77-38.9 mg/m³ were found in areas where Banbury mixers were loaded; 1.41-21.2 mg/m³ during milling; and 0.14-4.24 mg/m³ in the general air of milling rooms.

Pagnatto et al. (1961, 1979) reported a reduction in exposure to benzene during the proofing of fabric after substitution of benzene by other solvents. Exposure can occur both during the preparation of proofing compounds and during their application.

In 1960-1964, levels of 6-44 ppm were found in the churn room, 10-140 ppm at the saturator, and 3-39 ppm at the spreader. The solvent in use at that time contained 3-7.5% benzene. Substitution of a benzene-free solvent in 1964 reduced exposure to 'none detectable'. Exposure to other solvents may continue.

In a series of 'health hazard evaluations' by the US National Institute for Occupational Safety and Health (1977a, 1979, 1980), employee exposures at a rubber factory were surveyed. Biological data on 51 employees exposed to ethylenethiourea were evaluated, and exposures in compounding, milling and fabric-proofing operations were monitored. Air contamination ranged from non-detectable to a level of 77 $\mu g/m^3$, except for one man who loaded churns in a fabric-proofing operation who was exposed to 1100 $\mu g/m^3$ during a 15-min sampling period.

In a Finnish rubber factory, levels of 0.001-0.072 mg/m^3 ethylenethiourea were measured in the breathing zone of workers in milling and mixing operations, 0.004-0.006 mg/m^3 during calendering, 0.012-0.206 mg/m^3 during extruding and 0.051-0.081 during cleaning. Levels of 0.0001-0.011 mg/m^3 methylenebis-ortho-chloroaniline were measured in areas outside those in which its use was permitted (Enwald, 1982).

During an inspection of a tyre company by the US Occupational Safety and Health Administration (1980), personal samples were taken on a worker in the compounding area to determine his exposure to a number of organic materials: 0.01 mg/m^3 2-morpholinothiobenzothiazole, 0.26 mg/m^3 diphenylguanidine; 17.0 mg/m^3 polymerized 1,2-dihydro-2,2,4-trimethylquinoline and 3.4 mg/m^3 N-cyclohexyl-2-benzothiazole sulphoxide were measured.

At a factory where surgical, household and industrial gloves were manufactured from natural latex, gloves were dipped in a suspension of talc in a liquid containing ethanol, isopropanol and methyl isobutyl ketone. The average levels of the solvents found in breathing area samples, using a combustible gas indicator, was 40 ppm; maxima of 130 ppm ethanol and 110 ppm methyl isobutyl ketone were measured. Kitagawa indicator tubes were also used to sample for ethanol and ketones (measured as methyl ethyl ketone): at the talc slurry, 800, 500 and 400 ppm ethanol were found; and in the breathing zone, 80 ppm ketone were measured (The Industrial Commission of Ohio, 1971).

In an Egyptian study (Noweir et al., 1972) on three large tyre plants, total dust concentrations in area samples were 18-40 million particles per cubic foot (mppcf) in the storage area and 20-36 mppcf in the compounding area. In open-mixing, 20-50 mppcf particulates were found, while in the inner-tube building section of one plant, a total dust level of 11 mppcf was measured. The curing area was less dusty in terms of airborne particulate levels: 5 mppcf were found in two plants investigated.

Total dust concentrations in the air around core-winding machines for making golf-balls were 12.7-50.7 mg/m³ in personal samples. After a local exhaust system was installed, 2.4-8.6 mg/m³ were measured. During loading of storage hoppers, 88 mg/m³ total dust were measured; after an enclosure was fitted, <1 mg/m³ was found (Nutt, 1979).

Average concentrations of respirable dust measured in US studies in connection with medical investigations ranged from 0.47 to 1.63 mg/m³ (near a cureman) (Fine & Peters, 1976; Fine et al., 1976). In another plant, the average concentration of respirable dust ranged between 0.51 (in extruding) to 3.55 mg/m³ (in a rubber band area); 1.29 mg/m³ were found in a curing area.

The content of the atmosphere in the curing area may vary according to whether the process is manual or automatic (Burgess et al., 1977). Manual operators may experience concentrations of respirable dust six times higher than those of men working in automatic curing: mean concentrations dropped from 1.59 to 0.28 mg/m³ in a changeover from manual to automatic press operation. Carbon black particulates comprised 'a significant portion' of the respirable dust in processing areas.

Dust measurements by personal sampler in a Swedish tyre factory in 1976 (Gunnarsson, personal communication) showed total dust levels in the weighing and mixing department to be above the Swedish occupational standard for inert organic dust of 5 mg/m³.

The benzo[a]pyrene content in the weighing area of a non-specified rubber industry was 0.01-0.05 μg/m³ (0.03-0.20 μg/m³ total polycyclic aromatic hydrocarbons); that at a mixing station was 0.01-0.05 μg/m³ (0.06-1.2 μg/m³ total). The ratio in the air varied with the type of soot used in the process (Otto & Schmidt, 1978).

In the air at a mixing station of a tyre factory, 16.7 and 19.0 ng/m³ benzo[a]pyrene were found; the levels in air close to extruders were generally half or less than half (3.2-12.1 ng/m³) of those values. The air above conveyors contained 15.7-43.0 ng/m³; and the air in an inner tube department had 21.3-32.1 ng/m³. Air around curing presses contained levels of 3.7-12.8 ng/m³, and tyre trimming areas had from 'not detectable' to 56.8 ng/m³ (Nutt, 1976).

Oil mists were measured at various work areas in a Finnish rubber factory, and the maximum quantity of benzo[a]pyrene was calculated. At extruders, <0.016-0.096 μg/m³ were estimated; at calenders, <0.016-<0.248 μg/m³; and during milling, <0.016-<0.040 μg/m³ (Enwald, 1982).

The levels of benzo[a]pyrene taken inside factories are, in general, similar to those taken in the outside air (Nutt, 1976; Williams et al., 1980).

Gases and vapours have been investigated mostly in tyre and tube manufacturing industries, or in laboratory model systems that imitate field conditions. In one field study (Noweir et al., 1972), no nitrogen dioxide was detectable in most areas investigated; although air samples from curing area in two factories contained mean levels of 0.57 and 0.81 ppm. In mixing areas, hydrogen sulphide was found at concentrations of 0.22 ppm (closed mixing), 0.12 and 0.34 ppm (open mixing) in three different factories. Sulphur dioxide levels were 1.20 ppm (closed mixing) and 1.30 ppm (open mixing) in one factory and 0.61 ppm (open mixing) in a second factory. In the curing areas of two factories, mean concentrations of hydrogen sulphide were 0.46 and 0.34 ppm, and those of sulphur dioxide were 2.40 and 1.10 ppm, respectively.

In a laboratory model of tyre curing, Fraser and Rappaport (1976) demonstrated the presence of about 20 different chemicals in effluent air, including toluene, 4-vinylcyclohexene, ethylbenzene, 1,3-dimethylbenzene (xylene), 1,4-dimethylbenzene (xylene), styrene, tert-butylisothiocyanate, 1,5-cyclooctadiene, benzothiazole, N-sec-butylaniline, 1,5,9-cyclododecatriene, methylnaphthalene, 1,3-butadiene trimer, ethylnaphthalene and dimethylnaphthalene. Most of these compounds were probably derived from the raw elastomer used, or from an aromatic oil added to the mixture.

Some of the compounds were later identified in the air at the centre and at the periphery of tyre curing areas, where a similar rubber mixture was being used (Fraser & Rappaport, 1976; Rappaport & Fraser, 1977). Thus, mean concentrations of toluene were 1120 ppb in the centre and 1160 at the periphery of the curing area; those of 4-vinylcyclohexene were 71 ppb and 92 ppb; of ethylbenzene, 78 and 112 ppb; of styrene, 85 and 111 ppb; of 1,5-cyclooctadiene, 6 and 6 ppb; and of 1,5,9-cyclododecatriene, 7 and 16 ppb, respectively. Many unidentified chemicals were present in the air samples.

In a factory where rubber footwear was manufactured, employees in the compounding and doubling rooms were found to have been exposed to excessive concentrations of airborne particulates. Levels of zinc stearate, as measured near the lining calender and near the vulcanizers, were judged to be capable of producing intermittent, short-term sensory irritation. The levels of methylene chloride and of methylene-di(4-phenylisocyanate) produced under normal operating conditions at the polyurethane injection-moulding operation were judged to be non-toxic, although potentially toxic conditions could exist during maintenance procedures (Levy, 1976).

Workers in a tyre-manufacturing factory where a hexamethylene-tetramine-resorcinol resin system was used were exposed to resorcinol, formaldehyde and ammonia at concentrations of <0.3 mg/m^3, 0.05 mg/m^3 and 0.1 mg/m^3, respectively (Gamble et al., 1976).

Residual chloroprene levels in a typical press roll-building operation using polychloroprene were measured by taking air samples during the entire roll-building operation. No residual chloroprene and <3 ppm toluene were detected (National Institute for Occupational Safety & Health, 1977b).

The concentration of chloroprene monomer in solid polychloroprene rubber is less than 1 ppm by weight, but it may be much higher, up to 5000 ppm, in polychloroprene latices (Nutt, 1976). Atmospheric concentrations in area samples were 2-12 ppm during the compounding of latex, 3-6 ppm during the use of compounded latex, and 2-20 ppm during the production of dipped goods from polychloroprene latex. The concentrations in personal samples during use of compounded latex were 2-4 ppm.

Table 12. Summary of studies of specific exposures in the rubber industry

REFERENCE	MATERIAL	LEVEL	COMMENTS
Noweir et al. (1972)	Total dust	18-32 mppcf 20-36 mmpcf 20-50 mmpcf 11 mmpcf 5 mmpcf	storage compounding open mixing inner tube building curing
Nutt (1979)	Total dust	12.7-50.7 mg/m³ 2.4-8.6 mg/m³ 88 mg/m³ <1 mg/m³	Personal sample; core-winding " " " " (with exhaust) " " " loading " " " (with exhaust)
Gunnarsson	Total dust	>5 mg/m³	Personal samples; weighing, mixing
Fine et al. (1976)	Respirable dust	0.47-1.41 mg/m³ 0.51-3.55 mg/m³ 0.26-1.54 mg/m³ 0.24-0.78 mg/m³	tube curing extruder rubber-band curing, manual curing, automatic
Nutt (1976)	Benzo[a]pyrene	~ 0.02 µg/m³ up to 0.01 µg/m³ 0.02-0.04 µg/m³ 0.02-0.03 µg/m³ up to 0.01 µg/m³ up to 0.06 µg/m³	mixing, tyre extruder above conveyors inner tube building curing finishing
Otto & Schmidt (1978)	Benzo[a]pyrene	0.01-0.05 µg/m³	weighing, mixing
Williams et al. (1981)	Benzo[a]pyrene	0-32.3 µg/m³ 0-15 µg/m³ 0-8.8 µg/m³ 0-15.3 µg/m³	Banbury, tyre area milling curing inspection
Enwald (1982)	Benzo[a]pyrene	<0.016-0.096 µg/m³ <0.016-<0.248 µg/m³ <0.016-0.040 µg/m³	extruding calendering milling
Noweir et al. (1972)	Nitrogen dioxide Hydrogen sulphide Sulphur dioxide	570-810 ppb 220 ppb 120-340 ppb 340-460 ppb 1200 ppb 610-1300 ppb 1100-2400 ppb	curing mixing open mixing curing closed mixing open mixing curing
Fraser & Rappaport (1976)	Toluene 4-Vinylcyclohexene Ethylbenzene Styrene 1,5-Cyclooctadiene 1,5,9-Cyclododecatriene	1120-1160 ppb 71-92 ppb 78-112 ppb 85-111 ppb 6 ppb 7-16 ppb	curing curing curing curing curing curing
Sands & Benitez (1961)	Carbon black (total dust)	1.77-38.9 µg/m³ 1.41-21.2 µg/m³ 0.41-4.24 µg/m³	mixing milling area sample; milling
Industrial Commission of Ohio (1971)	Ethanol Methyl isobutyl ketone	40 ppm 40 ppm	dipping dipping

Table 12 (condt)

REFERENCE	MATERIAL	LEVEL		COMMENTS
Pagnatto et al. (1961, 1979)	Benzene	6-44 ppm 10-140 ppm 3-39 ppm		mixing) saturating) 1960-1964 spreading)
Nutt (1976)	Chloroprene	2-12 ppm 3-6 ppm 2-20 ppm		compounding building dipping
Occupational Safety & Health Administration (1980)	2-Morpholinothiobenzothiazole Diphenylguanidine Polymerized 1,2-dihydro-2,2,4- trimethylquinoline N-Cyclohexyl-2-benzothiazole sulphoxide	0.01 mg/m³ 0.26 mg/m³ 17.0 mg/m³ 3.4 mg/m³		compounding compounding compounding compounding
Enwald (1982)	Ethylenethiourea	0.001-0.072 mg/m³ 0.004-0.006 mg/m³ 0.012-0.206 mg/m³ 0.051-0.081 mg/m³		milling, mixing calendering extruding maintenance
	Methylenebis-ortho- chloroaniline	0.001-0.011 mg/m³		general air

4. Biological monitoring

Biological monitoring of carcinogens and mutagens is in a phase of rapid development. Many of the findings presented here are based upon a small number of measurements, and more experience is needed before any definite conclusion about their importance can be made. However, because of the long latency periods preceding the diagnosis of cancer, methods of biological monitoring can be used to identify worker exposure. An overview of the present possibilities and future perspectives of biological monitoring in the identification of cancer risk in individuals exposed to carcinogens has been published elsewhere (Vainio et al., 1981).

4.1 Chemicals and their metabolites in biological fluids

Only a few substances that are known to cause cancer in humans have been analysed in biological samples, including arsenic, benzene, chromium and nickel (Vainio et al., 1981).

Within the rubber industry, exposure to benzene has been monitored via excretion of phenol in the urine (Pagnatto et al., 1961, 1979) (see above).

In a study on human volunteers (Kummer & Tordoir, 1975), 19 volunteers were given 10 mg N-phenyl-2-naphthylamine containing 8 ng 2-naphthylamine (0.8 mg/kg bw). From 0.4-3 μg 2-naphthylamine were found in 24-hour urine samples from 7 subjects, 6 of whom were non-smokers. In 4 workers exposed to N-phenyl-2-naphthyl-amine dusts (approximate intake, 40 mg), which were estimated to contain 32 ng 2-naphthylamine, 3-8 μg 2-naphthylamine were found in 24-hour urine samples.

2-Naphthylamine was found at a level of 3-4 μg in 24-hour samples of urine from two volunteers who ingested 50 mg N-phenyl-2-naphthylamine containing 0.7 μg 2-naphthylamine, and from workers (unspecified number) estimated to have inhaled 30 mg N-phenyl-2-naphthylamine (Moore et al., 1977).

4.2   Thioethers in urine

Alkylated amino acid residues have been measured in urine in a number of studies (Jones, 1973; Ehrenberg et al., 1974; van Doorn et al., 1981). Alkyl derivatives of cysteine or N-acetyl-cysteine have been demonstrated in the urine of rubber workers (Vainio et al., 1978) and of workers exposed to methyl chloride (van Doorn et al., 1980). The levels at which these thioethers and alkylcysteines are found in urine provide indirect informa-tion about exposure to alkylating and arylating compounds; how-ever, this method does not permit the identification of specific compounds.

The thioether content of the morning urine of rubber workers and of radial-tyre builders was higher than that of the urine of clerks. Women excreted higher levels than men. The highest level of thioethers was found in the urine of female workers in the belt department; high levels were also found in workers in the calendering department, in raw material stores and in chemical mixing sections; and lower levels were seen in workers in the dispatching station and offices (Vainio et al., 1978; Kilpikari, 1981).

4.3 Mutagenicity in urine

Mutagenicity has been detected in the urine of humans (Siebert & Simons, 1973; Yamasaki & Ames, 1977; McCoy et al., 1978; Falck et al., 1980) and of rats (Bos et al., 1980; Reddy et al., 1980; Tanaka et al., 1980) exposed to mutagens.

The mutagenic activity of the urine of workers in the tyre-manufacturing department of a rubber factory was investigated using the bacterial fluctuation test, with Escherichia coli WP2 and Salmonella typhimurium TA98 as the indicator organisms. The urine of both smokers and non-smokers exhibited significantly higher mutagenic activity than that of non-occupationally exposed controls (Falck et al., 1980). The extent of mutagenic activity in the urine of workers varied according to job category, in the following descending order: cleaners at the mixing and weighing department > vulcanizers of tyres > mixers of chemicals > vulcanizers of boots (Vainio et al., 1982).

4.4 Sister chromatid exchanges in peripheral lymphocytes

The frequency of sister chromatid exchange (SCE) in cultured blood lymphocytes is significantly higher in those from people exposed to mutagenic and carcinogenic materials (Funes-Cravioto et al., 1977; Husgafvel-Pursiainen et al., 1980; Lambert et al., 1982).

The frequency of SCE in cultured peripheral lymphocytes of rubber workers who smoked was higher than that in unexposed smokers. Workers in chemical weighing and mixing departments had higher frequencies of SCEs in their lymphocytes than did their unexposed, matched (age, sex, smoking habits) controls (Vainio et al., 1982).

5. Summary

Analytical techniques have seldom been employed in the past to survey atmospheric contamination in the rubber industry, so that there are few reported data on individual materials. The most data are available on levels of total particulates and solvents.

The handling, weighing and mixing of raw materials in the rubber industry have always been visibly dusty processes, and the areas in which they are carried out have been the main focus of sampling for particulate exposure. Current monitoring data indicate that exposures to greater than the recommended limits are not uncommon; and anecdotal information suggests that in the past exposures were to considerably higher levels. Most industrial hygiene measurements are still compared with established limits for carbon black or with general dust standards, and the implications of exposure to potentially more toxic materials are rarely evaluated.

Heating and curing of rubber compounds generates a visible fume, the inhalation of which may constitute a significant health hazard. This fume has a complex chemical composition, which makes detailed analysis very difficult. For the UK industry, it has been suggested that the solvent-soluble fraction of total particulates should be used as an indicator of fume contamination in the areas in which the samples were taken. Such monitoring has been put into practice.

Recent findings of nitrosamines in the rubber industry indicate widespread contamination by several nitrosamines at the $\mu g/m^3$ level. The levels of N-nitrosomorpholine and, in some studies, N-nitrosodimethylamine, were associated with the use of N-nitrosodiphenylamine, secondary amines and the presence of nitrogen oxides in the work environment. Under some conditions, the levels of N-nitrosodimethylamine and N-nitrosomorpholine exceeded 100 $\mu g/m^3$.

The mixing of solvents may be considered to fall into the category of handling of raw materials, although it is often done in facilities separate from the main factory. While the toxic effects of over-exposure to solvents have been recognized for many decades, and individual companies have probably monitored workers' exposure, little published data were available prior to the early 1960s. Other jobs for which data are now available include building, preparation for curing and product finishing in the tyre industry, and the spreading of proofing compounds in the coated-fabrics industry.

The data in this section are presented separately for specific processing areas, so that they can be used as indicators of the exposures in individual job categories or areas.

It is evident from this review of the industrial hygiene data that studies should be carried out to evaluate the individual components of particulates. The analytical techniques are available to increase the data base, and research must be made into a clearer understanding of the work place environment in the rubber industry.

Very few data obtained by biological monitoring were available to the Working Group. The findings are limited to reports of excess levels of thioethers in the urine of tyre-manufacturing workers, an increased level of mutagenic activity in the urine of workers in mixing and weighing and vulcanization departments, and an increased prevalence of sister chromatid exchange in peripheral lymphocytes of rubber workers involved in mixing and weighing of compounds.

6. References

Bos, R.P., Brouns, R.M.E., van Doorn, R., Theuws, J.L.G. & Henderson, P.T. (1980) The appearance of mutagens in urine of rats after the administration of benzidine and some other aromatic amines. Toxicology, 16, 113–122

Burgess, W.A., DiBerardinis, L., Gold, A. & Treitman, R. (1977) Exposure to air contaminants in tire building (Abstract no. 39). Rubber Chem. Technol., 51, 379–381

van Doorn, R., Borm, P.J.A., Leijdekkers, C.-M., Henderson, P.T., Reuvers, J. & van Bergen, T.J. (1980) Detection and identification of S-methylcysteine in urine of workers exposed to methyl chloride. Int. Arch. occup. environ. Health, 46, 99–109

van Doorn, R., Leijdekkers, C.-M., Bos, R.P., Brouns, R.M.E. & Henderson, P.T. (1981) Detection of human exposure to electrophilic compounds by assay of thioether detoxication products in urine. Ann. occup. Hyg., 24, 77–92

Ehrenberg, L., Hiesche, K.D., Osterman-Golkar, S. & Wennberg, I. (1974) Evaluation of genetic risks of alkylating agents: Tissue doses in the mouse from air contaminated with ethylene oxide. Mutat. Res., 24, 83–103

Enwald, E. (1982) How safe is it to work with rubber? In: Proceedings of the Scandinavian Rubber Conference, Helsinki, May, Trelleborg, Scandinavian Rubber Society (in press)

Fajen, J.M., Carson, G.A., Rounbehler, D.P., Fan, T.Y., Vita, R., Goff, U.E., Wolf, M.H., Edwards, G.S., Fine, D.H., Rheinhold, V. & Biemann, K. (1979) N-Nitrosamines in the rubber and tire industry. Science, 205, 1262–1264

Falck, K., Sorsa, M., Vainio, H. & Kilpikari, I. (1980) Mutagenicity in urine of workers in rubber industry. Mutat. Res., 79, 45–52

Fine, L.J. & Peters, J.M. (1976) Respiratory morbidity in rubber workers. I. Prevalence of respiratory symptoms and disease in curing workers. Arch. environ. Health, 31, 5–9

Fine, L.J., Peters, J.M., Burgess, W.A. & DiBerardinis, L.J. (1976) Studies of respiratory morbidity in rubber workers. Part IV. Respiratory morbidity in talc workers. Arch. environ. Health, 31, 195-200

Fraser, D.A. & Rappaport, S. (1976) Health aspects of the curing of synthetic rubbers. Environ. Health Perspect., 17, 45-53

Funes-Cravioto, F., Kolmodin-Hedman, B., Lindsten, J., Nordenskjöld, M., Zapata-Gayon, C., Lambert, B., Norberg, E., Olin, R. & Swensson, A. (1977) Chromosome aberrations and sister-chromatid exchange in workers in chemical laboratories and a rotoprinting factory and in children of women laboratory workers. Lancet, ii, 322-325

Gamble, J.F., McMichael, A.J., Williams, T. & Battigelli, M. (1976) Respiratory function and symptoms: an environmental-epidemiological study of rubber workers exposed to a phenol-formaldehyde type resin. Am. ind. Hyg. Assoc. J., 37, 499-513

Husgafvel-Pursiainen, K., Mäki-Paakkanen, J., Norppa, H. & Sorsa, M. (1980) Smoking and sister chromatid exchange. Hereditas, 92, 247-250

The Industrial Commission of Ohio (1971) Report re: Affiliated Hospital Products, Inc., Columbus, OH, Division of Safety and Hygiene

Jones, A.R. (1973) The metabolism of biological alkylating agents. Drug Metab. Rev., 2, 71-100

Kilpikari, I. (1981) Correlation of urinary thioethers with chemical exposure in a rubber plant. Br. J. ind. Med., 38, 98-100

Kummer, R. & Tordoir, W.F. (1975) Phenyl-betanaphthylamine (PBNA), another carcinogenic agent? T. soc. Geneesk., 53, 415-419

Lambert, B., Lindblad, A., Holmberg, K. & Francesconi, D. (1982) Use of sister chromatid exchange to monitor human populations for exposure to toxicologically harmful agents. In: Wolff, S., ed., Sister Chromatid Exchange, New York, John Wiley & Sons (in press)

Levy, B.S.B. (1976) Health Hazard Evaluation/Toxicity Determination. Report H.H.E. 75-15-250, Converse Rubber Company, Malden, Massachusetts (PB-249 430), Washington DC, National Technical Information Service

McCoy, E.C., Hankel, R., Robbins, K., Rosenkranz, H.S., Giuffrida, J.G. & Bizzari, D.V. (1978) Presence of mutagenic substances in the urines of anesthesiologists (Abstract). Mutat. Res., 53, 71

McGlothlin, J.D., Wilcox, T.C., Fajen, J.M. & Edwards, G.S. (1981) A health hazard evaluation of nitrosamines in a tire manufacturing plant. In: Choudhary, G., ed., Chemical Hazards in the Workplace. Measurement and Control (ACS Symposium Series 149), Washington DC, Americal Chemical Society, pp. 283-299

Moore, R.M., Jr, Woolf, B.S., Stein, H.P., Thomas, A.W. & Finklea, J.F. (1977) Metabolic precursors of a known human carcinogen. Science, 195, 344

National Institute for Occupational Safety & Health (1977a) Health Hazard Evaluation Determination. Report no. 77-67-499, St Clair Rubber Company, Marysville, Michigan, Cincinnati, OH

National Institute for Occupational Safety & Health (1977b) Survey Report of Cincinnati Rubber Manufacturing Company, Norwood, Ohio (PB-278 792), Washington DC, National Technical Information Service [Chem. Abstr., 89, 220163h]

National Institute for Occupational Safety & Health (1978) Criteria for a Recommended Standard ... Occupational Exposure to Carbon Black, Cincinnati, OH

National Institute for Occupational Safety & Health (1979) Interim Report No. 1, Health Hazard Evaluation Project No. HHE 79-75. St Clair Rubber Company, Marysville, Michigan, Cincinnati, OH

National Institute for Occupational Safety & Health (1980) Interim Report No. 1, Health Hazard Evaluation Project No. HHE 79-126. St Clair Rubber Company, Marysville, Michigan, Cincinnati, OH

Noweir, M.H., El-Dakhakhny, A.-A. & Osman, H.A. (1972) Exposure to chemical agents in rubber industry. J. Egypt. publ. Health Assoc., 47, 182-201

Nutt, A. (1976) Measurement of some potentially hazardous materials in the atmosphere of rubber factories. Environ. Health Perspect., 17, 117-123

Nutt, A.R. (1979) Control of dusts and fumes - Is there a problem? In: BRMA Ventilation Symposium, 1979, Birmingham, British Rubber Manufacturers' Association, Ltd, pp. 11-20

Nutt, A. (1981) The impact of new sampling techniques on industry. In: Health and Safety in the Plastics and Rubber Industries, University of Warwick, 1980, London, The Plastics and Rubber Institute, pp. 21.1-21.6

Occupational Safety & Health Administration (1977) Test for Hazardous Substance - 527 (Carbon Black) (29CFR 1910.1000), Washington DC, US Department of Labor

Occupational Safety & Health Administration (1980) Citation and Notification of Penalty No. 59410, Report No. 089 McCreary Tire & Rubber, Washington DC, US Department of Labor

Otto, J. & Schmidt, E. (1978) Workplace concentrations of poly-cyclic aromatic hydrocarbons (Ger.). Z. ges. Hyg., 24, 896-898

Pagnatto, L.D., Elkins, H.B., Brugsch, H.B. & Walkley, J.E. (1961) Industrial benzene exposure from petroleum naphtha: I. Rubber coating industry. Am. ind. Hyg. Assoc. J., 22, 417-421

Pagnatto, L.D., Elkins, H.B. & Brugsch, H.G. (1979) Benzene exposure in the rubber coating industry - a follow-up. Am. ind. Hyg. Assoc. J., 40, 137-146

Parkes, H.G., Whittaker, B. & Willoughby, B.G. (1975) The Monitoring of the Atmospheric Environment in UK Tyre Manufacturing Work Areas, Birmingham, British Rubber Manufacturers' Association, Ltd

Rappaport, S.M. & Fraser, D.A. (1977) Air sampling and analysis in a rubber vulcanization area. Am. ind. Hyg. Assoc. J., 38, 205-210

Reddy, T.V., Benjamin, T., Grantham, P.H., Weisburger, E.K. & Thorgeirsson, S.S. (1980) Mutagenicity of urine from rats after administration of 2,4-diaminoanisole. Mutat. Res., 79, 307-317

Ringenburg, V. & Fajen, J.M. (1980) Surveys for N-Nitroso Compounds at B.F. Goodrich, Woodburn, Indiana 46797, Cincinnati, OH, National Institute for Occupational Safety & Health

Siebert, D. & Simon, U. (1973) Cyclophosphamide: Pilot study of genetically active metabolites in the urine of a treated human patient. Induction of mitotic gene conversions in yeast. Mutat. Res., 19, 65-72

Spiegelhalder, B. & Preussmann, R. (1982) Nitrosamines and rubber. In: Bartsch, H., O'Neill, I.K., Castegnaro, M. & Okada, M., eds, N-Nitroso Compounds: Occurrence and Biological Effects (IARC Scientific Publications No. 41), Lyon, International Agency for Research on Cancer (in press)

Tanaka, K.-I., Marui, S. & Mii, T. (1980) Mutagenicity of extracts of urine from rats treated with aromatic amines. Mutat. Res., 79, 173-176

Vainio, H., Savolainen, H. & Kilpikari, I. (1978) Urinary thioether of employees of a chemical plant. Br. J. ind. Med., 35, 232-234

Vainio, H., Sorsa, M., Rantanen, J., Hemminki, K. & Aitio, A. (1981) Biological monitoring in the identification of the cancer risk of individuals exposed to chemical carcinogens. Scand. J. Work Environ. Health, 7, 241-251

Vainio, H., Falck, K., Mäki-Paakkanen, J. & Sorsa, M. (1982) Possibilities for identification of genotoxic risks in the rubber industry: use of uFinary mutagenicity assay and chromosomal SCEs. In: Armstrong, B. & Bartsch, H., eds, Environmental Host Factors in Carcinogenesis (IARC Scientific Publications No. 39), Lyon, International Agency for Research on Cancer (in press)

Van Ert, M.D., Arp, E.W., Harris, R.L., Symons, M.J. & Williams, T.M. (1980) Worker exposures to chemical agents in the manufacture of rubber tires: Solvent vapor studies. Am. ind. Hyg. Assoc. J., 41, 212-219

Wassermann, M. (1960) Present-day trends in industrial hygiene in agriculture (Abstract). In: Abstracts. Thirteenth International Congress on Occupational Health, New York City, 1960

Williams, T.M., Harris, R.L., Arp, E.W., Symons, M.J. & Van Ert, M.D. (1980) Worker exposure to chemical agents in the manufacture of rubber tires and tubes: Particulates. Am. ind. Hyg. Assoc. J., 41, 204-211

Yamasaki, E. & Ames, B.N. (1977) Concentration of mutagens from urine by adsorption with the nonpolar resin XAD-2: Cigarette smokers have mutagenic urine. Proc. natl Acad. Sci. USA, 74, 3555-3559

ENVIRONMENTAL MONITORING TECHNIQUES

Various techniques have been developed to optimize engineering controls and to estimate worker exposure through the measurement of concentrations. Results of such methods can be confounded by factors such as poor work practices and personal hygiene, periodic fluctuation in emission of contaminants, changes in process, and the limitations of the sampling equipment available. Additionally, environmental monitoring cannot adequately evaluate skin absorption.

1.   Sampling methods

Personal: A sampling device (i.e., filter, cyclone or adsorption tube) is attached to the lapels in the area of the breathing zone of the workers. The concentration measured by personal samplers may be higher than that measured by fixed sampling devices, and personal sampling permits a more exact evaluation of the actual inhalation of substances.

Area: The work place air is sampled using a static sampling train. This method gives an indication of the concentration in a particular work area.

Process: This is a static sampling method located at the point closest to the process generating the contamination. It does not indicate actual personal exposure but does indicate the contaminant.

2.   Components of sampling systems

Pumps: These devices are designed to pull a defined volume of air through a sample collector. Pumps are all electrical; however, most of those used for personal sampling are battery operated.

Direct reading: Such devices are designed to give an immediate indication of the concentration of a specific contaminant or contaminants. They may be indicator tubes, sophisticated electronic monitoring devices designed to measure a specific contaminant, portable gas chromatographs, sensitized tapes (for isocyanates), portable infra-red spectrophotometers or direct reading dust monitors.

Particulate samplers: These are used to capture dusts and aerosols. A size-selective sampler may be used to separate respirable particles (which can penetrate deep into the lung) from coarser, non-respirable particles. Sampling for respirable particulate is generally done when dusts that cause lung disease are present. Sampling for 'total particulate' (both respirable and non-respirable) is generally done when the dusts are of unknown or systemic toxicity, when both ingestion and inhalation may occur.

Solid adsorbent tubes: These are used to sample gas phase contaminants and are comprised of charcoal, MgAl silica, silica gel, etc.

3.   Analytical methods

These include specific chemical methods and instrumental methods, e.g., atomic absorption, infra-red spectroscopy and gas chromatography, in combination with various detectors such as chemiluminescence.

This section includes information on chemicals for which some data on carcinogenic, mutagenic or teratogenic effects were available to the Working Group. The selection of chemicals included in this section is not the result of an exhaustive screening of the literature on all chemicals used or formed in the rubber industry. Some of the chemicals have already been considered in previous <u>IARC Monographs</u>, and, for these, reference to the pertinent Monograph is given (see also Appendices 2 and 3). For a number of chemicals, information on carcinogenicity, mutagenicity or teratogenicity was derived from the literature and was not critically analysed or evaluated in the same way as that for chemicals previously considered in <u>IARC Monographs</u>. This section should therefore be read more as an introduction than as an exhaustive and complete review.

1.   Carcinogenic, mutagenic and teratogenic effects

1.1   Accelerators, antioxidant and curing agents

Of the organic peroxides used as curing agents, dicumyl peroxide, bis(2,4-dichlorobenzoyl)peroxide and α,α'-bis(<u>tert</u>-butylperoxyisopropyl)benzene were reported to be skin irritants, while <u>tert</u>-butylperoxide was not. Their acute toxicity in animals has been summarized by Holmberg and Sjöstrom (1977), but virtually no evaluable data are available on their carcinogenic, mutagenic or teratogenic effects. Hydrogen peroxide was reported to be carcinogenic to mouse duodenum when administered at a concentration of 0.4% in drinking water for 108 weeks (Ito <u>et al.</u>, 1981). It was also shown to induce DNA repair in <u>Escherichia coli</u> (Rosenkranz, 1973) and mutations in <u>Saccharomyces cerevisiae</u> (Thacker, 1975).

The accelerators and curing agents commonly used are thiuram compounds, including tetramethylthiuram disulphide (thiram, TMTD), tetraethylthiuram disulphide (disulfiram, TETD) and tetramethylthiuram monosulphide (TMTM). (See also Appendix 1).

TMTD and TETD were evaluated for carcinogenicity in an IARC Monograph (IARC, 1976b). The two carcinogenicity studies in experimental animals and the one case report of human thyroid cancer were considered an insufficient basis for evaluating the carcinogenicity of TMTD; the data for TETD were also too limited to evaluate carcinogenicity. In one study of oral administration to mice, the incidence of liver-cell tumours was increased in males of two strains, and the number of lung tumours was increased in males of one strain. Both TMTD and TETD react with nitrite to form carcinogenic nitrosodialkylamines. TETD is metabolized in rats and man to diethyldithiocarbamate, glucuronide and sulphate conjugates, diethylamine and carbon disulphide.

These compounds were investigated in a series of reactivity studies in vitro (Hemminki et al., 1980). TMTM, TMTD, TETD, zinc and copper dimethyldithiocarbamates, zinc, cadmium and tellurium diethyldithiocarbamates, and zinc dibutyldithiocarbamate were incubated with synthetic nucleophiles, 4-(para-nitrobenzyl)-pyridine and deoxyguanosine. The thiuram compounds were not reactive; copper dimethyldithiocarbamate, cadmium and tellurium diethyldithiocarbamate and zinc dibutyldithiocarbamate reacted slowly with both deoxyguanosine and 4-(para-nitrobenzyl)pyridine. There seemed to be no correlation between mutagenicity in Escherichia coli WP2 and chemical reactivity.

In a series of mutagenicity tests on rubber accelerators (Hedenstedt et al., 1979), TMTD and TMTM were mutagenic but TETD was non-mutagenic to Salmonella typhimurium. TMTD was the most active of the thiurams. Five out of nine tested dithiocarbamates were also mutagenic, ziram being the most active.

4,4'-Dithiomorpholine, zinc ethylphenyldithiocarbamate, N,N'-dicyclohexyl-para-phenylenediamine, N,N'-diphenyl-para-phenylenediamine, 4,4'-diaminodiphenylmethane, 6-ethoxy-1,2-di-hydro-2,2,4-trimethylquinoline and N-methyl-N,4-dinitrosoaniline were all direct or indirect mutagens for S. typhimurium in another study (Hedenstedt, 1982). TMTD was also found to be mutagenic in another study on S. typhimurium TA100 (Shirasu et al., 1977).

TMTD, TMTM and TETD (in order of decreasing toxicity) produced deaths and malformations in chicken embryos (Korhonen et al., 1982a). The dithiocarbamates investigated were cadmium and zinc diethyldithiocarbamate, zinc ethylphenyldithiocarbamate, zinc dibutyldithiocarbamate, copper dimethyldithiocarbamate, tellurium diethyldithiocarbamate and piperidine pentamethylenedithiocarbamate. The cadmium and zinc salts were particularly embryotoxic (Korhonen et al., 1982b).

Ethylenethiourea has been judged to be carcinogenic in rats (IARC, 1974). It was also teratogenic in two studies in rats (Khera, 1973; Ruddick & Khera, 1975). When tested on chicken embryos, together with 1,3-dibutylthiourea, 1,3-diphenylthiourea, tetramethylthiourea, trimethylthiourea, 1,3-diethylthiourea and carbon disulphide, ethylenethiourea was the least embryotoxic compound in the series. Carbon disulphide was inactive at the concentrations tested. Tetramethylthiourea and 1,3-diphenylthiourea were the most active teratogens in this test system; ethylenethiourea was a weak teratogen (Korhonen et al., 1982c).

1.2 Solvents

Solvents that have been used or are used in the rubber industry include benzene, trichloroethylene, 1,1,1-trichloroethane and methylene chloride; 1,4-dioxane is used as a stabilizer in solvents. Generally, these compounds are not chemically reactive and do not appear to react with macromolecules, but their metabolites may do so.

Benzene is a known clastogen and has been considered to be carcinogenic in humans and rodents (IARC, 1982). It was teratogenic in rats (Kuna & Kapp, 1981). 1,4-Dioxane is carcinogenic in rats and guinea-pigs (IARC, 1976b).

The evidence for the carcinogenicity of trichloroethylene and 1,1,1-trichloroethane is limited; and the data on methylene chloride were inadequate for evaluation (IARC, 1979c). 1,1,1-Trichloroethane induced mutations in E. coli in the presence of a liver microsomal activation system; the increase was small but statistically significant (Norpoth et al., 1980). The data reported in the literature regarding the mutagenicity of trichloroethylene are conflicting. However, in the presence of a rodent liver activation system, a technical-grade product slightly increased mutagenicity in E. coli (Greim et al., 1975); and a product 99.5% pure increased mutagenicity in S. typhimurium TA100 (Bartsch et al., 1979). Irreversible binding of ^{14}C-trichloroethylene to mouse liver constituents, in vitro and in vivo, has been described (Uehleke & Poplawski-Tabarelli, 1977).

Dichloromethane is weakly mutagenic in S. typhimurium TA98 and TA100, both in the presence and absence of a liver activation system (Jongen et al., 1978). Covalent binding and metabolism to carbon monoxide, both in vivo and in vitro, have been described (Ahmed et al., 1980).

Studies on the teratogenicity of trichloroethylene, 1,1,1-trichloroethane, methylene chloride and 1,4-dioxane were either inconclusive or failed to demonstrate skeletal or visceral mal-formations (IARC, 1976b, 1979c).

Dimethylformamide, also used in the rubber industry, is metabolized in rats to N-methylformamide (Barnes & Ranta, 1972), which is teratogenic and embryotoxic to rats (Stula & Krauss, 1977). Ethylene dichloride, which has been used as a solvent in the rubber industry, is carcinogenic to mice and rats and is mutagenic to S. typhimurium with or without metabolic activation (IARC, 1979c).

In human whole blood cultures, low concentrations (0.0125-0.05%) of a rubber solvent refined from a straight-run petroleum distillate of paraffin-based crude oil (consisting of a mixture of paraffins, monocycloparaffins, monoolefins, benzene and alkyl benzenes) caused an increased frequency of chromatid gaps and breaks; high concentrations (>0.05%) caused increases in the frequency of chromosome breaks. Concentrations up to a toxic level failed to produce sister chromatid exchanges (Altenburg et al., 1979).

1.3 Monomers

Small amounts of monomers, e.g., acrylonitrile, butadiene, chloroprene, ethylene, propylene, styrene, vinyl acetate, vinyl chloride and vinylidene chloride, may remain in solid rubber and could be released into the work environment. Most of these mono-mers do not bind directly with cellular macromolecules, but their metabolites may do so. Metabolic activation of acrylonitrile, chloroprene, styrene and vinyl chloride leads to reaction pro-ducts which are mutagenic in S. typhimurium and in other bacte-rial test systems. In the case of acrylonitrile, chloroprene and vinyl chloride, a low mutagenic response was obtained in S. typhimurium and E. coli without metabolic activation (IARC, 1979b). Chloroprene, styrene and vinyl chloride also produce clastogenic effects.

There is <u>sufficient evidence</u> for the carcinogenicity of acrylonitrile and vinyl chloride in experimental animals, and <u>limited evidence</u> for the carcinogenicity of styrene. The data were inadequate for an evaluation of chloroprene. Vinyl chloride is carcinogenic to humans, and there is <u>limited evidence</u> that acrylonitrile is too (IARC, 1979b,c). (See also Appendix 3.)

Acrylonitrile, chloroprene, styrene and vinyl chloride are teratogenic to experimental animals, and there is a suspicion that styrene and vinyl chloride have teratogenic effects in humans (IARC, 1979a,b)

Epichlorohydrin is used in the manufacture of elastomers. It reacts directly with macromolecules and it is mutagenic, clastogenic and carcinogenic in mice and rats (IARC, 1976a; Laskin <u>et al.</u>, 1980). No adequate epidemiological observations on the carcinogenicity of epichlorohydrin to humans have been published (IARC, 1976a, 1979b).

1.4 Talc

French chalk (talc) is widely used as an antitacking agent. It has been used in many processes and is still used in substantial quantities. It is a major component of environmental dusts encountered in the rubber industry. Its composition is variable, being dependent upon the source of supply; for the most part, talc particles are 'platey' in character. Some talcs, however, may contain asbestos fibres, which are carcinogenic in both humans and animals (IARC, 1977). Prolonged and excessive exposure to talc has been shown to give rise to a number of documented cases of respiratory disease. (See section VI, .2.2).

1.5 Carbon blacks

Assessment of possible hazards from carbon black is difficult, because different preparations contain variable amounts of many compounds, some of which have still not been identified. The chemical composition and physical properties differ with methods of preparation and the nature of the starting material and, probably, from day to day.

The most probable carcinogenic hazard is associated with the 'benzene extractables'. The material, extracted from furnace black, consists mainly of aromatic hydrocarbons and sulphur compounds. Some compounds have been identified by computerized gaschromatographic mass spectrometry and high-resolution mass spectrometry (Lee & Hites, 1976). Among them, benz[a]anthracene, benzo[a]pyrene and indeno(1,2,3-cd)pyrene are known carcinogens (IARC, 1973); chrysene has been described as an initiating agent, and pyrene and fluoranthene as cocarcinogens for mouse skin (Van Duuren, 1976). Oxygen derivatives (Gold, 1975) and nitro derivatives (Fitch & Smith, 1979) of polycyclic compounds have also been found in extracts of commercial carbon blacks. Benzo[a]-pyrene was found in benzene extracts of all types of carbon black examined (Troitskaya et al., 1975). The amounts of some polycyclic hydrocarbons found in the benzene extracts of furnace carbon blacks are shown in Table 13 (from Locati et al., 1979).

Existing data indicate that the known carcinogens present in carbon blacks are strongly adsorbed but can be eluted by biological fluids. Although Neal et al. (1962) reported that polycyclic hydrocarbons, including benzo[a]pyrene, in furnace and channel blacks are not eluted by human blood plasma or gastric juice, Kutscher et al. (1967) found that bovine serum elutes 10-20% of benzo[a]pyrene from various types of carbon blacks within periods ranging from 4-60 hours depending upon the particle size. When a commercial carbon black (500-nm particle size) was incubated with sterile human plasma, several polycyclic aromatic hydrocarbons, including benzo[a]pyrene, were extracted within 16-192 hours. Elution of benzo[a]pyrene from fine-particle carbon black (80 nm) was more difficult, but 65% was extracted within eight days (Falk et al., 1958).

The rates of elution by benzene and the amounts of material extractable from carbon black vary with the type of carbon. Thus extraction of two carbon blacks which contained over 0.1% of extractable material, was almost complete in 150 hours (Locati et al., 1979). In a study using three organic solvents for extraction of adsorbates from five rubber-grade oil-furnace blacks, toluene was found to be a better extractant than benzene and both to be superior to cyclohexane (Taylor et al., 1980).

Table 13. Polycyclic aromatic hydrocarbons (PAH) identified in five types of carbon black. Values expressed as percent of benzene extract; mean value and range of 5 samples for each black type[a]

PAH	Sample				
	A	B	C	D	E
Phenanthrene and/or anthracene	0.07 (<0.05-0.1)	absent	<0.05	absent	0.2 (0.1-0.5)
Fluoranthene	4.1 (3.8-4.3)	3.7 (3.4-3.9)	3.5 (2.9-4.3)	4.1 (3.4-6.4)	4.3 (3.9-5.2)
Benzo[d,e,f]dibenzo-thiophene + benzo[a]-acenaphthylene	<0.05	<0.3	<0.3	absent	<0.05
Pyrene	22.2 (21.3-24.9)	23.2 (21.6-24.0)	16.5 (13.4-18.7)	17.2 (14.3-18.1)	17.2 (14.3-20.1)
Benzo[g,h,i]-fluoranthene	7.2 (5.9-7.6)	6.3 (5.6-7.2)	6.9 (6.5-7.3)	4.6 (4.2-5)	7.8 (7.5-8.1)
Cyclopenta[cd]-pyrene	10.2 (5.6-14.7)	<0.3	7.0 (6.8-7.3)	4.4 (4.2-5)	6.5 (5.2-7.8)
Benzofluoranthenes (total)	0.7 (0.4-1.1)	absent	<0.3	1.2 (0.9-1.4)	0.6 (0.4-0.9)
Benzopyrenes (total)	1.4 (1.1-1.9)	0.5 (<0.3-0.7)	1.1 (0.4-2.1)	2.6 (1.5-3.2)	2.7 (2.0-3.9)
Dimethylcyclopentapyrene and/or dimethyl-benzofluoranthene	2.5 (2.0-3.5)	0.5 (<0.3-0.7)	0.9 (0.3-1.3)	1.9 (1.7-2.3)	1.4 (1.1-1.7)
Indenopyrene	1.7 (1.5-2.2)	0.5 (<0.3-0.7)	0.1 (abs.-0.3)	2.3 (2.1-2.5)	2.9 (2.7-3.1)
Benzo[g,h,i]perylene	11.7 (10.9-13.8)	6.2 (5.5-8.5)	8.7 (8.2-9.5)	13.5 (12-16.5)	13.6 (12.8-17)
Anthanthrene	3.2 (2.8-3.5)	-	0.8 (<0.3-1.2)	2.3 (1.9-3.3)	3.5 (2.8-5.5)
Benzoacridine derivative	<0.05	absent	absent	absent	0.2 (abs.-0.5)

Table 13 (contd)

PAH	Sample				
Isomer of coronene	6.3 (5.1-7.2)	1.1 (abs.-2.2)	0.1 (abs.-0.3)	0.5 (abs.-1)	5.1 (4.6-5.7)
Coronene	7.2 (4.1-10)	1.2 (<0.3-3.2)	3.8 (3.5-4.4)	8.9 (8.5-9.8)	11.7 (9.5-13.8)
TOTAL	78.5	43.8	50.05	63.5	77.5

[a] From Locati et al. (1979)

Methylene chloride extracts of soots prepared by burning either kerosene or equal parts of pyridine, decaline and ortho-xylene or thiophene, were assayed in S. typhimurium in the presence of liver supernatant from Aroclor-induced rats for the induction of 8-azaguanine-resistant mutants. Mutation frequencies decreased in the following order: kerosene soot > furnace blacks > nitrogen-containing soot > sulphur-containing soot (Kaden et al., 1979). Several nitrated polycyclic aromatic hydrocarbons were mutagenic in S. typhimurium and induced unscheduled DNA repair in cultured human (HeLa) cells (Campbell et al., 1981). Samples of furnace blacks used as photocopy toners were found to be mutagenic in S. typhimurium, partly because of the presence in them of nitroaromatics (Rosenkranz et al., 1980; Löfroth et al., 1980).

Studies on the carcinogenicity of carbon blacks, by oral, skin, s.c. or inhalation exposure (Nau et al., 1958a,b, 1960, 1962, 1976), provided no evidence of carcinogenic effects; but the studies were inadequate in terms of number of animals and duration.

Furnace black (but not channel black) when suspended in tri-caprylin induced sarcomas upon injection into mice. As it was not carcinogenic when implanted alone, it is probable that it became so when polycyclic aromatic hydrocarbon carcinogens were eluted by the tricaprylin. Injection of benzene extracts of furnace black also induced sarcomas (Steiner, 1954).

When benzene-extractable materials from channel and furnace blacks were administered to mice by s.c. injection, skin application or feeding, malignant tumours were produced (Nau et al., 1958a,b, 1960). Malignant tumours were also produced following s.c. injections of cotton-seed oil in which the carbon blacks had been suspended for 1-6 months (Nau et al., 1960).

When 3-methylcholanthrene was adsorbed onto carbon black, its carcinogenic effect following s.c. administration to rats was reduced in comparison to that produced when the same dose was given alone (von Haam et al., 1958).

In a retrospective cohort study of workers involved in the manufacture of carbon black, no excess mortality from malignant neoplasms was noted; but the number of deaths considered was small (Robertson & Ingalls, 1980)

1.6   Aromatic amines

The metabolism and the nature of reactive intermediates formed from aromatic amines and their interaction with cellular macromolecules have been reviewed by Boyland (1958), Miller and Miller (1969), Clayson and Garner (1976), Miller (1978), Irving (1979) and Kriek and Westra (1979).

The carcinogenic or genotoxic activity of all aromatic amines that have been studied in detail is dependent on metabolic activation in vivo. Differences in these metabolic pathways largely account for the differences seen in tissue- and species-susceptibilities to cancer induction. The carcinogenicity of aromatic amines or amides is dependent on their oxidation to N-hydroxy derivatives, while the carcinogenicity of aromatic nitro compounds is linked to their reduction to hydroxylamines. Further conversion of the N-hydroxylamine or N-hydroxyamide to reactive intermediates can occur in several ways, including (1) esterification of the N-hydroxy group, (2) non-enzymic protonation of the nitrogen of the hydroxylamine, and (3) oxidation to a free radical of arylhydroxamic acids. Following generation of such reactive electrophilic intermediates in tissues or cells, macromolecular binding to nucleic aids and proteins has been observed. As a consequence, mutations (and other genotoxic effects, including malignant transformation) have been induced in a variety of cells and organisms when the reactive intermediates or the parent

amines were assayed in the presence of a mammalian drug metabo-
lizing system. In many cases, arylamidated and arylaminated
products were formed with nucleic acid bases.

A great number of aromatic amines have now been studied for
carcinogenicity, and considerable data have been reported in the
first 27 volumes of the IARC Monographs. However, many of the
aromatic amines considered in that series could not be evaluated
for carcinogenicity, due to the inadequacy of experiments in
animals and/or the lack of data concerning man. (See also
Appendix 2.)

Naphthylamine-acetaldehyde condensates, of which the most
important was known by the trade name 'Nonox S', were introduced
around 1928 as antioxidants in the rubber product manufacturing
industry. They were used in the UK and other countries (but
apparently not in the US) for the production of tyres, tubes, air
bags, electric cables and miscellaneous rubber goods, and were
present in rubber compounds in concentrations of up to 1%. (It
was the opinion of the members of the Working Group that concentrations of up to 4% may have been present in some products,
particularly in air bags.) Their use was discontinued in the UK
in 1949. Although the manufacturing process has changed several
times, early products contained up to 2.5% 1-naphthylamine and up
to 0.25% 2-naphthylamine. Exposure to Nonox S in rubber factories
has been associated with an increase in the incidence of bladder
cancer in workers (Veys, 1969).

4-Aminobiphenyl, benzidine and 2-naphthylamine are known to
be carcinogenic for humans (IARC, 1979b). There is sufficient
evidence of the carcinogenicity of 2,4-diaminotoluene and 4,4'-
methylenebis(2-chloroaniline) in experimental animals. For
1-naphthylamine, 2,5-diaminotoluene, 4,4'-diaminodiphenylmethane
and N-phenyl-2-naphthylamine, the available data were inadequate
to assess carcinogenicity in experimental animals or in humans.
(See Appendix 3.)

The experimental animal species most frequently used to
investigate the carcinogenicity of aromatic amines are the dog
and the hamster, in which the urinary bladder is the main target
organ, as in humans. Aromatic amines have been shown to be carcinogenic in other rodent species, but the urinary bladder was not
necessarily the target organ.

Methods of analysis for aromatic amines of major industrial importance have been summarized (Egan et al., 1981).

1.7   Mineral oils, tar products and polycyclic aromatic hydrocarbons

Mineral oils (e.g., coal-tar oils, petrolatum) and tar products (e.g., bitumen, pitch) are widely used in the rubber industry as extenders. The amount of mineral oils (rich in aromatics), in tyres, for example, increased over past years up to about 20% or even more, since they are cheap and provide desirable properties to the finished rubber. Extenders such as the high-boiling mineral oil distillates (so-called aromatic oils), obtained from residues of solvent-refining and the manufacture of lubricating and cutting oils, contain relatively large quantities of polycyclic aromatic hydrocarbons (PAH), and 30% and more of the oil may consist of 4-6-ring PAHs. (See also section VI, 1.5.)   PAHs may also be formed when tars and mineral oils are heated.

Although mineral oils and tar products vary in composition depending on their origin, the methods of production, etc., they all induce carcinogenic effects in mammals, including man. Their carcinogenicity may be dependent on the presence of carcinogenic PAHs (IARC, 1979b).

Benzo[a]pyrene is the carcinogenic PAH most widely investigated; benz[a]anthracene, benzo[b]fluoranthene, benzo[j]fluoranthene, chrysene, dibenz[a,h]anthracene, dibenzo[a,h]pyrene, dibenzo[a,i]pyrene and indeno[1,2,3-cd]pyrene) have also been considered by an IARC Working Group (IARC, 1973).

Mineral oils containing different amounts of PAHs have been found to be mutagenic in the Salmonella typhimurium/microsome test (Hermann et al., 1982).

1.8   Nitroso compounds

N-Nitrosodi-n-butylamine,   N-nitrosodiethylamine,   N-nitrosodimethylamine, N-nitrosomorpholine, N-nitrosopiperidine and N-nitrosopyrrolidine have been shown to be carcinogenic in various animal species, after administration by various routes. These compounds are metabolized to reactive metabolites, which are mutagenic in various experimental systems (IARC, 1978). There is

limited evidence for the carcinogenicity of N-nitrosodiphenylamine in rats; but it was not mutagenic in prokaryote or euka-
ryote cells (IARC, 1982), although it is a transnitrosating agent
in vivo (Ohshima et al., 1982). No carcinogenic effects were
observed when dinitrosopentamethylenetetramine was tested in rats
by oral administration and i.p. injection (IARC, 1976a); and in a
cell-transformation assay, negative results were also obtained
(Styles, 1978). The data on the carcinogenicity of N-methyl,N-4-
dinitrosoaniline were considered to be inadequate for evaluation
(IARC, 1972). para-Nitroso-N,N-dimethylaniline has produced
oesophageal tumours in rats (Goodall et al., 1968).

1.9 Phthalate and adipate esters

Among the phthalic acid esters used in the rubber industry,
di(2-ethylhexyl) phthalate has been most extensively investigated
for its toxicological properties and is the most widely used. It
inhibits mitochondrial function and causes peroxisome prolifera-
tion, hepatomegaly and testicular atrophy in rodents. Various
mutagenicity tests in bacteria and mammalian cells showed negative or contradictory results. Long-term administration of di-
(2-ethylhexyl) phthalate to rats and mice resulted in hepato-
cellular tumours. Di(2-ethylhexyl) adipate produced hepato-
cellular tumours in mice; but di(n-butyl) phthalate was apparently negative when tested for carcinogenicity in mice and rats
(IARC, 1982).

1.10 Curing fumes and other emissions

The compounds present in the air during vulcanization
(curing fumes) are mainly produced by the volatilization of
rubber chemicals and their impurities and of the products of
chemical reactions occurring during curing. (See also Sections IV
and V.)

Air samples from industrial curing of acrylonitrile-
butadiene styrene copolymer, ethylene-propylene rubber and chloroprene rubber were mutagenic in S. typhimurium (Hedenstedt,
1982). In laboratory model systems, the curing of ethylene propylene rubber and chloroprene rubber produced mutagenic gases and
vapours. On the basis of these and other series of tests of condensates from cured rubber material, it was concluded that its
mutagenicity was dependent to a large extent on the composition
of the polymer (Hedenstedt, 1982).

In other model systems, in which mixing and curing conditions were simulated (Hedenstedt et al., 1981), air samples from
the curing of styrene-butadiene rubber and from the mixing and
curing of chloroprene rubber and ethylene-propylene rubber were
mutagenic to S. typhimurium.

No experimental data are available concerning the long-term
toxicity of curing fumes.

2.   Effects in humans (other than cancer)

In this part, some effects in humans are described which are
indicative of exposures that occurred within the working or
general environment. Some of the data may be useful in assessing
that exposure levels were sufficiently high to produce the ad-
verse effect. However, such effects may have no relation per se
to the existence of a carcinogenic risk.

2.1   Dermatological effects

Dermatological effects resulting from exposure to rubber and
rubber chemicals have been known for years in rubber goods manufacture (Cronin, 1980) and have been described in consumers.
Non-specific dermatological reactions to rubber gloves and to
footwear were reported many years ago (Downing, 1933; Marcussen,
1943). 'Accelerator agents', especially mercaptobenzothiazole,
were described as the specific cause (Bonnevie & Marcussen,
1945). Shortly thereafter, seven cases of dermatitis of the eyelids were reported, due to the use of eyelash curlers and to the
presence in them of the antioxidant, N-phenyl-2-naphthylamine
(Curtis, 1945). In a case report of 42 individuals with dermatitis due to rubber gloves, mercaptobenzothiazole, TMTD and dipentamethylenethiuram disulphide were identified as the causative
agents (Wilson, 1960). Of 100 cases of 'shoe dermatitis', 94%
were attributed to exposure to mercaptobenzothiazole or TMTD or
both (Cronin, 1966). Another report indicated that TMTD was responsible for a number of cases of rubber-glove dermatitis (van
Ketel, 1968). Another series of 104 cases were attributed to
exposure to thiuram accelerators or mercaptobenzothiazole
(Wilson, 1969). N-Isopropyl-N'-phenyl-para-phenylenediamine has
been reported to be responsible for 23 cases of dermatitis
following exposure to rubberized fabrics (Batschvarov & Minkov,

1968) and for dermatitis due to contact with automobile tyres (Jordan, 1971). It has also been reported to produce cross-sensitivity to the hair dye, para-aminodiphenylamine (Schønning & Hjorth, 1969).

Alkyl phenols and hydroquinone have been reported to cause leucodermas in rubber workers (Calnan, 1973). Phenylenediamines in rubber products are common causes of dermatitis (te Lintum & Nater, 1974; Nater, 1975), and a cross-reactivity occurs between different phenylenediamines (Rudzki et al., 1976). 4,4'-Dithiodimorpholine, another rubber chemical, has been reported to be a skin sensitizer (Heydenreich & Ølholm-Larsen, 1976). Sensitivity to N-isopropyl-N'-phenyl-para-phenylenediamine, N-phenyl-N-cyclohexyl-para-phenylenediamine and N-dimethyl-1,3-butyl-N'-phenyl-para-phenylenediamine has been reported in workers handling tyres. All subjects sensitive to the first were also sensitive to the second, and 37% of them to para-phenylenediamine. The last-mentioned was the most powerfully allergenic compound (Herve-Bazin et al., 1977).

Disulfiram (TETD) and thiram (TMTD), like most dithio-carbamates, alter ethanol metabolism (van Logten, 1972); there has been a report that in three patients with eczema from rubber gloves the condition was aggravated after consumption of ethanol (van Ketel, 1968).

Superficial keratitis has been observed in rubber workers exposed to ethyl isothiocyanate (Groves & Smail, 1969).

The International Contact Dermititis Research Group has proposed the following patch-test allergens in relation to exposure to rubber chemicals:

N-cyclohexylbenzothiazylsulphenamide
hydroquinone monobenzylether
1,3-diphenylguanidine
phenyl-β-naphthylamine
N-phenyl-N'-isopropyl-para-phenylenediamine
4,4'-dihydroxydiphenyl
2-mercaptobenzimidazole
hexamethylenetetramine
tetramethylthiuram monosulphide
bis(diethyldithiocarbamato)zinc
mercaptobenzothiazole
tetramethylthiuram disulphide
phenylcyclohexyl-para-phenylenediamine
diphenyl-para-phenylenediamine
dibenzothiazyldisulphide
morpholinylmercaptobenzothiazole
tetraethylthiuram disulphide
dipentamethylenethiuram disulphide
di-β-naphthyl-para-phenylenediamine
bis(dibutyldithiocarbamato)zinc (Malten et al., 1976).

2.2   Respiratory effects

In a study of 239 Egyptian rubber workers in three factories, chronic bronchitis and chronic bronchial asthma were found among mixing and compounding workers exposed to dust and rubber additives, while workers exposed only to by-product gases had bronchial asthma (Noweir et al., 1972; Osman et al., 1972).

In a Swedish report (Fristedt et al., 1968), five cases of talcosis were described in one rubber factory. The mean average exposure to respirable dust (37-66 million particles per cubic foot) was twice to three times above the occupational standard at that time, which was 20 million particles per cubic foot.

The substitution for talc of powder with a fine particle size and containing a high content of crystalline silica in a rubber processing plant resulted in the development of silicosis in a number of exposed workers. The average time of exposure was 6.8 years (Gaubatz & Gaubatz-Trott, 1973).

Workers exposed to curing fumes had a higher prevalence of chronic bronchitis than controls. Respiratory morbidity was related to both intensity and length of exposure to fumes. In addition, forced vital capacity was significantly decreased in curing workers; and those workers re-examined one year later suffered an excessive loss in pulmonary function compared with those not exposed (Fine & Peters, 1976a,b).

Sixty-five men exposed to dust in the processing area of three rubber factories had a higher prevalence of chronic productive coughs and a decrease in the ratio of forced expiratory volume:forced vital capacity when compared with controls. The effects on pulmonary function were related to length of exposure. The authors concluded that exposures to processing dusts at the level measured produced chronic respiratory disease (Fine & Peters, 1976c).

Eighty talc workers were also studied in the three rubber manufacturing plants. Although exposure to talc was below the current threshold limit value (20 million particles per cubic foot), workers exposed for 10 years had statistically significantly decreased forced expiratory volume and an increase in respiratory morbidity, despite the absence of changes in chest X-rays (Fine et al., 1976).

Rubber workers exposed to the hexamethylenetetramine-resorcinol adhesive system had an excess of acute respiratory symptoms and statistically insignificant reductions in forced expiratory volume and forced vital capacity. However, statistically significant decreases in pulmonary function were seen over a six-hour period of a work shift (Gamble et al., 1976).

A questionnaire on respiratory symptoms was answered by 1820 of 2856 white male production workers. The data were analysed according to where the individuals worked in rubber production. The prevalence of respiratory symptoms was high in those workers currently involved in milling, tube building, tube curing and tube inspection (McMichael et al., 1976). Another study of chronic respiratory disease in the rubber industry was based on a cohort on 4302 male rubber workers, of whom 73 terminated their employment with pulmonary disability. These 73 workers had spent significantly longer in curing preparation, curing and finishing and inspection work areas, each of which implied exposure to particulate material and/or to solvents. The authors concluded that a significant risk of developing a pulmonary disability was associated with smoking and exposure to dust and fumes, and in particular to talc and carbon black (Lednar et al., 1977).

Two further studies (Weeks et al., 1981a,b) revealed that employment in curing departments was associated with shortness of breath, chest tightness, wheeze, reduced forced expiratory volume and forced vital capacity and a decline in the ratio of forced expiratory volume:forced vital capacity. In addition, tingling and numbness occurred in the extremities. All of these associations became stronger with increase in duration of employment in the curing department. Exposure to respirable particulates causes not only increased symptoms of respiratory disease but also nausea and abdominal pain. Workers exposed to emissions from heated uncured rubber reported chest tightness on return to work.

At a US tyre factory, 210 workers (172 men and 38 women) developed a syndrome related to exposure to the volatile products released from a synthetic rubber formulation, first used in 1960. The factory employed approximately 2200 workers at the time of the outbreak, about 600 of whom were repeatedly exposed to the new formulation in their daily work. Symptoms occurred most frequently in workers in the Banbury-calender and tyre-building areas, where 32% and 22%, respectively, of the workers were afflicted. The symptoms included severe respiratory irritation, weakness, weight loss and general malaise. Fever and radiographic and pulmonary function abnormalities were also noted in many of those affected. More than 17% of the affected employees were permanently disabled. A similar syndrome was reported in at least four other factories in which the adhesive system had been introduced. After the system was modified, in late 1962, the prevalence of symptoms remained low, and no new cases appeared (doPico et al., 1975).

Chronic lung diseases (pneumoconiosis, pulmonary fibrosis, bronchitis and emphysema) occur in workers exposed to carbon black (National Institute for Occupational Safety & Health, 1978); and a higher incidence of pneumoconiosis has been reported in those exposed to channel black than in those exposed to thermal or furnace black (Troitskaya et al., 1975).

2.3 Effects on reproduction

Data on hospitalized patients who had had miscarriages (spontaneous abortions) were analysed in conjunction with membership files of the Union of Rubber and Leather Workers (about 10 000 women) and records of the personnel of a rubber factory (about 1600 women) in Finland. Spontaneous abortions were calculated in two ways for each population analysed: rate (no. of spontaneous abortions x 100/no. of pregnancies) and ratio (no. of spontaneous abortions x 100/no. of births). The two frequencies were slightly increased for all Union members, as compared with all Finnish women. Moreover, age-standardized frequency was higher when the pregnancy occurred during Union membership than when it occurred before or after joining the Union. The frequency of spontaneous miscarriages among Union members employed only in the rubber industry was higher among those employed for 3 to 35 months than for those employed for longer periods of time. The employees of the rubber factory had slightly fewer spontaneous abortions on average than did the community population. However, women employed for 3 to 23 months had markedly higher frequencies of spontaneous abortion than those employed for longer times (Hemminki et al., 1982). [Because the data in these two studies present a conflicting picture with respect to the relation between rubber work and spontaneous abortions, no conclusions can be drawn.]

3. Summary

The number and diversity of chemicals used or formed and the multiplicity of exposures experienced within the rubber industry make it difficult to attribute a particular toxic effect to a given exposure.

Carbon blacks and mineral oils are major constituents in such products as rubber tyres. Data on the carcinogenicity of carbon blacks in experimental animals are inconclusive. Carbon blacks contain varying amounts of polycyclic aromatic compounds, some of which are carcinogenic and which may become bioavailable through elution. Solvent extracts of carbon blacks have been found to be mutagenic and carcinogenic in experimental systems. The mutagenicity and carcinogenicity of mineral oils are also dependent upon the chemical composition of the oils, and are possibly related to the high levels of polycyclic aromatic compounds they contain.

The toxicity of curing fumes from vulcanization processes probably depends on a number of factors, among which the composition of the rubber, temperature and presence or absence of oxygen may be important. Some curing fumes have been found to be mutagenic in bacteria. Certain thiuram compounds and dithiocarbamates are mutagenic to Salmonella typhimurium. Ethylenethiourea is carcinogenic and teratogenic to rats; and other thioureas were teratogenic to chicken embryos.

Many of the solvents that are used in the rubber industry are mutagenic and carcinogenic in experimental systems. Benzene, the use of which as a solvent has been reduced in the rubber industry, causes a variety of disorders of the haematopoietic system and is considered to be carcinogenic in man and in rodents.

Among the monomers to which workers may be exposed in the rubber industry, vinyl chloride has been shown conclusively to be carcinogenic to humans; and there is limited evidence in humans and animals that acrylonitrile, epichlorohydrin and styrene are carcinogenic. These monomers and chloroprene are also mutagenic and teratogenic in experimental systems.

Some N-nitroso compounds, N-nitrosodimethylamine, N-nitrosodiethylamine, N-nitrosodi-n-butylamine, N-nitrosomorpholine, N-nitrosopiperidine and N-nitrosopyrrolidine, are formed during rubber processing and occur in work atmospheres; they are also mutagenic and carcinogenic in experimental systems. N-Nitrosodiphenylamine, which is used as a retardant, is not mutagenic but is a nitrosating agent in vivo and is carcinogenic in rats when administered at high dose levels.

The aromatic amines, 4-aminobiphenyl, benzidine and 2-naphthylamine, are known to be carcinogenic in humans, and their use has been withdrawn in some countries. Other aromatic amines are widely used in the rubber industry. There is some evidence that N-phenyl-2-naphthylamine can be partly biotransformed to 2-naphthylamine in humans. A number of antioxidants that are naphthylamine-acetaldehyde condensates containing 1- and 2-naphthylamine as impurities are carcinogenic in humans and have been withdrawn from use in the rubber industry in some countries. There is <u>sufficient evidence</u> for the carcinogenicity in exper- imental animals of 2,4-diaminotoluene and 4,4'-methylenebis(2- chloroaniline), but they are still used.

Di(2-ethylhexy) phthalate and di(2-ethylhexyl) adipate, which are used as plasticizers, are reported to be carcinogenic in rodents.

Peroxides in use in the rubber industry have not generally been well studied with regard to possible mutagenic and carcino- genic effects. However, hydrogen peroxide has been found to be mutagenic and was reported to produce intestinal cancer in one study in mice.

A number of health effects other than cancer, including allergic dermatitis and impaired respiratory function, have been observed in rubber workers.

4. References

Ahmed, A.E., Kubic, V.L., Stevens, J.L. & Anders, M.W. (1980) Halogenated methanes: metabolism and toxicity. Fed. Proc., 39, 3150-3155

Altenburg, L.C., Ray, J.H., Smart, C.E. & Moore, F.B. (1979) Rubber solvent: a clastogenic agent that fails to induce sister-chromatid exchanges. Mutat. Res., 67, 331-341

Barnes, J.R. & Ranta, K.E. (1972) The metabolism of dimethylformamide and dimethylacetamide. Toxicol. appl. Pharmacol., 23, 271-276

Bartsch, H., Malaveille, C., Barbin, A. & Planche, G. (1979) Mutagenic and alkylating metabolites of halo-ethylenes, chlorobutadienes and dichlorobutenes produced by rodent or human liver tissue. Evidence for oxirane formation by P450-linked microsomal mono-oxygenases. Arch. Toxicol., 41, 247-277

Batschvarov, B. & Minkov, D.M. (1968) Dermatitis and purpura from rubber in clothing. Trans. St John's Hosp. Dermatol. Soc., 54, 178-182

Bonnevie, P. & Marcussen, P.V. (1945) Rubber products as a widespread cause of eczema. Report of 80 cases. Acta dermato-veneral., 25, 163-178

Boyland, E. (1958) The biochemistry of cancer of the bladder. Br. med. Bull., 14, 153-158

Calnan, C.D. (1973) Occupational leukoderma from alkyl phenols. Proc. R. Soc. Med., 66, 258-260

Campbell, J., Crumplin, G.C., Garner, J.V., Garner, R.C., Martin, C.N. & Rutter, A. (1981) Nitrated polycyclic aromatic hydrocarbons: potent bacterial mutagens and stimulators of DNA repair synthesis in cultured human cells. Carcinogenesis, 2, 559-565

Clayson, D.B. & Garner, R.C. (1976) Carcinogenic aromatic amines and related compounds. In: Searle, C.E., ed., Chemical Carcinogens (ACS Monograph No. 173), Washington DC, American Chemical Society, pp. 366-461

Cronin, E. (1966) Shoe dermatitis. Br. J. Dermatol., 78, 617-625

Cronin, E. (1980) Contact Dermatitis, Edinburgh, Churchill Livingstone, pp. 714-770

Curtis, G.H. (1945) Contact dermatitis of eyelids caused by an antioxidant in rubber fillers of eyelash curlers. Report of seven cases. Arch. Dermatol. Syphilol., 52, 262-265

Downing, J.G. (1933) Dermatitis from rubber gloves. New Engl. J. Med., 208, 196-198

Egan, H., Fishbein, L., Castegnaro, M., O'Neill, I.K. & Bartsch, H., eds (1981) Environmental Carcinogens. Selected Methods of Analysis, Vol. 4, Some Aromatic Amines and Azo Dyes in the General and Industrial Environment (IARC Scientific Publications No. 40), Lyon, International Agency for Research on Cancer

Falk, H.L., Miller, A. & Kotin, P. (1958) Elution of 3,4-benzpyrene and related hydrocarbons from soots by plasma proteins. Science, 127, 474-475

Fine, L.J. & Peters, J.M. (1976a) Respiratory morbidity in rubber workers. I. Prevalence of respiratory symptoms and disease in curing workers. Arch. environ. Health, 31, 5-9

Fine, L.J. & Peters, J.M. (1976b) Respiratory morbidity in rubber workers. II. Pulmonary function in curing workers. Arch. environ. Health, 31, 10-14

Fine, L.J. & Peters, J.M. (1976c) Studies of respiratory morbidity in rubber workers. III. Respiratory morbidity in processing workers. Arch. environ. Health, 31, 136-140

Fine, L.J., Peters, J.M., Burgess, W.A. & DiBerardinis, L.J. (1976) Studies of respiratory morbidity in rubber workers. IV. Respiratory morbidity in talc workers. Arch. environ. Health, 31, 195-200

Fitch, W.L. & Smith, D.H. (1979) Analysis of adsorption proper-
    ties and adsorbed species on commercial polymeric carbons.
    Environ. Sci. Technol., 13, 341-346

Fristedt, B., Mattsson, S.B. & Schütz, A. (1968) Talcosis by
    exposure to granular talc in a rubber industry (Nor.). Nord.
    Hyg. Tidskr., 49, 66-71

Gamble, J.F., McMichael, A.J., Williams, T. & Battigelli, M.
    (1976) Respiratory function and symptoms: an environmental-
    epidemiological study of rubber workers exposed to a
    phenol-formaldehyde type resin. Am. ind. Hyg. Assoc. J., 37,
    499-513

Gaubatz, E. & Gaubatz-Trott, H. (1973) Pneumoconiosis in workers
    in a rubber-processing plant. Radiological and histological
    studies (Ger.). Prax. Pneumol., 27, 740-742

Gold, A. (1975) Carbon black adsorbates: Separation and identifi-
    cation of a carcinogen and some oxygenated polyaromatics.
    Anal. Chem., 47, 1469-1472

Goodall, C.M., Lijinsky, W. & Smillie, A.C. (1968) Oncogenicity
    of p-nitroso-N,N-dimethylaniline in rats. Proc. Univ. Otago
    med. School, 46, 68-70

Greim, H., Bonse, G., Radwan, Z., Reichert, D. & Henschler, D.
    (1975) Mutagenicity in vitro and potential carcinogenicity
    of chlorinated ethylenes as a function of metabolic oxirane
    formation. Biochem. Pharmacol., 24, 2013-2017

Groves, J.S. & Smail, J.M. (1969) Outbreak of superficial
    keratitis in rubber workers. Br. J. Ophthalmol., 53, 683-687

von Haam, E., Titus, H.L., Caplan, I. & Shinowara, G.Y. (1958)
    Effect of carbon blacks on carcinogenic compounds. Proc.
    Soc. exp. Biol. Med., 98, 95-98

Hedenstedt, A. (1982) Genetic health risks in the rubber
    industry: Mutagenicity studies on rubber chemicals and
    process vapours. In: International Symposium on Prevention
    of Occupational Cancer, Helsinki, Finnish Institute of
    Occupational Health (in press)

Hedenstedt, A., Rannug, U., Ramel, C. & Wachtmeister, C.A. (1979) Mutagenicity and metabolism studies on 12 thiuram and dithiocarbamate compounds used as accelerators in the Swedish rubber industry. Mutat. Res., 68, 313-325

Hedenstedt, A., Ramel, C. & Wachtmeister, C.A. (1981) Mutagenicity of rubber vulcanization gases in Salmonella typhimurium. J. Toxicol. environ. Health, 8, 805-814

Hemminki, K., Falck, K. & Vainio, H. (1980) Comparison of alkylation rates and mutagenicity of directly acting industrial and laboratory chemicals. Epoxides, glycidyl ethers, methylating and ethylating agents, halogenated hydrocarbons, hydrazine derivatives, aldehydes, thiuram and dithiocarbamate derivatives. Arch. Toxicol., 46, 277-285

Hemminki, K., Niemi, M.-L., Kyrrönen, P., Kilpikari, I. & Vainio, H. (1982) Spontaneous abortions and reproductive selection mechanisms in the rubber and leather industry in Finland. Br. J. ind. Med. (in press)

Hermann, M., Durand, J.P., Charpentier, J.M., Chaude, O., Hofnung, M., Petroff, N., Vandecasteele, J.-P. & Weill, N. (1982) Correlations of mutagenic activity with polynuclear aromatic hydrocarbons content of various mineral oils. In: Fourth International Symposium on Polynuclear Aromatic Hydrocarbons, Columbus, OH (in press)

Herve-Bazin, B., Gradiski, D., Duprat, P., Marignac, B., Foussereau, J., Cavelier, C. & Bieber, P. (1977) Occupational eczema from N-isopropyl-N'-phenylparaphenylenediamine (IPPD) and N-dimethyl-1,3-butyl-N'-phenylparaphenylenediamine (DMPPD) in tyres. Contact Dermatitis, 3, 1-15

Heydenreich, G. & Ølholm-Larsen, P. (1976) 4,4'-Dithiodimorpholine, a new rubber sensitizer. Contact Dermatitis, 2, 292-293

Holmberg, B. & Sjöström, B. (1977) A Toxicological Survey of Chemicals Used in the Swedish Rubber Industry, Stockholm, National Board of Occupational Safety & Health, pp. 3-4

IARC (1972) IARC Monographs on the Evaluation of Carcinogenic Risk of Chemicals to Man, Vol. 1, Lyon, International Agency for Research on Cancer, pp. 141-144

IARC (1973) IARC Monographs on the Evaluation of Carcinogenic Risk of Chemicals to Man, Vol. 3, Certain Polycyclic Aromatic Hydrocarbons and Heterocyclic Compounds, Lyon, International Agency for Research on Cancer

IARC (1974) IARC Monographs on the Evaluation of Carcinogenic Risk of Chemicals to Man, Vol. 7, Some Anti-thyroid and Related Substances, Nitrofurans and Industrial Chemicals, Lyon, International Agency for Research on Cancer, pp. 45-52

IARC (1976a) IARC Monographs on the Evaluation of Carcinogenic Risk of Chemicals to Man, Vol. 11, Cadmium, Nickel, Some Epoxides, Miscellaneous Industrial Chemicals and General Considerations on Volatile Anaesthetics, Lyon, International Agency for Research on Cancer, pp. 241-256

IARC (1976b) IARC Monographs on the Evaluation of Carcinogenic Risk of Chemicals to Man, Vol. 12, Some Carbamates, Thiocarbamates and Carbazides, Lyon, International Agency for Research on Cancer

IARC (1977) IARC Monographs on the Evaluation of Carcinogenic Risk of Chemicals to Man, Vol. 14, Asbestos, Lyon, International Agency for Research on Cancer

IARC (1978) IARC Monographs on the Evaluation of the Carcinogenic Risk of Chemicals to Humans, Vol. 17, Some N-Nitroso Compounds, Lyon, International Agency for Research on Cancer

IARC (1979a) IARC Monographs on the Evaluation of the Carcinogenic Risk of Chemicals to Humans, Vol. 19, Some Monomers, Plastics and Synthetic Elastomers, and Acrolein, Lyon, International Agency for Research on Cancer

IARC (1979b) IARC Monographs on the Evaluation of the Carcinogenic Risk of Chemicals to Humans, Supplement 1, Chemicals and Industrial Processes Associated with Cancer in Humans, Lyon, International Agency for Research on Cancer

IARC (1979c) IARC Monographs on the Evaluation of the Carcino-
    genic Risk of Chemicals to Humans, Vol. 20, Some Halogenated
    Hydrocarbons, Lyon, International Agency for Research on
    Cancer

IARC (1982) IARC Monographs on the Evaluation of the Carcinogenic
    Risk of Chemicals to Humans, Vol. 27, Some Aromatic Amines,
    Anthraquinones and Nitroso Compounds, and Inorganic
    Fluorides Used in Drinking-water and Dental Preparations,
    Lyon, International Agency for Research on Cancer

IARC (1982) IARC Monographs on the Evaluation of the Carcinogenic
    Risk of Chemicals to Humans, Vol. 29, Some Industrial
    Chemicals and Dyestuffs, Lyon, International Agency for
    Research on Cancer (in press)

Irving, C.C. (1979) Species and tissue variations in the meta-
    bolic activation of aromatic amines. In: Griffin, A.C. &
    Shaw, C.R., eds, Carcinogens: Identification and Mechanisms
    of Action, New York, Raven Press, pork, Raven Press, pp. 211-227

Ito, A., Watanabe, H., Naito, M. & Naito, Y. (1981) Induction of
    duodenal tumors in mice by oral administration of hydrogen
    peroxide. Gann, 72, 174-175

Jongen, W.M.F., Alink, G.M. & Koeman, J.H. (1978) Mutagenic
    effect of dichloromethane on Salmonella typhimurium. Mutat.
    Res., 56, 245-248

Jordan, W.P. (1971) Contact dermatitis from N-isopropyl-N-phenyl-
    paraphenylenediamine. "Volkswagen dermatitis". Arch.
    Dermatol., 103, 85-87

Kaden, D.A., Hites, R.A. & Thilly, W.G. (1979) Mutagenicity of
    soot and associated polycyclic aromatic hydrocarbons to
    Salmonella typhimurium. Cancer Res., 39, 4152-4159

van Ketel, W.G. (1968) Rubber, alcohol and eczema (Dutch).
    Dermatologica, 136, 442-444

Khera, K.S. (1973) Ethylenethiourea: teratogenicity study in rats
    and rabbits. Teratology, 7, 243-252

Korhonen, A., Hemminki, K. & Vainio, H. (1982a) Application of the chicken embryo in testing for embryotoxicity. I. Thiurams. Scand. J. Work environ. Health (in press)

Korhonen, A., Hemminki, K. & Vainio, H. (1982b) Embryotoxicity of industrial chemicals on the chicken embryo. II. Dithiocarbamates. Teratogenesis Carcinog. Mutagenesis (in press)

Korhonen, A., Hemminki, K. & Vainio, H. (1982c) Embryotoxicity of industrial chemicals on the chicken embryo. III. Thiourea derivatives. Acta pharmacol. toxicol. (in press)

Kriek, E. & Westra, J.G. (1979) Metabolic activation of aromatic amines and amides and interactions with nucleic acids.   In: Grover, P.L., ed., Chemical Carcinogens and DNA, Vol. II, Boca Raton, FL, CRC Press Inc., pp. 1–28

Kuna, R.A. & Kapp, R.W., Jr (1981) The embryotoxic/teratogenic potential of benzene vapor in rats. Toxicol. appl. Pharmacol., 57, 1–7

Kutscher, W., Tomingas, R. & Weisfeld, H.P. (1967) Studies on the hazards from carbon black with particular consideration to its carcinogenic activity – Report 5 – Elution of 3,4-benzopyrene by blood serum and some protein factors in the serum (Ger.). Arch. Hyg., 151, 646–655

Laskin, S., Sellakumar, A.R., Kuschner, M., Nelson, N., LaMendola, S., Rusch, G.M., Katz, G.V., Dulak, N.C. & Albert, R.E. (1980) Inhalation carcinogenicity of epichlorohydrin in noninbred Sprague-Dawley rats. J. natl Cancer Inst., 65, 751–757

Lednar, W.M., Tyroler, H.A., McMichael, A.J. & Shy, C.M. (1977) The occupational determinants of chronic disabling pulmonary disease in rubber workers. J. occup. Med., 19, 263–268

Lee, M.L. & Hites, R.A. (1976) Characterization of sulfur-containing polycyclic aromatic compounds in carbon blacks. Anal. Chem., 48, 1890–1893

te Lintum J.C.A. & Nater, J.P. (1974) Allergic contact dermatitis caused by rubber chemicals in dairy workers. Dermatologica, 148, 42–46

Locati, G., Fantuzzi, A., Consonni, G., Li Gotti, I. & Bonomi, G. (1979) Identification of polycyclic aromatic hydrocarbons in carbon black with reference to cancerogenic risk in tire production. Am. ind. Hyg. Assoc. J., 40, 644-652

Löfroth, G., Hefner, E., Alfheim, I. & Møller, M. (1980) Mutagenic activity in photocopies. Science, 209, 1037-1039

van Logten, M.J. (1972) De Dithiocarbamaat-Alcohol-Reactie bij de Rat [The Dithiocarbamate-Alcohol Reaction in the Rat], Terborg, The Netherlands, Bedrijf, FA. Lammers

Malten, K.E., Nater, J.P. & van Ketel, W.G. (1976) Patch Testing Guidelines, Nijmegen, Dekker & van de Vegt

Marcussen, P.V. (1943) Rubber footwear as a cause of foot eczema. Acta dermatol. Venerol., 23, 331-342

McMichael, A.J., Gerber, W.S., Gamble, J.F. & Lednar, W.M. (1976) Chronic respiratory symptoms and job type within the rubber industry. J. occup. Med., 18, 611-617

Miller, E.C. (1978) Some current perspectives on chemical carcinogenesis in humans and experimental animals: Presidential address. Cancer Res., 38, 1479-1496

Miller, J.A. & Miller, E.C. (1969) The metabolic activation of carcinogenic aromatic amines and amides. In: Homburger, F., ed., Progress in Experimental Tumor Research, Vol. 11, Basel, Karger, pp. 273-301

Nater, J.P. (1975) High sensitivity to rubber (Ger.). Berufs-Dermatosen, 23, 161-168

National Institute for Occupational Safety & Health (1978) Criteria for a Recommended Standard...Occupational Exposure to Carbon Black   (DHEW (NIOSH) Publication No. 78-204), Washington DC, US Government Printing Office

Nau, C.A., Neal, J. & Stembridge, V. (1958a) A study of the physiological effects of carbon black. I. Ingestion. Arch. ind. Health, 17, 21-28

Nau, C.A., Neal, J. & Stembridge, V. (1958b) A study of the physiological effects of carbon black. II. Skin contact. Arch. ind. Health, 18, 511-520

Nau, C.A., Neal, J. & Stembridge, V.A. (1960) A study of the physiological effects of carbon black. III. Adsorption and elution potentials; subcutaneous injections. Arch. environ. Health, 1, 512-533

Nau, C.A., Neal, J., Stembridge, V.A. & Cooley, R.N. (1962) Physiological effects of carbon black. IV. Inhalation. Arch. environ. Health, 4, 415-431

Nau, C.A., Taylor, G.T. & Lawrence, C.H. (1976) Properties and physiological effects of thermal carbon black. J. occup. Med., 18, 732-734

Neal, J., Thornton, M. & Nau, C.A. (1962) Polycyclic hydrocarbon elution from carbon black or rubber products. Arch. environ. Health, 4, 598-606

Norpoth, K., Reisch, A. & Heinecke, A. (1980) Biostatistics of Ames-test data. In: Norpoth, K.H. & Garner, R.C., eds, Short-term Test Systems for Detecting Carcinogens, New York, Springer, pp. 312-322

Noweir, M.H., El-Dakhakhny, A.A. & Osman, H.A. (1972) Exposure to chemical agents in rubber industry. J. Egypt. publ. Health Assoc., 47, 182-201

Ohshima, H., Béréziat, J.C. & Bartsch, H. (1982) Measurement of endogenous N-nitrosation in rats and humans by monitoring urinary and faecal excretion of N-nitrosamino acids. In: Bartsch, H., O'Neill, I.K., Castegnaro, M. & Okada, M., eds, N-Nitroso Compounds: Occurrence and Biological Effects (IARC Scientific Publications No. 41), International Agency for Research on Cancer (in press)

Osman, H.A., Wahdan, M.H. & Noweir, M.H. (1972) Health problems resulting from prolonged exposure to chemical agents in rubber industry. J. Egypt. publ. Health Assoc., 47, 290-311

doPico, G.A., Rankin, J., Chosy, L.W., Reddan, W.G., Barbee, R.A., Gee, B. & Dickie, H.A. (1975) Respiratory tract disease from thermosetting resins. Study of an outbreak in rubber tire workers. Ann intern. Med., 83, 177-184

Robertson, J. McD. & Ingalls, T.H. (1980) A mortality study of carbon black workers in the United States from 1935 to 1974. Arch. environ. Health, 35, 181-186

Rosenkranz, H.S. (1973) Sodium hypochlorite and sodium perborate: preferential inhibitors of DNA polymerase-deficient bacteria. Mutat. Res., 21, 171-174

Rosenkranz, H.S., McCoy, E.C., Sanders, D.R., Butler, M., Kiriazides, D.K. & Mermelstein, R. (1980) Nitropyrenes: Isolation, identification, and reduction of mutagenic impurities in carbon black and toners. Science, 209, 1039-1043

Ruddick, J.A. & Khera, K.S. (1975) Pattern of anomalies following single oral doses of ethylenethiourea to pregnant rats. Teratology, 12, 277-282

Rudzki, E., Ostaszewski, K., Grzywa, Z. & Kozlowska, A. (1976) Sensitivity to some rubber additives. Contact Dermatitis, 2, 24-27

Schønning, L. & Hjorth, N. (1969) Cross sensitization between hair dyes and rubber chemicals. Berufs-Dermatosen, 17, 100-106

Shirasu, Y., Moriya, M., Kato, K., Lienard, F., Tezuka, H. & Teramoto, S. (1977) Mutagenicity screening on pesticides and modification products: a basis of carcinogenicity evaluation. In: Hiatt, H.H., Watson, J.D. & Winston, J.A., eds, Origins of Human Cancer, Book A, Cold Spring Harbor, NY, Cold Spring Harbor Laboratory, pp. 267-285

Steiner, P.E. (1954) The conditional biological activity of the carcinogens in carbon blacks, and its elimination. Cancer Res., 14, 103-110

Stula, E.F. & Krauss, W.C. (1977) Embryotoxicity in rats and rabbits from cutaneous application of amide-type solvents and substituted ureas. Toxicol. appl. Pharmacol., 41, 35–55

Styles, J.A. (1978) Mammalian cell transformation in vitro. Br. J. Cancer, 37, 931–936

Taylor, G.T., Redington, T.E., Bailey, M.J., Buddingh, F. & Nau, C.A. (1980) Solvent extracts of carbon black – determination of total extractables and analysis for benzo(α)pyrene. Am. ind. Hyg. Assoc. J., 41, 819–825

Thacker, J. (1975) Inactivation and mutation of yeast cells by hydrogen peroxide. Mutat. Res., 33, 147–156

Troitskaya, N.A., Velichkovsky, B.T., Bikmullina, S.K., Sazhina, T.G., Gorodnova, N.V. & Andreeva, T.D. (1975) Substantiation of the maximum permissible concentration of industrial carbon black in the air of workrooms (Russ.). Gig. Tr. Prof. Zabol., 3, 32–36

Uehleke, H. & Poplawski-Tabarelli, S. (1977) Irreversible binding of ^{14}C-labelled trichloroethylene to mice liver constituents in vivo and in vitro. Arch. Toxicol., 37, 289–294

Van Duuren, B.L. (1976) Tumor-promoting and co-carcinogenic agents in chemical carcinogenesis. In: Searle, C.E., ed., Chemical Carcinogens (ACS Monograph No. 173), Washington DC, American Chemical Society, pp. 24–51

Veys, C.A. (1969) Two epidemiological inquiries into the incidence of bladder tumors in industrial workers. J. natl Cancer Inst., 43, 219–226

Weeks, J.L., Peters, J.M. & Monson, R.R. (1981a) Screening for occupational health hazards in the rubber industry. Part I. Am. J. int. Med., 2, 125–142

Weeks, J.L., Peters, J.M. & Monson, R.R. (1981b) Screening for occupational health hazards in the rubber industry. Part II: Health hazards in the curing department. Am. J. int. Med., 2, 143–151

Wilson, H.T.H. (1960) Rubber-glove dermatitis. <u>Br. med. J.</u>, <u>ii</u>, 21-23

Wilson, H.T.H. (1969) Rubber dermatitis. An investigation of 106 cases of contact dermatitis caused by rubber. <u>Br. J. Dermatol.</u>, <u>81</u>, 175-179

1.   Introduction

1.1   Types of epidemiological studies

Most of the epidemiological reports available for review were retrospective follow-up studies of cohorts of rubber workers or were case-control studies of people with cancer. In follow-up studies, the rate of occurrence of, or death from, cancer is compared with the rate in a control population – typically, the general population. In case-control studies, people with specific cancers are compared with people without that cancer as to their occupational history in the rubber industry.

The Working Group noted that the cohorts in the follow-up studies are of two distinct types with regard to intake characteristics:

(a) Census cohort: This type of cohort, typified by the studies of the UK Employment Medical Advisory Service (Baxter & Werner, 1980) and of the University of North Carolina (McMichael et al., 1974), consists of workers actively employed at one point in time or of a combination of active and retired workers. The cohort is closed, in that no new workers are entered after the initial cohort has been defined.

(b) Active intake cohort: This type of cohort, typified by the studies of the British Rubber Manufacturers' Association (Parkes et al., 1982), consists of all workers newly employed over a certain period of time. The studies from Harvard University (Monson & Nakano, 1976a) are a combination of the two types.

A limitation of the census type of cohort is that people who have had short-term exposure are particularly likely not to be included. The susceptibility of such people to occupational carcinogens may differ from that of people who were included in the census.

A characteristic of the active intake type of cohort is that a relatively high proportion of person-years during early years of follow-up are included. Because occupational cancer is not likely to occur during those early years, their inclusion tends to dilute any real excess that may subsequently occur. This does not constitute a necessary limitation, for analyses can take into account the occurrence of cancer according to years after initial exposure.

Frequently, in follow-up studies, the rate of death in the study population is less than that in the general population. This difference has been termed the 'healthy worker effect'. The lower death rate, which is most pronounced early in the follow-up period, occurs because only relatively healthy persons enter into the employment force. The effect is likely to be more pronounced in active intake cohort studies, in which people are followed from initial employment.

The Working Group considered these differences in the characteristics of the various cohorts and concluded that they represented no important difficulties in evaluating the available data.

1.2 Information on work history

In the follow-up studies, varying detail was available on the work experience of members of the cohort. Some studies disposed of complete work histories from company records; some had access to summary work histories from union records; some had information only on the job at enrolment into the study; some could take into account only the most representative or usual job.

In studies in which information on more than one job or exposure was available for each individual, non-mutually-exclusive analyses may have been done: Each worker may have been entered into more than one analysis of cancer occurrence among people ever employed in different work areas. In studies in which information on only one job was available for each individual, that job may not have been the appropriate characterization of the individual.

The Working Group considered these differences in the detail of work history available in the follow-up studies and concluded that they represented no important difficulties in evaluating the available data. However, they recommended that future analyses take a person's complete work history into account, whenever possible.

In case-control studies conducted within the general population, a person's work history may have been characterized only as 'rubber worker'. When such studies show no association between work in the rubber industry and a specific cancer, a causal association may have been masked by inadequate information on exposure. When case-control studies show a positive association, judged to be causal, it is likely to be an underestimate of the true measure among some subgroups.

Case-control studies may have been conducted in geographic areas where the prevalence of work in the rubber industry was low. Very few of the cases (and of the controls) may have been found to be rubber workers. In the event that no positive association is found between rubber work and a specific cancer, studies of this type should be judged to provide only weak evidence that no association exists.

1.3   Measures of disease frequency

In occupational cohort studies, standardized mortality (or morbidity) ratios (SMRs) are typically computed. [A SMR is the number of deaths observed in a group divided by the number expected in the same group, the resultant quotient being multiplied by 100. The expected numbers, which are customarily based on the mortality experience of a general population, are usually standardized for age and calender time.] An alternative way of presenting the information incorporated within the SMR is to report the observed and expected numbers of deaths (or cases). In analyses in which rates of cancer are computed internally for two subgroups of a study population, the ratio of the two rates is referred to as the risk ratio (RR). The RR is also usually standardized for age and calender time (SRR).

In case-control studies, disease rates are not usually computed, because the size of the population that gave rise to the cases is unknown. In such situations, the RR is based on the frequency of exposure among the cases and among the controls.

In this monograph, the data are reported as presented by the author. For practical purposes, in the evaluation of these data, SMRs, RRs, observed/expected ratios, and SRRs may be considered to be equivalent.

1.4 Information used

In the preparation of this monograph, a number of case reports, population surveys and descriptive epidemiological studies on workers in the rubber industry were considered. The summary of the evidence underlying the final evaluation does not include those studies in which no quantitative estimate of possible excess cancer in rubber workers could be made. Population surveys were also discounted, because more specific information was available from cohort and case-control studies. Data from early epidemiological studies that are included in or superseded by later studies have not been included. Certain early studies of historical interest are cited in Section II.

In selecting data for inclusion in the body of this text, no absolute criteria were used. While, in general, associations based on fewer than five exposed persons with cancer were not included, there were occasional exceptions.

The characteristics of the epidemiological studies considered are summarized in Table 14; and the essential data from each study are shown in Table 15, at the end of this section.

2. Studies of British rubber workers

2.1 Early studies

As part of his investigation of bladder cancer in the dyestuffs industry (Case et al., 1954a), Case reviewed the bladder cancer mortality experience of the county borough which includes Birmingham. He was impressed with the frequency with which death certificates relating to bladder cancer also related to employment in the rubber industry. He therefore undertook a formal evaluation of bladder cancer among rubber workers and, in a single publication (Case & Hosker, 1954), reported the results of two independent investigations. The first of these was a national survey of mortality from bladder cancer. Among rubber workers during the period 1936-1951, 26 deaths from bladder cancer occurred, whereas, on the basis of the estimated number and age of the men employed in the rubber industry (which information was available from various governmental publications) and national bladder cancer mortality rates, it was estimated that 15.9 bladder cancer deaths would have been expected. The second investigation was based on hospital reports. These permitted estimation of the number of new cases of bladder cancer that would be expected among men engaged in 'rubber occupations' in Greater Birmingham, a centre of the rubber industry. During the period 1936-1950, 22 cases were observed, and 4.0 were expected.

Although Case's studies could not incriminate any specific etiologic agent, it was inferred that the excess of bladder cancer was attributable to an antioxidant that contained about 2.5% of free naphthylamine, including 2-naphthylamine, a known bladder carcinogen. This antioxidant was removed from the manufacturing process in the UK in 1949 (Case, 1966).

The investigation of Case and Hosker rests in part on relatively crude information; however, it contains no identified source of bias. Alternative causes of bladder cancer, apart from the occupational exposure, were not considered but are unlikely to explain the observed excesses.

Following that study, another was carried out in the British electric-cable industry, since rubber had long been used to insulate power cables, and during 1935-1949 antioxidants containing 1- and 2-naphthylamines as residual contaminants had been used in compounding the rubber (Davies, 1965). Investigations of the work force in one large cable factory showed that of 30 male workers with more than 10 years' exposure to rubber compounding and milling in general, and to the naphthylamine-containing antioxidants in particular, six had developed bladder tumours. Four of these cases were fatal, whereas 0.2 deaths were expected on the basis of national age-specific rates. All four deaths occurred in people under the age of 60.

2.2 <u>Studies by the Employment Medical Advisory Service</u> (renamed Health and Safety Executive)

A detailed census of active workers in the British rubber and cablemaking industries was taken on 1 February 1967. Some 40 867 men, aged 35 years and over, who had worked for at least one year were enumerated. The census covered 381 factories (including both the major rubber factories investigated by the British Rubber Manufacturers' Association and many smaller ones) and 13 sections of the industry, including tyres, remoulds, cables, adhesives, clothing, belting, hose, flooring and footwear.

The study population was subdivided into one of three groups, as follows:

(A) started work before 1 January 1950 in a factory where the suspect antioxidant had been used (12 779 men)

(B) started work on or after 1 January 1950 in a factory where the suspect antioxidants had been used (18 118 men)

(C) worked in factories where purportedly the suspect antioxidants had never been used (9970 men).

The results have been reported (Fox <u>et al.</u>, 1974; Fox & Collier, 1976) and consolidated in a report with 10 years of follow-up (Baxter & Werner, 1980). The data presented are from the latest report. The numbers of deaths observed are compared with those expected on the basis of age-sex-specific mortality rates for England and Wales. In some analyses, social class and regional variation in mortality patterns were controlled. Each man was classified by his occupation at the date of the census; no previous or ulterior information about job category was available. Essentially, the population defined was a survivor group, not necessarily representative of the three situations defined in A, B, C above. The study was initially set up to examine the bladder cancer situation in the UK rubber industry; but the total mortality pattern, and especially that due to cancer, was examined.

(<u>a</u>) <u>Bladder cancer</u>

Overall in group A, 36 deaths were observed and 25.0 were expected. For the tyre sector within group A, there were 13 cases observed and 13.4 expected; for the non-tyre sectors there were 23 observed and 11.6 expected. Within groups B and C no differences were observed between the tyre and non-tyre sectors. Overall for group B, there were 24 deaths observed and 22.3 expected. For group C, there were 13 deaths observed and 13.4 expected.

For men in group A in the non-tyre sectors, there were excesses in those working in cable and electrical goods (6 observed; 1.9 expected) and in mouldings, motor accessories and mechanicals (13 observed; 5.5 expected). When certain other occupational categories for non-tyre sectors were combined (i.e., extruding, component building, inspection with painting, and operating staff), there were 15 deaths observed and 6.0 expected. When these same occupational categories were added together for groups A, B and C, there were 29 deaths observed and 17.3 expected.

When the whole study population was taken into account, there were 73 observed deaths due to bladder cancer and 57.6 expected between 1967 and 1976.

(<u>b</u>) <u>Other cancers</u>

When groups A, B and C are taken together, there were 1748 deaths from malignant neoplasms observed and 1603.9 expected (SMR = 109) during the observation period. Excesses of cancer at specific sites were as follows (observed/expected numbers): stomach, 216/176.4; colon, 107/93.2; and trachea, bronchus and lung, 822/716.5. There was no excess of leukaemia (33/33.8).

In the tyre sector of the industry, the observed/expected numbers of deaths from selected types of cancer were: stomach (91/73.9) and lung (326/299.4). There was considerable variation among the 12 factories studied, but there were excesses of lung cancer in 10 of the factories and of stomach cancer in eight.

In the non-tyre sector, the numbers were 125/117.1 for stomach cancer and 496/465.0 for lung cancer. Within the entire cohort, stomach cancer did not occur in excess in workers in the early part of the production line (23/24.5). The largest excess occurred among site workers (23/16.7). Lung cancer occurred in excess among men mixing latex (18/10.8) and in those handling finished goods (77/63.8).

[This study is continuing.]

2.3 Studies by the British Rubber Manufacturers' Association

Veys (1969) reported on bladder tumour incidence at a rubber factory. The study, subsequently extended (Veys, 1980, 1981), showed that there were more than twice as many bladder tumour registrations as expected among 2081 men working at the factory between 1946-1949 and followed up to 1970 (23 observed, 10.3 expected). The men had been exposed to an antioxidant containing residual 1- and 2-naphthylamine (0.25% of the latter) until it was removed from processing in October 1949. At a second rubber tyre factory, there were twice as many bladder tumour registrations among 3867 men employed between 1945-1949 and followed up for the next 20 years (26 observed, 13.2 expected).

Among 2846 men newly engaged at one of the factories after 1 January 1950 and followed for varying periods up to 1970, six cases were observed whereas 4.5 were expected. Most of the cases of bladder cancer occurred in men working in chemical stores, mixing and milling, calendering and maintenance.

Another study by the British Rubber Manufacturers' Association (Parkes et al., 1982) was undertaken to discover whether the withdrawal of the 2-naphthylamine contaminant in 1949 had effectively removed the bladder cancer hazard, and at the same time to reveal any other specific hazards. An active intake cohort of 36 696 men who had entered any one of 13 factories between 1946 and 1960 inclusive and had worked there for at least one year were divided into three entry groups and followed up to the end of 1975. (Eighteen percent of the population of the Employment Medical Advisory Service study were included in this study.) By 31 December 1975, all but 5.3% had been traced. Five of the factories were in Scotland, for which Scottish mortality data were used to calculate expected deaths; and the remainder were in England, for which the data on England and Wales were used. All of the following data are derived from workers who entered the study on the tenth anniversary of their employment.

The all-neoplasms SMR was 107 (1335/1251.0) for the whole industry (England and Scotland), but there was considerable variation among factories. The SMR was 122 for both lung cancer (633/517.4) and stomach cancer (173/141.8). There was an excess of thyroid cancer (5/2.2), mostly confined to the first quinquennial group (1946-1950) and to workers in the Scottish factories. An excess of leukaemia (31/28.1) was confined to the third quinquennial group (1956-1960) in England and Wales (7/2.9). The SMR for cancer of the oesophagus was 120 (38/31.8) in the whole industry: the excess was found in the first entry group in England and Wales (22/15.8).

There was essentially no overall excess of bladder cancer (23/22.6) in the rubber industry in England and Wales for the first quinquennial group, who might have been exposed to the suspect aromatic-amine bladder carcinogens. However, when that group was examined by individual occupational categories, there were excesses in those in extruding (5/1.8) and in curing (5/2.8). For the two groups who entered employment after January 1950, when the suspect antioxidants had been removed, there were no excesses (8/14.1).

The lung cancer excess in workers in the tyre sector was mostly confined to those in the first quinquennial group (349/282.4). When workers were examined by job category, excesses were seen in those employed in component building (136/104.4), curing (45/36.7), inspection (17/8.3), handling of finished goods (32/19.5) and maintenance (69/61.2). In workers in the non-tyre sector, there were excesses in all three quinquennial intakes (117/73.7); when the men were examined by job category, the excesses reflected the same pattern as for those in tyres, but appeared in addition among those working in rubber compounding (15/6.7) and in extruding (15/6.9).

In workers in the tyre sector, stomach cancer mortality was raised in the first group (92/78.6) and in the third group (19/11.4). When the data were examined by job category, the excesses related, in contrast to lung cancer, to the earliest stages of processing – rubber compounding (13/7.2), extruding (12/7.7), and in site workers (14/6.0). For the non-tyre sector, 32 were observed whereas 20.6 were expected. The numbers are small, but the excesses were again in workers in rubber compounding (4/1.8), extruding (4/1.9), component building (6/3.2) and maintenance (4/2.1).

3.   Studies of rubber workers in the US

3.1   Studies from the Harvard School of Public Health

The data available to investigators at the Harvard School of Public Health derive mainly from a mortality study of workers at a rubber plant in Akron, Ohio (Monson & Nakano, 1976a,b; Monson & Fine, 1978; Delzell & Monson, 1981, 1982). In the initial phase of this study, 13 571 white male production workers who were working at the plant on or after 1 January 1940, and who had worked for at least five years at the plant through June 1971, were followed from January 1940 through June 1974. During that period, 980 deaths from cancer were observed, whereas 1046.4 were expected on the basis of US age-time-specific rates (SMR = 94). Excesses of specific cancers were (observed/expected numbers): stomach – 98/93.9; bladder – 48/39.5; and leukaemia – 55/43.0.

Among this group of workers, bladder cancer occurred to excess only among those who had started working before 1935 (43/30.7), mainly among those who had worked at least 35 years (17/10.0), and only among those who had died after 1954 (40/29.6). Leukaemia occurred in excess only among men who had started work before 1935 (46/30.7) and who had worked at least 25 years (37/23.1).

In the second phase of the study, cancer morbidity between 1964 and 1974 was ascertained by a review of Akron-area hospital tumour registries (Monson & Fine, 1978). The rates of cancer were measured among workers in specific areas of the rubber plant. Account was taken of the years an individual had worked in a specific area. The following excesses of specific cancers in specific jobs were seen (observed/expected), based on a minimum of eight cases; the minimum lengths of exposure on which the figures are based are noted:

> stomach cancer: compounding, mixing, milling, testing
> (5 yrs) – 13/5.9;
> large-intestinal cancer: compounding, mixing, milling,
> testing (5 yrs) – 17/8.5;
> lung cancer: tyre curing (5 yrs) – 31/14.1; tyre moulding
> (5 yrs) – 10/5.0; fuel cell/deicer manufacture (ever
> employed) – 46/29.1;
> pancreatic cancer: tyre curing (5 yrs) – 8/3.2;
> bladder cancer: tyre building (5 yrs) – 16/10.7;

prostatic cancer: machine maintenance (ever employed) –
22/12.7;
skin cancer: tyre assembly (5 yrs) – 12/1.9;
brain cancer: tyre assembly (5 yrs) – 8/2.0;
lymphoma: tyre building (5 yrs) – 8/3.2;
leukaemia: calendering (5 yrs) – 8/2.2; tyre curing (15 yrs)
– 8/2.6; tyre building (5 yrs) – 12/7.5

In the third phase of this study, mortality follow-up
extended through 30 June 1978 (Delzell & Monson, 1981), and
people who had worked from two to five years in the plant since
1940 were included. Between July 1974 and June 1978, there were
259 deaths from cancer observed and 253.9 expected among white
males.

In the total mortality data for white male union members of
one factory (between 1 January 1940 and 30 June 1978, 1352 deaths
from cancer were observed and 1408.3 were expected (SMR = 96).
For bladder cancer, there were 60 deaths observed and 51.3
expected; for leukaemia, there were 68 deaths observed and 56.2
expected.

Data were also presented for black male union members, for
salaried men, salaried women and for female production workers
(Monson & Nakano, 1976b; Delzell & Monson, 1981). The following
observed and expected numbers for cancer mortality represent
follow-up from 1 January 1940 through 30 June 1978: non-white
union members: 63/78.8; salaried men: 203/278.1; female production workers: 241/313.0; and salaried women: 78/98.7.

Delzell and Monson (1982) also compared mortality among
processing workers and non-processing workers and the US white
male population; similar results were obtained in relation to
each comparison population. Processing workers were divided into
'front processing' (compounding, mixing and milling operations)
and 'back processing' (extrusion, calendering, cement mixing and
rubberized fabric operations). Among front processing workers,
there was excess mortality from the following cancers (observed/-
expected numbers): all digestive cancer – 51/34.0; stomach cancer
– 15/7.1; and large-intestinal cancer – 19/11.2. Among back
processing workers, there was excess mortality from biliary and
liver cancer – 9/3.8 – and leukaemia – 14/8.2. Among front
processing workers, the excesses of stomach and large-intestinal
cancer were seen mainly in men who had started work in front

processing before 1950 (33/16.6). Most of the excess did not occur until at least 20 years after first employment (29/13.6). Among back processing workers, the excess of leukaemia was seen mainly in men who had started work in back processing before 1950 (13/6.2), and who had worked at least five years (10/4.5). Most of the excess did not occur until at least 25 years after first employment (10/3.6).

[The data available to the Harvard investigators permitted assessment of follow-up from 1940. Thus, the excesses seen tend to reflect associations with working in the 1920s and 1930s. This must be kept in mind in comparing these data with those from other studies.]

A recent study (Delzell et al., 1982) on a plant in south-western Connecticut covers 1792 white male workers employed after 1947, who were alive on 1 January 1954 and had had more than two years' employment in the industry. This population was followed up from 1 January 1954 to 31 December 1976 (for mortality) and to 31 December 1977 (for cancer registration). The population is a young one (81% of the person-years below 55). Overall, there were 90 cases of cancer observed and 97.6 expected, on the basis of incident rates from the Connecticut Tumor Registry. An overall excess of mortality from cancer of the pancreas (6/2.8) was observed in that section of the population who had started work before 1950 (5/2) and who had worked between 10 and 24 years in the plant (5/1.7).

3.2 Studies from the University of North Carolina

This research derived predominantly from two retrospective mortality follow-up studies at the Akron, Ohio, plants of two large tyre and rubber companies. Each study population, defined on a census basis, comprised active and retired male employees who were at least 40 years old and were alive on 1 January 1964.

In the first study population, of 6678 production workers, 351 cancer deaths occurred over a nine-year follow-up period, whereas 336.9 were expected on the basis of US male age-race-specific rates (McMichael et al., 1974). Types of cancers for which observed numbers exceeded expected ones were: stomach (39 observed/20.9 expected), large-intestinal (39/31.8), prostatic (49/34.4), lymphosarcoma (14/6.2) and leukaemia (16/12.5). With regard to bladder cancers, 9 cases were observed versus 12.3

expected. For this and all five other, smaller plants within the same company, the proportional mortality ratio during 1964–1972 was elevated for cancers of the stomach, prostate and the lymphatic and haematopoietic systems.

In subsequent case–control analyses within this population (McMichael et al., 1976a,b), the detailed job histories of seven specific cancer case groups were compared with those of an age-stratified random sample of workers without cancer. Positive associations entailing at least five cases exposed in a specific job category for at least five years, were found for:

> stomach cancer: compounding and mixing – RR 2.0 (5 exposed cases); tubing (extrusion) – 2.3 (5);
> colorectal cancer: tubing (extrusion) – 2.2 (7); maintenance – 1.8 (9);
> respiratory cancer: receiving and shipping – 1.9 (11); compounding and mixing – 1.4 (12); mill-mixing – 2.1 (5); tubing (extrusion) – 1.4 (8); reclaim – 2.3 (10);
> prostatic cancer: compounding and mixing – 1.6 (5); calendering and plystock – 2.4 (9); janitoring, trucking, etc. – 3.5 (16);
> lymphatic and haematopoietic cancers: compounding and mixing – 1.4 (5); inspection and finishing – 2.0 (6); synthetic plant – 6.2 (6).

In a case–control study based upon all seven US plants within the same company, the relation between lymphatic and haematopoietic cancers and exposure to solvents was evaluated (McMichael et al., 1975): 88 cases were compared with 264 controls, matched individually for sex, race, plant and age at death. Seventy job groupings were categorized independently by industrial hygienists as to estimated solvent exposure (high, medium, light or none). Only lymphatic leukaemia was judged to be associated with exposure to solvents, with an overall relative risk of 3.3, based on 12 exposed cases. A dose–response relationship was observed.

Wolf et al. (1981) conducted a case–control study of 72 deaths from leukaemia that had occurred among the employees of four rubber companies between 1964 and 1973. These cases overlap largely with those studied by McMichael et al. (1975), but the method of assessing work experience differed. The results obtained are similar to those of the earlier report.

A case-control study, in which 88 cases of prostatic cancer from within the same study population (followed to 1975) were compared with 258 individually matched controls (Goldsmith et al., 1980), further examined the relationship between prostatic cancer and 20 specific job categories. For job exposures longer than five years, two job categories in the compounding and mixing area showed relative odds of 2.0 and 3.0; these were 'service to batch preparation' and 'batch preparation', respectively. The odds ratios were based on 6 and 11 exposed cases, respectively.

In a case-control study of stomach cancer, for which subjects were drawn from the two companies studied by the group at the University of North Carolina, 100 cases and 400 individually matched controls were compared with respect to their detailed work experience (Blum et al., 1979). Job categories that were positively associated with stomach cancer (RR >1.2, at least 15 exposed cases) were batch preparation, calendering, tyre building, curing preparation, maintenance and other preparation. Further, individual jobs were independently categorized as to estimated exposure to polycyclic hydrocarbons, N-nitrosamines, carbon black and talc: Non-statistically significant positive associations with stomach cancer were observed with two or more years' exposure to the first three substances. For two or more years of talc exposure, the RR was 2.5 (16 exposed cases) in one company, and 1.3 (26 exposed cases) in the other. The possibility that asbestiform materials are present in talc was noted. (See IARC, 1977.)

In the second follow-up study, 8418 white male active and retired production workers were followed from 1 January 1964 through 31 December 1973 (Andjelkovich et al., 1976). The authors observed 457 cancer deaths, whereas 470.2 were expected on the basis of age-specific rates for US white males. Types of cancer for which observed numbers of deaths exceeded expected were: stomach – 34/27.6; large-intestinal – 53/45.7; pancreatic – 34/27.9; prostatic – 50/45.9; bladder – 21/18.1; lymphatic and haematopoietic – 52/41.9.

In a more detailed analysis of the same study population (Andjelkovich et al., 1977) mortality was assessed according to a worker's most representative department, which was the work area in which the employee was judged to have worked the longest. Positive associations, based on at least five deaths, were found for:

stomach cancer: milling - 6 observed/1.6 expected;
prostatic cancer: general service - 10/4.7; and
leukaemia: general service - 6/2.4.

In a third report (Andjelkovich et al., 1978), the equivalent mortality experience of 1649 white female production
employees was determined from 1 January 1964 to 31 December 1973.
During that period, 62 cancer deaths were observed, whereas 61.7
were expected; the following excesses of specific cancers
(observed/expected numbers) were seen: stomach - 4/2.6; large-
intestinal - 11/8.0; rectal - 4/2.0; and lung - 9/4.7. No details
of relationships to detailed work experience were provided.

Investigators from the University of North Carolina and
Harvard University conducted a collaborative case-control study
of bladder cancer in five US tyre and rubber companies (Checkoway
et al., 1981).   Cases were 220 men with bladder cancer, identified from death certificates and Akron area hospital records;
controls were 440 men individually matched to cases for race,
year of birth and company. Detailed work histories within the
rubber industry were compared. Three work areas were associated
with bladder cancer (RR, number of exposed cases): milling - 1.9,
26; calender operation (but not extruding) - 2.2, 18; and final
inspection of tyres - 1.5, 50. The associations with milling and
calendering were stronger for men with longer durations of exposure. The association with milling occurred mainly in one
company, while the association with calender operation was seen
mainly in a second. [This study makes it possible to evaluate the
association between specific job categories and bladder cancer in
the US rubber industry. No clear-cut localization of excess
bladder cancer risk was identified. The associations seen tended
to be present within one company only.]

In view of earlier suggestions (Mancuso et al., 1968; Monson
& Nakano, 1976a) of an excess of brain cancer in tyre assembly
and curing workers, Symons et al. (1982) examined all available
data from the mortality studies by the University of North
Carolina. In the published studies, 32 cases were observed where
38.2 were expected; in four previously unpublished 'technical
reports', 8 cases were observed where 9.1 were expected. Despite
this overall deficit of cases, a case-control study was then
conducted within one of the original study populations. Twenty-
two people with cancer of the brain or other parts of the central
nervous system, who had died between 1952 and 1971, were compared

with a large, individually matched control group for any differences in exposure at work in tyre assembly or related jobs. No positive association was evident (odds ratios, 0.5 and 1.1).

4.   Other studies of rubber workers

Bovet and Lob (1980) studied the mortality experience of a population of rubber workers in Switzerland, following them from 1 January 1955 to 31 December 1975; workers in a munitions factory served as a comparison population. Using expected numbers based on death rates in the general population, excesses of the following types of cancer were found in the rubber workers: urinary bladder (4/1.1), stomach (8/4.6) and glioblastomas (2/0.9). An excess of urinary bladder cancer (5/2.6) was also found in the munitions workers.

Kilpikari (1982) investigated cancer mortality among 784 male workers in a Finnish rubber plant (tyre, tube and footwear manufacture), by following them from 1 January 1953 (or from date of first employment) to death or to 31 December 1976. Seven fatal cancers were observed and 6.8 expected.

5.   Other case-control studies

5.1   Bladder cancer

Between 1 January 1967 and 30 June 1968, 722 new cases of cancer of the lower urinary tract were identified in the Boston and Brockton Standard Metropolitan Statistical Areas (Cole et al., 1971). Interviews were conducted with 470 patients with transitional or squamous-cell carcinoma of the lower urinary tract and with 500 controls from the general population. Lifetime occupational histories were obtained for 461 cases and for 485 controls (Cole et al., 1972). Of the men (controlled for age and cigarette smoking), 51 had had an occupation in the rubber industry, representing a RR of 1.6. If only the men's usual occupations were considered, 19 of the cases were in rubber workers, giving a RR of 1.7.

In Canada, occupational histories were obtained from 480 men with bladder cancer and from 480 controls matched for age and neighbourhood (Howe et al., 1980). Five of the patients and one of the controls reported having been rubber workers.

In Finland, occupational histories were obtained from 180 patients with bladder cancer and from 180 age- and sex-matched controls (Tola et al., 1980). Two of the patients and none of the controls had had as their predominant occupation work in the rubber industry; 12 of the patients and five of the controls had been employed at some time in leather or rubber industries.

[The Canadian and Finnish studies were done in areas where rubber factories were uncommon. The data show an association between work in the rubber industry in general and bladder cancer.]

5.2   Tumours of the central nervous system

Data on brain tumours from the Swedish Cancer Registry for the years 1961–1973 were analysed in a case–control fashion (Englund et al., 1981). A further analysis, incorporating 1960 census data on the sex and age structure of the population, enabled calculation of the expected numbers of brain tumours for people in various occupations and industries. The analysis showed, for the rubber industry, a relative risk of 1.2, based on 30 observed brain tumours. Additionally, there was an elevated age-adjusted annual incidence rate of 17 per 100,000 (33 cases) for all brain tumours in workers in the rubber industry, in comparison with 12 per 100 000 in the general population; for glioblastomas only, the rates were 10 per 100 000 in the rubber industry and 5 per 100 000 in the general population.

TABLE 14.

CHARACTERISTICS OF THE EPIDEMIOLOGICAL STUDIES REVIEWED

[a] Intake period for case-control studies or surveys;
follow-up period for cohort studies

NA - not available

Table 14. Characteristics of the epidemiological studies reviewed

Reference	Type of study	No. of subjects	Period[a]	Total no. of deaths (all causes) Obs.	Exp.	Comments
Andjelkovich et al. (1976)	Cohort	8418	1964-1973	2373	2524.5	
Andjelkovich et al. (1977)	Cohort	8418	1964-1973	-	-	Analysis by occupational title group of the same population as in above reference
Andjelkovich et al. (1978)	Cohort	1649	1964-1973	279	270.9	Women only
Baxter & Werner (1980)	Cohort	40 867	1967-1976	5773	5912.5	
Blum et al. (1979)	Case-control within cohort	101 cases 393 controls	1964-1973			Stomach cancer
Bovet & Lob (1980)	Cohort	931	1959-1975	115	143.9	
Case & Hosker (1954)	Survey		1936-1951			Mortality survey of bladder cancer
	Survey		1936-1950			Incidence survey of bladder cancer
Case (1966)	Survey		1936-1965			Mortality survey of bladder cancer
Checkoway et al. (1981)	Case-control	220 cases 440 controls	1940-1974			Bladder cancer
Cole et al. (1972)	Case-control	461 cases 485 controls	1967-1968			Bladder cancer
Davies (1965)	Cohort	139	1946-1964	NA	NA	Information on bladder cancer only
Delzell & Monson (1981)	Cohort	29 087	1940-1978	9388	11 355.7	

Reference	Type of study	No. of subjects	Period[a]	Total no. of deaths (all causes)		Comments
				Obs.	Exp.	
Delzell & Monson (1982)	Cohort	2666	1940-1978	1131	1281.7	
Delzell et al. (1982)	Cohort	1792	1954-1976	249	280.3	Mortality and cancer incidence (tyre manufacture)
Englund et al. (1982)	Survey					Brain cancer
Fox et al. (1974)	Cohort	40 867	1967-1971	2029	2085.0	Same cohort as Baxter & Werner (1980)
Fox & Collier (1976)	Cohort	40 867	1972-1974	2018	1970.8	Same cohort as Baxter & Werner (1980)
Goldsmith et al. (1980)	Case-control within cohort	88 cases 258 controls	1964-1974			Prostatic cancer
Howe et al. (1980)	Case-control	480 cases 480 controls	1974-1976	NA	NA	Bladder cancer
Kilpikari et al. (1981)	Cohort	1331	1953-1976	NA	NA	
Kilpikari (1981)	Cohort	784	1953-1976	29	42.6	
McMichael et al. (1974)	Cohort	6678	1964-1972	1783	1798.5	
McMichael et al. (1975)	Case-control within cohort	88 cases 264 controls	1964-1973			Leukaemia

Reference	Type of study	No. of subjects	Period[a]	Total no. of deaths (all causes) Obs.	Exp.	Comments
McMichael et al. (1976a)	Case-control within cohort	6678	1964-1973	1983	2023.5	Many different cancers Relative risks of various job categories compared with those of all other workers
McMichael et al. (1976b)	Cohort	18 903	1964-1973	5106	5431.9	Results of case-control studies are also reported (lung, bladder, stomach, prostate)
Monson & Nakano (1976a)	Cohort	13 571	1940-1974	5069	6186.9	
Monson & Nakano (1976b)	Cohort	10 529	1940-1974	1846	2642.2	
Monson & Fine (1978)	Cohort	13 570	1940-1976	NA	NA	Incident study of 1359 cases of cancer
Parkes et al. (1982)	Cohort	33 815	1946-1975	4882	4841.5	Follow-up began on tenth anniversary of employment
Symons et al. (1982)	(see 'comments')					Review of data, some previously unpublished, on brain and nervous system cancer mortality
Tola et al. (1980)	Case-control	180 cases 180 controls	1975-1976			Bladder cancer
Veys (1980)	Cohort	3867	1945-1970	NA	NA	Incident study of bladder cancer
	Cohort	2081	1946-1970	NA	NA	Incident study of bladder cancer
Wolf et al. (1981)	Case-control within cohort	72 cases 286 controls	1964-1973			Leukaemias

TABLE 15

SUMMARY OF DATA FROM EPIDEMIOLOGICAL STUDIES CONSIDERED

[a] Exposure: U   Unspecified (total group)
               T   Tyre
               NT   Non-tyre
               S   Solvent
               P1   Raw materials handling, weighing and mixing
               P2   Milling
               P3   Extruding and calendering
               P4   Component assembly and building
               P5   'Curing' or vulcanization
               P6   Inspection and finishing
               P7   Storage and dispatch
               P8   General service

[b] SMR - Standardized mortality (or morbidity) ratio. When the
expected number is not given, the SMR is a standardized rate
ratio.

RR - Relative risk

Observed = number of exposed cases in case-control studies

NA - not available

Table 15. Summary of data from epidemiological studies considered

Reference	Type of study	Exposure[a]	Results[b]				Comments
			SMR	RR	Observed	Expected	
(a) Bladder							
Andjelkovich et al. (1976)	Cohort	U	116		21	18.1	
Andjelkovich et al. (1978)	Cohort	U	204		2	1.0	Women only
Baxter & Werner (1980)	Cohort	U	144		36	25.0	Group A: men employed before 1950 in factories that used known carcinogenic compounds
		U	108		24	22.3	Group B: men employed in 1950 or later in factories that used known carcinogenic compounds
		U	97		13	13.4	Group C: men employed in factories that never had used known carcinogenic compounds
	Cohort	U	127		73	57.6	
		P1,P2	87		6	6.9	
		P3	116		8	6.9	
		P4	176		13	7.4	
		P5	80		7	8.6	
		P6	125		5	4.0	
		P7	143		7	4.9	
Bovet & Lob (1980)	Cohort	U	362		4	1.1	
Case (1966)	Survey	U	204		20	9.8	Deaths occurring in 1952-1956
		U	245		27	11.0	Deaths occurring in 1957-1961
		U	231		25	10.8	Deaths occurring in 1962-1965
Case & Hosker (1954)	Survey	U	164		26	15.9	Mortality survey, deaths occurring in 1936-1951
	Survey	U	550		22	4.0	Incidence survey, cases reported in 1936-1950

Reference	Type of study	Exposure[a]	Results[b]				Comments
			SMR	RR	Observed	Expected	
(a) Bladder (contd)							
Checkoway et al. (1981)	Case-control	P1		1.1	36		
		P2		1.9	26		
		P3		1.3	94		[RR estimated by Working Group]
		P4		1.0	60		
		P5		1.1	72		
		P6		1.5	50		[RR estimated by Working Group]
Cole et al. (1972)	Case-control	U		1.6		51	
Davies (1965)	Cohort	NT	2000		4	0.2	Cable workers
Delzell & Monson (1981)	Cohort	U	115		78	67.8	All study groups combined
Delzell et al. (1982)	Cohort	T	63		1	1.6	Mortality
	Cohort	T	41		3	7.4	Incidence
Fox et al. (1974)	Cohort	U	130		11	8.5	Group A)
	Cohort	U	97		7	7.2	Group B) see Baxter & Werner (1981)
	Cohort	U	114		5	4.4	Group C)
Fox & Collier (1976)	Cohort	U	205		16	7.8	Group A)
	Cohort	U	188		13	6.9	Group B) see Baxter & Werner (1981)
	Cohort	U	190		8	4.2	Group C)
Howe et al. (1980)	Case-control	U		5.0	NA		5 matched pairs of cases exposed, control not / 1 matched pair of controls exposed, case not
Kilpikari et al. (1981)	Cohort	U	670		2	0.3	

Reference	Type of study	Exposure[a]	Results[b]				Comments
			SMR	RR	Observed	Expected	
(a) Bladder (contd)							
McMichael et al. (1974)	Cohort	U	73		9	12.3	
McMichael et al. (1976a)	Case-control	P1, P2		1.8	3		[RR and observed number estimated by Working Group]
Monson & Fine (1978)	Cohort	P4 P6 P7	150 150 110		16 5 4		Incidence
Monson & Nakano (1976a)	Cohort	U	122		48	39.5	
Parkes et al. (1982)	Cohort	U P1,P2 P3 P4 P5 P6 P7 P8	84 87 190 96 132 63 30 93		36 4 8 14 7 1 1 4	42.9 4.6 4.2 14.6 5.3 1.6 3.3 4.3	
Tola et al. (1980)	Case-control	U	NA	–	2		2 cases and 0 controls worked in rubber industry
Veys (1980)	Cohort Cohort	T T	197 223		26 23	13.2 10.3	Two factors. Exposure to 2-naphthylamine
(b) Stomach							
Andjelkovich et al. (1976)	Cohort	U	123		34	27.7	
Andjelkovich et al. (1977)	Cohort	P1 P2	479 369		3 6	0.6 1.6	

(b) Stomach (contd)

Reference	Type of study	Exposure[a]	Results[b]				Comments
			SMR	RR	Observed	Expected	
Andjelkovich et al. (1978)	Cohort	U	155		4	2.6	Women only
Baxter & Werner (1980)	Cohort	U	122		216	176.4	
		P1,P2	94		23	24.5	
		P3	112		24	21.5	
		P4	86		20	23.3	
		P5	59		16	27.0	
		P6	129		16	12.4	
		P7	102		17	16.7	
Blum et al. (1979)	Case-control	(see 'comments')		1.1	45		'Two or more years' exposure to polycyclic hydrocarbons'
				1.5	57		'Two or more years' exposure to nitrosamines'
				1.4	37		'Two or more years' exposure to carbon black'
				1.9	42		'Two or more years' exposure to talc' [RR estimated by Working Group)
Bovet & Lob (1980)	Cohort	U	175		8	4.6	
Delzell & Monson (1981)	Cohort	U	95		139	146.8	All study groups combined
Delzell & Monson (1982)	Cohort	P1,P2	186		15	8.1	[SMRs estimated by Working Group]
		P3,P5	110		10	9.1	
Delzell et al. (1982)	Cohort	T	100		3	3.0	Mortality
		T	59		3	5.1	Incidence
Fox & Collier (1976)	Cohort	T	113		25	22.2	

Reference	Type of study	Exposure[a]	Results[b]				Comments
			SMR	RR	Observed	Expected	
(b) Stomach (contd)							
McMichael et al. (1974)	Cohort	U	187		39	20.9	
McMichael et al. (1976a)	Case-control	P1,P2,P3		2.1	12		[RR and observed number estimated by Working Group]
Monson & Fine (1978)	Cohort	P1,P2,P3 P4	220 140		13 4		Incidence
Monson & Nakano (1976a)	Cohort	U	104		98	93.9	
Parkes et al. (1982)	Cohort	U P1,P2 P3 P4 P5 P6 P7 P8	129 169 145 124 110 176 59 213		183 26 20 61 20 9 6 26	141.8 15.4 13.8 49.3 18.2 5.1 10.2 12.2	
(c) Lung							
Andjelkovich et al. (1976)	Cohort	U	83		116	139.8	
Andjelkovich et al. (1977)	Cohort	(see 'comments')	434		3	0.7	Workers with synthetic latex
Andjelkovich et al. (1978)	Cohort	U	190		9	4.7	Women only

(c) Lung (contd)

Reference	Type of study	Exposure[a]	Results[b] SMR	RR	Observed	Expected	Comments
Baxter & Werner (1980)	Cohort	U P1,P2 P3 P4 P5 P6 P7	115 87 89 103 95 87 121		822 82 75 94 101 42 77	716.5 94.3 84.5 91.7 106.2 48.3 63.8	
Bovet & Lob (1980)	Cohort	U	47		5	10.6	
Delzell & Monson (1981)	Cohort	U	84		438	523.2	All study groups combined
Delzell et al. (1982)	Cohort	T T	99 126		15 24	15.2 19.0	Mortality Incidence
Fox et al. (1974)	Cohort	T	134		131	97.8	
Fox & Collier (1976)	Cohort	T	127		117	91.8	
Kilpikari et al. (1981)	Cohort	U	150		3	2	Cancer of respiratory organs
McMichael et al. (1974)	Cohort	U	83		91	109.3	
McMichael et al. (1976a)	Case-control	P1,P2,P3		1.7	35		[RR and observed number estimated by Working Group]
Monson & Fine (1978)	Cohort	P5 P8	210 160		41 46		[SMRs estimated by Working Group] Incidence
Monson & Nakano (1976a)	Cohort	U	92		234	253.1	

Reference	Type of study	Exposure[a]	Results[b]		Observed	Expected	Comments
			SMR	RR			
(c) Lung (contd)							
Monson & Nakano (1976b)	Cohort	NT	333		3	0.9	Women only
Parkes et al. (1982)	Cohort	U	123		638	517.4	
		P1,P2	123		71	57.7	
		P3	119		62	52.2	
		P4	126		230	182.8	
		P5	127		88	69.3	
		P6	186		36	19.4	
		P7	149		54	36.2	
		P8	131		51	38.9	
(d) Lymphatic and haematopoietic							
Andjelkovich et al. (1976)	Cohort	U	124		52	41.9	
Andjelkovich et al. (1977)	Cohort.	P8	246		6	2.4	Leukaemia only
Andjelkovich et al. (1978)	Cohort	U	92		5	5.4	Women only
Baxter & Werner (1980)	Cohort	T	95		33	34.7	
		NT	80		44	55.1	
Delzell & Monson (1981)	Cohort	U	107		202	189.1	All study groups combined
Delzell & Monson (1982)	Cohort	P1,P2	161		7	4.4	Leukaemia only
		P3,P4	180		9	5.0	[SMRs estimated by Working Group]
Delzell et al. (1982)	Cohort	T	45		1	2.2	Mortality (leukaemia only)
			100		3	3.0	Incidence
Fox & Collier (1976)	Cohort	T	143		6	4.2	

Reference	Type of study	Exposure[a]	Results[b]				Comments
			SMR	RR	Observed	Expected	
(d) Lymphatic and haematopoietic (contd)							
Kilpikari et al. (1981)	Cohort	U	130		2	1.6	
McMichael et al. (1974)	Cohort	U	160		30	18.7	
McMichael et al. (1975)	Case-control	S		3.3	12		Lymphatic leukaemia
McMichael et al. (1976a)	Case-control	P1,P2,P6,P8		2.9	21		[RR and observed number estimated by Working Group]
Monson & Fine (1978)	Cohort	P3 P4 P5	360 233 310		8 20 8	—	[SMR estimated by Working Group] Incidence
Monson & Nakano (1976a)	Cohort	U	113		106	93.4	
Parkes et al. (1982)	Cohort	U	110		31	28.1	Leukaemia only
Wolf et al. (1981)	Case-control	S P1 P2 P3 P5 P8		0.8 1.1 0.7 0.6 0.9 1.4	69 10 5 2 13 36		[RR estimated by Working Group]
(e) Prostate							
Andjelkovich et al. (1976)	Cohort	U	109		50	45.9	
Andjelkovich et al. (1977)	Cohort	P8	212		10	4.7	

Reference	Type of study	Exposure[a]	Results[b] SMR	Results[b] RR	Observed	Expected	Comments
(e) Prostate (contd)							
Baxter & Werner (1980)	Cohort	T NT	105 95		21 34	20.0 35.7	
Delzell & Monson (1981)	Cohort	U	102		121	118.6	White male union members only
Delzell et al. (1982)	Cohort	T	57 88		2 9	3.5 10.2	Mortality Incidence
Goldsmith et al. (1980)	Case-control P1			2.8	14		
McMichael et al. (1974)	Cohort	U	142		49	34.4	
McMichael et al. (1976a)	Case-control P1,P3,P8			2.5	30		[RR and observed number estimated by Working Group]
Monson & Fine (1978)	Cohort	P6 P7 P8	760 240 180		4 4 22		[SMR estimated by Working Group] Incidence
Monson & Nakano (1976a)	Cohort	U	92		82	89.0	White male union members only
Parkes et al. (1982)	Cohort	U	66		30	45.4	
(f) Colon							
Andjelkovich et al. (1976)	Cohort	U	116		53	45.7	
Andjelkovich et al. (1977)	Cohort	(see 'comments')	629		4	0.6	Workers with special products

(f) Colon (contd)

Reference	Type of study	Exposure[a]	Results[b]				Comments
			SMR	RR	Observed	Expected	
Andjelkovich et al. (1978)	Cohort	U	137		11	8.0	Women only
Baxter & Werner (1980)	Cohort	T NT	113 116		40 67	35.4 57.9	
Delzell & Monson (1981)	Cohort	U	96		197	205.1	All study groups combined
Delzell & Monson (1982)	Cohort	P1,P2 P3,P5	180 100		? 12	10.6 12.0	[SMRs estimated by Working Group]
Delzell et al. (1982)	Cohort	T	196 121		9 12	4.6 9.9	Mortality Incidence
McMichael et al. (1974)	Cohort	U	123		39	31.8	
McMichael et al. (1976a)	Case-control	P3,P8		2.0	16		Colorectal cancer [RR and observed number estimated by Working Group]
Monson & Fine (1978)	Cohort	P1,P2,P3 P4	200 230		17 9	NA NA	Incidence
Monson & Nakano (1976a)	Cohort	U	101		104	103.1	
Parkes et al. (1982)	Cohort	U	91		67	73.7	

(g) Brain

Reference	Type of study	Exposure[a]	Results[b]				Comments
			SMR	RR	Observed	Expected	
Andjelkovich et al. (1976)	Cohort	U	92		8	8.7	
Baxter & Werner (1980)	Cohort	T	73		10	13.7	
		NT	52		11	21.1	
Bovet & Lob (1980)	Cohort	U	220		2	0.9	
Delzell & Monson (1981)	Cohort	U	97		50	51.8	All study groups combined
Delzell et al. (1982)	Cohort	T	100		0	1.7	Mortality
					2	2.0	Incidence
Englund et al. (1982)	Survey	U		1.4	33		[RR estimated by Working Group]
Fox & Collier (1976)	Cohort	T	95		4	4.2	
McMichael et al. (1974)	Cohort	U	68		4	5.9	
Monson & Fine (1978)	Cohort	P4	410		8		Incidence
Monson & Nakano (1976a)	Cohort	U	80		20	25.1	
Parkes et al. (1982)	Cohort	U	85		35	41.1	
Symons et al. (1982)	(see 'comments')	U	87		8	9.2	Review of data, some previously unpublished, from four different cohort studies
	Case-control	P4		1.1	5		[RR estimated by Working Group]

Reference	Type of study	Exposure[a]	Results[b]				Comments
			SMR	RR	Observed	Expected	
(h) Pancreas							
Andjelkovich et al. (1976)	Cohort	U	122		34	27.9	
Andjelkovich et al. (1978)	Cohort	U	88		3	3.4	Women only
Baxter & Werner (1980)	Cohort	T NT	107 85		29 37	27.1 43.6	
Delzell & Monson (1981)	Cohort	U	77		88	114.0	All study groups combined
Delzell et al. (1982)	Cohort	T	214 188		6 6	2.8 3.2	Mortality Incidence
McMichael et al. (1974)	Cohort	U	86		17	19.8	
Monson & Fine (1978)	Cohort	P5 P8	300 250		6 8		Incidence
Monson & Nakano (1976a)	Cohort	U	88		53	60.3	
(i) Others							
Baxter & Werner (1980)	Cohort	U	80		35	44.0	Oesophageal cancer
Delzell & Monson (1981)	Cohort	U	105		36	34.3	Oesophageal cancer
Kilpikari et al. (1981)	Cohort	U	140		7	5.1	'Cancer of digestive organs'
Monson & Fine (1978)	Cohort	P4	650		12		Skin cancer incidence

Reference	Type of study	Exposure[a]	Results[b]				Comments
			SMR	RR	Observed	Expected	
(i) Others							
Monson & Nakano (1976b)	Cohort	NT	167		13	7.8	Cervical cancer
Parkes et al. (1982)	Cohort	U	182		4	2.2	Thyroid cancer
Parkes et al. (1982)	Cohort	U	126		40	31.8	Oesophageal cancer

6. Summary

Evidence of increased cancer rates in rubber workers arose when Case reported a substantial excess of bladder cancer among rubber workers in the UK, particularly in Birmingham. Among British rubber workers, the death rate from bladder cancer during 1936-1951 was almost double that of the general population. A subsequent study of workers in the British cable-making industry also indicated an increase in bladder cancer risk. A study of bladder cancer incidence in two British tyre manufacturing plants showed a doubling of the rates: excesses were related particularly to exposures in milling, mixing, calendering and maintenance jobs. In two further mortality follow-up studies in the UK it was reported that excesses of bladder cancer mortality were virtually confined to workers first employed before 1950.

Subsequent to preliminary observations of cancer in the rubber industry by Mancuso in the US, follow-up studies of mortality were carried out among rubber workers in the Akron, Ohio, factories of three large rubber companies; these showed either an overall deficit of bladder cancer (one factory) or a small excess (two factories). In the largest of the three factories, the excess was greatest among workers first employed before 1935 and among those who had worked for more than 35 years. A case-control study of bladder cancer in rubber workers in Akron, Ohio, showed an approximate doubling in risk for milling and calendering workers in one factory.

In the follow-up studies of rubber workers in both the US and the UK, excess mortality from a number of other cancers has been reported. Some excesses were found in an entire factory population, and others in rubber workers in specific job categories. Within the US, these follow-up studies prompted a number of site-specific case-control studies of cancer within the same population of rubber workers.

Each of three US follow-up studies of male rubber workers within specific factories revealed more deaths than expected from cancers of the stomach and of the large intestine. In one of the studies, the excesses were noted primarily in workers in jobs early in the production line, where exposures are chiefly to particulates but also to some fume from uncured rubber. A case-control analysis of stomach cancer in the second of these studies showed a positive association with work early in the production line and with that in curing preparation and in maintenance. Further analysis, according to estimated exposure to specific agents, showed a positive association with exposure to talc. In one study in the UK, mortality from stomach cancer was increased among all workers, but particularly among men in jobs early in the production process. In a second study in the UK, excess mortality from stomach cancer was also observed among all workers, but not among particular occupations.

Excess mortality from lung cancer was found in one UK study in workers primarily in the non-tyre sector. In a second UK study, an excess of lung cancer was found among workers in many occupations in the tyre and non-tyre sectors. Excess cases of lung cancer in the US follow-up studies were associated with work in compounding and mixing, extrusion, tyre curing, rubber reclaim, and fuel-cell and de-icer manufacture.

Cancer of the prostate was associated with compounding and mixing and with calender operation in one US study and with general service and maintenance jobs in two. A case-control study on one factory revealed an excess of prostatic cancer in 'batch preparation' jobs within the compounding and mixing area.

Mortality from brain cancer was increased in tyre-building workers in one of three US study populations; a case-control study within another of these populations showed no such association.

Excesses of cancers of the lymphatic and haematopoietic systems were noted in the US, and an excess of leukaemia was noted in one of the UK studies. In one of the three US study populations, an excess of leukaemia was highest in workers in compounding and mixing, tyre inspection and synthetic rubber manufacture; in a second US population, the excess was highest in workers in calendering, tyre building and tyre curing. Similar, though weaker, associations were found for lymphomas. A case-control study of malignancies of the lymphatic and haematopoietic systems, drawing upon all seven US plants of one company, showed an increased risk of lymphatic leukaemia in workers in jobs entailing exposure to solvents.

An association was found between tyre building and the incidence of cancer of the skin in the one study in which incidence data were obtained.

Excesses of cancer at the following sites have been reported among rubber workers: thyroid, oesophagus, liver, pancreas and cervix. These excesses were isolated findings, were inconsistent or were based on observation of small numbers of exposed workers.

Most of the epidemiological evidence comes from studies in the UK and the US. Studies carried out in Canada, Finland, Sweden and Switzerland were either not specifically related to the rubber industry or were based on small numbers of subjects. Their results are in general in accordance with those of the British and US studies.

7. References

Andjelkovich, D., Taulbee, J. & Symons, M. (1976) Mortality experience of a cohort of rubber workers, 1964–1973. J. occup. Med., 18, 387–394

Andjelkovich, D., Taulbee, J., Symons, M. & Williams, T. (1977) Mortality of rubber workers with reference to work experience. J. occup. Med., 19, 397–405

Andjelkovich, D., Taulbee, J. & Blum, S. (1978) Mortality of female workers in a rubber manufacturing plant. J. occup. Med., 20, 409–413

Baxter, P.J. & Werner, J.B. (1980) Mortality in the British Rubber Industries 1967–76, London, Her Majesty's Stationery Office

Blum, S., Arp., E.W., Jr, Smith, A.H. & Tyroler, H.A. (1979) Stomach cancer among rubber workers: an epidemiologic investigation. In: Dusts and Diseases, Park Forest South, IL, Pathotox Publishers, pp. 325–334

Bovet, P. & Lob, M. (1980) Mortality from malignant tumours in workers in a rubber factory in Switzerland. Epidemiological study, 1955–1975 (Fr.). Schweiz. med. Wochenschr., 110, 1277–1287

Case, R.A.M. (1966) Tumours of the urinary tract as an occupational disease in several industries. Ann. R. Coll. Surg. Engl., 39, 213–235

Case, R.A.M. & Hosker, M.E. (1954) Tumour of the urinary bladder as an occupational disease in the rubber industry in England and Wales. Br. J. prev. soc. Med., 8, 39–50

Case, R.A.M., Hosker, M.E., McDonald, D.B. & Pearson, J.T. (1954) Tumours of the urinary bladder in workmen engaged in the manufacture and use of certain dyestuff intermediates in the British chemical industry. Part I. The role of aniline, benzidine, alpha-naphthylamine, and beta-naphthylamine. Br. J. ind. Med., 11, 75–104

Checkoway, H., Smith, A.H., McMichael, A.J., Jones, F.S., Monson, R.R. & Tyroler, H.A. (1981) A case-control study of bladder cancer in the United States rubber and tyre industry. Br. J. ind. Med., 38, 240-246

Cole, P., Monson, R.R., Haning, H. & Friedell, G.H. (1971) Smoking and cancer of the lower urinary tract. New Engl. J. Med., 284, 129-134

Cole, P., Hoover, R. & Friedell, G.H. (1972) Occupation and cancer of the lower urinary tract. Cancer, 29, 1250-1260

Davies, J.M. (1965) Bladder tumours in the electric-cable industry. Lancet, ii, 143-146

Delzell, E. & Monson, R.R. (1981) Mortality among rubber workers. III. Cause-specific mortality, 1940-1978. J. occup. Med., 23, 677-684

Delzell, E. & Monson, R.R. (1982) Mortality among rubber workers. V. Processing workers. J. occup. Med. (in press)

Delzell, E., Louik, C., Lewis, J. & Monson, R.R. (1982) Mortality and cancer morbidity among workers in the rubber tire industry. Am. J. int. Med. (in press)

Englund, A., Ekman, G. & Zabrielski, L. (1982) Occupational categories among brain tumour cases recorded in the cancer registry in Sweden. Ann. N.Y. Acad. Sci. (in press)

Fox, A.J. & Collier, P.F. (1976) A survey of occupational cancer in the rubber and cablemaking industries: analysis of deaths occurring in 1972-74. Br. J. ind. Med., 33, 249-264

Fox, A.J., Lindars, D.C. & Owen, R. (1974) A survey of occupational cancer in the rubber and cablemaking industries: results of five-year analysis, 1967-71. Br. J. ind. Med., 31, 140-151

Goldsmith, D.F., Smith, A.H. & McMichael, A.J. (1980) A case-control study of prostate cancer within a cohort of rubber and tire workers. J. occup. Med., 22, 533-541

Howe, G.R., Burch, J.D., Miller, A.B., Cook, G.M., Esteve, J., Morrison, B., Gordon, P., Chambers, L.W., Fodor, G. & Winsor, G.M. (1980) Tobacco use, occupation, coffee, various nutrients, and bladder cancer. J. natl Cancer Inst., 64, 701-713

IARC (1977) IARC Monographs on the Evaluation of Carcinogenic Risk of Chemicals to Man, Vol. 14, Asbestos, Lyon, International Agency for Research on Cancer

Kilpikari, I. (1982) Mortality among male rubber workers in Finland. Arch. environ. Health (in press)

Mancuso, T.F., Ciocco, A. & El-Attar, A.A. (1968) An epidemiological approach to the rubber industry. A study based on departmental experience. J. occup. Med., 10, 213-232

McMichael, A.J., Spirtas, R. & Kupper, L.L. (1974) An epidemiologic study of mortality within a cohort of rubber workers, 1964-72. J. occup. Med., 16, 458-464

McMichael, A.J., Spirtas, R., Kupper, L.L. & Gamble, J.F. (1975) Solvent exposure and leukemia among rubber workers: an epidemiologic study. J. occup. Med., 17, 234-239

McMichael, A.J., Spirtas, R., Gamble, J.F. & Tousey, P.M. (1976a) Mortality among rubber workers: relationship to specific jobs. J. occup. Med., 18, 178-185

McMichael, A.J., Andjelkovic, D.A. & Tyroler, H.A. (1976b) Cancer mortality among rubber workers: an epidemiologic study. Ann. N.Y. Acad. Sci., 271, 125-137

Monson, R.R. & Fine, L.J. (1978) Cancer mortality and morbidity among rubber workers. J. natl Cancer Inst., 61, 1047-1053

Monson, R.R. & Nakano, K.K. (1976a) Mortality among rubber workers. I. White male union employees in Akron, Ohio. Am. J. Epidemiol., 103, 284-296

Monson, R.R. & Nakano, K.K. (1976b) Mortality among rubber workers. II. Other employees. Am. J. Epidemiol., 103, 297-303

Parkes, H.G., Veys, C.A., Waterhouse, J.A.H., Cook, D. & Peters, A.T. (1982) Cancer mortality in the British rubber industry. Br. J. ind. Med. (in press)

Symons, M.J., Andjelkovich, D.A., Spirtas, R. & Herman, D.R. (1982) Brain and central nervous system cancer mortality in US rubber workers. Ann. N.Y. Acad. Sci. (in press)

Tola, S., Tenho, M., Korkala, M.-L. & Järvinen, E. (1980) Cancer of the urinary bladder in Finland. Association with occupation. Int. Arch. occup. environ. Health, 46, 43–51

Veys, C.A. (1969) Two epidemiological inquiries into the incidence of bladder tumors in industrial workers. J. natl Cancer Inst., 43, 219–226

Veys, C.A. (1980) Developing opportunities for research in occupational medicine. J. Soc. occup. Med., 30, 19–26

Veys C.A. (1981) Bladder cancer in rubber workers: The story reviewed and updated. Plastics Rubber Process. Appl., 1, 207–212

Wolf, P.H., Andjelkovich, D., Smith, A. & Tyroler, H. (1981) A case-control study of leukemia in the US rubber industry. J. occup. Med., 23, 103–108

1.   Summary

Because of the diversity and changeability of exposures within the rubber industry, the multiple exposures experienced by many workers within the industry, and the lack of historical industrial hygiene data, most epidemiological studies of cancer in rubber workers have not been exposure-specific or have used job categories as a substitute for exposure categories. In some studies no attempt was made to subdivide factory populations.

The difficulty of identifying etiological factors in cancer causation is compounded by the need to estimate exposures that occurred several decades ago in relation to cancer occurring currently, and by frequent incongruities between the boundaries of process-defined jobs and the actual exposure to agents of interest. A further difficulty arises from the frequent lack of information about non-occupational risk factors for cancer, such as smoking and diet, which may vary among occupational subgroups of rubber workers. Such internal differences are less likely to exist, however, than are differences between populations of rubber workers and comparison populations.

When cancer excesses have been related with some consistency to specific jobs within the rubber industry, the available industrial hygiene data on the agent to which cases were probably exposed, together with evidence of any toxicological effects of those agents, assist in evaluating the etiological plausibility of the epidemiological finding.

Cancer of the urinary bladder, clearly excessive in British rubber workers employed before 1950, particularly those in jobs likely to entail exposure to aromatic amines, seems not be increased in employees who entered since that date. No clear evidence exists for a comparable bladder cancer excess in US rubber workers. Although based on small numbers, there is some evidence that an excess of bladder cancer was present in rubber workers in other countries where such studies were carried out. While the withdrawal in 1949 of certain antioxidants containing 2-naphthylamine from the UK rubber industry seems likely to have accounted substantially for the subsequent decline in bladder cancer there, a more general awareness of the carcinogenic potential of some aromatic amines, and general improvements in industrial hygiene practices, may also have contributed.

Among US rubber workers, excess malignancies of the lymphatic and haematopoietic systems, particularly lymphatic leukaemia, have been associated with jobs entailing exposure to solvents. Benzene, considered to be a human carcinogen, was once used as a solvent within the rubber industry and may still be present as a contaminant of other organic solvents.

Stomach cancer, consistently elevated in studies of US and British rubber workers, appears to be associated with jobs early in the production line, including compounding and mixing, milling and extrusion.

Lung cancer is positively related to a variety of jobs within the rubber industry. Attribution to specific factors in the workers' environment cannot be made.

Mortality from prostatic cancer was found to be moderately elevated in several studies, and some association was found with compounding and mixing jobs. In general, the etiology of pro-static cancer is not understood. The only occupational risk factor suggested to date is cadmium; compounds of cadmium are occasionally included in a rubber batch.

The lack of consistent associations between specific jobs and cancer of the large intestine does not permit a causal relationship to be inferred.

Isolated or small excesses of some other cancers (e.g., thyroid, oesophagus, brain, skin and pancreas) do not yet justify the drawing of etiological inferences. However, some toxicological and epidemiological information suggests possible mechanisms for the causation of cancers at certain sites. The strong association of skin cancer with tyre building, in the one incident study done to date, raises the possibility that skin carcinogenesis occurs via contact with mineral extender oils in the uncured rubber. Experimental evidence in animals that ethylenethiourea is carcinogenic for the thyroid should be noted. So also should suggestions, from epidemiological studies, of excesses of cancers of the brain and pancreas in workers in the petrochemical industry.

Many materials that occur in the work atmosphere in rubber factories are experimental mutagens or carcinogens; these include mineral oils, carbon black (extracts), curing fumes, some monomers, solvents, nitroso compounds and aromatic amines, thiurams and dithiocarbamate compounds, ethylenethiourea, di(2-ethylhexyl) phthalate, di(2-ethylhexyl) adipate and hydrogen peroxide. However, experimental toxicological information on chemicals that are used or formed is restricted to a small fraction of all chemicals used: most compounds have not been investigated for their possible mutagenic or carcinogenic effects. Studies with exposure indicators, such as mutagenic activity in urine, thioether excretion and sister chromatid exchange, point to the possibility that rubber workers are exposed to mutagens.

The combination of chemical exposures that occurs in the rubber industry is probably more relevant to the cancer pattern observed than are single compounds or groups of compounds. The variety of exposures increases the likelihood that there are interactive effects between two or more such agents, and, in turn, that there is interaction with non-occupational factors.

2. Evaluation

The Working Group examined the combined evidence from epidemiological data about the extent and distribution of cancer within the rubber industry and from relevant industrial hygiene and toxicological information to evaluate the carcinogenic risks within the rubber industry. The evaluation has been made in terms of the three degrees of evidence prescribed for this Monograph series – sufficient, limited, inadequate.

Primary consideration was given to the quality of the epidemiological research, and to the strength and consistency of the reported cancer associations within the industry. In further evaluating the likelihood of an occupational causation for these cancer excesses, judgements were made about the types of exposures experienced by groups of workers, and the evidence that such exposures have carcinogenic effects.

The Working Group thus made the following assessment: (Listing does not imply that that cancer hazard is universal in all rubber factories in all countries, nor that the degree of evidence applies to all situations.)

STRENGTH OF CURRENTLY AVAILABLE EVIDENCE
FOR PAST OR PRESENT CANCER EXCESSES IN THE RUBBER INDUSTRY

Strength of evidence	Type of cancer	Presumed agent or job category
<u>Sufficient</u> for excess occurrence in rubber workers and for causal association with occupational exposures	Bladder Leukaemia	Aromatic amines Solvents
<u>Sufficient</u> for excess occurrence in rubber workers; and <u>limited</u> for causal association with occupational exposures	Stomach Lung	Compounding, mixing and milling Various
<u>Limited</u> for excess occurrence in rubber workers and for causal association with occupational exposures	Skin	Tyre building
<u>Limited</u> for excess occurrence in rubber workers; and inadequate for causal association with occupational exposures	Colon Prostate Lymphoma	
Inadequate for excess occurrence in rubber workers and for causal association with occupational exposures	Brain Thyroid Pancreas Oesophagus	

Accelerator – material added to a rubber compound to increase the rate of vulcanization and to permit vulcanization to proceed at lower temperatures and with greater efficiency. Chemicals which increase the speed of reaction between sulphur and rubber, and can decrease the quantity of sulphur necessary for vulcanization. They can considerably improve the physical and technical properties of the vulcanisate

Activator – material added to a rubber mixture to activate and increase the efficacy of the accelerator

Antidegradant – a substance, which when added to rubber in a small quantity retards ageing and protects from internal and external influences. Of 3 types: (1) antioxidants (vide infra); (2) antiozonants (vide infra); and (3) specialized additives which protect against, e.g., light, harmful metals (copper and manganese inhibitors), flexing fatigue, heat and weather

Antioxidant – a substance which protects against the destructive effects of oxygen, by retarding or preventing atmospheric oxidation

Antiozonant – a substance which protects against the destructive effect of ozone

Banbury – a machine widely used in the rubber industry to mix rubber with various compounding ingredients. It is enclosed and has massive rotors driven by powerful motors capable of kneading the highly viscous rubber mix. It is usually loaded at the top with local exhaust ventilation and discharged onto a mill located on a lower floor

Bead – ring-shaped, rubber-coated wire which ensures a seal between the tyre and the rim of the wheel

Blowing agent – product which decomposes into gaseous substances at high temperatures or which evolves gases, and thus causes rubber compounds to expand during vulcanization. Used for the production of cellular and hollow rubber articles

Bonding agent – a substance used to improve the adhesion of rubber to textiles or metals, especially steel. May be incorporated into the rubber mix or applied in a dip bath. Of major importance in steel-reinforced tyres. Also used to improve adhesion between silicone rubber articles

Calender – machine used to produce smooth, uniform rubber sheeting and to coat and friction textiles. Consists of 2-5 chilled cast-iron or steel rolls, 500-2000 mm in length. The nip between the rolls may be adjusted; the rolls are hollow and may be heated or cooled

Cement – a term used mainly in the US for an adhesive consisting of rubber dissolved in a suitable solvent

Channel black – a carbon black made from gaseous hydrocarbons (usually natural gas), by partial burning in sooty flames impinging on a cool surface such as channel iron

Clastogen – a substance that causes chromosomal damage

Coagulant – material that causes the precipitation or coagulation of latex

Component building – (see Tyre building)

Compounding – the incorporation of ingredients and ancillary substances necessary for mixing, processing and vulcanization and for achieving the required physical properties such as hardness and modulus of the vulcanized product

Conditioning agent – (see Lubricant)

Cord – textile- or steel-reinforcement used to give rubber articles, such as tyres, strength in a specific direction

Curing – (see Vulcanization)

Deflashing – part of the finishing process, in which 'flash' (roughness or extrusions of cured rubber articles) is removed, by hand, by machine (roller trim), by buffing or by low-temperature tumbling (whereby the flash is made brittle and removed in a tumbler)

Die-cut – cut out of a sheet of material using a metal block on which the pattern or contour is engrained

Dipping – process in which a rubber solution or latex compound is deposited on a mould by dipping. After the solvent has been evaporated, a film remains, which is vulcanized

Ebonite – rubber heated for long periods of time with large amounts of sulphur to produce a hard product, termed variously 'ebonite', 'vulcanite' or 'hard rubber'

Elastomer – natural and synthetic, vulcanizable product, which reveals elastic properties after cross-linking, can be stretched to at least double its length at room temperature and, on removal of the tension, quickly return to its original length

Extender oil – an oil added primarily to high-Mooney cold styrene-butadiene rubber to reduce cost and aid processing. The aromatic extender oils contain relatively large amounts of polynuclear aromatic hydrocarbons.

Extruder – machine for forming continuous, long lengths of rubber or plastic compounds by forcing them through an opening (die) which is the shape of the profile required

Fillers – mostly particulate constituents of a compound; added in large quantities to rubber to improve physical properties or to lower volume cost

Fume – in this monograph, used to refer to vapours, smokes and aerosols rising from heated processes

Furnace black – carbon black produced by incomplete combustion of liquid or gaseous hydrocarbons at 1200–1600°C in special furnaces

Green rubber – uncured, compounded rubber

Hopper – a box, tank or other container for loose material or liquid which is passed or fed into some other container

Jacket – the insulation around a cable

<u>Latex</u> – a colloidal suspension of natural or synthetic polymers;
the sap of rubber-yielding plants; or a polydispersed
colloidal system of rubber particles in an aqueous phase

<u>Lubricant</u> – compound for reducing friction between two sliding
surfaces. Solids include graphite, molybdenite, talc;
plastics include fatty acids and soaps, sulphur-treated
bitumen and residues from petroleum distillation. Liquids
include oils from animal, vegetable or mineral sources.

<u>Masterbatch</u> – an intermediate compounded rubber mixture, usually
lacking one or more compounding ingredients

<u>Mastication</u> – plasticization of rubber by mechanical and thermal
means on open rolls or in an internal mixer, in which
reaction with oxygen causes scission of the molecular chains

<u>Mezzanine</u> – a low storey between two main storeys of a building

<u>Mill</u> (<u>mixing rolls</u>) – a machine consisting of two hollow steel
rolls which contain cooling or heating systems and are
placed in a frame in a horizontal or diagonal position. The
rolls move in opposite directions at different speeds, the
rear roll moving faster. Raw rubber is processed between the
rolls by mechanical friction and plasticized. A band of
rubber is formed around the front roll, its thickness
depending on the gap between the rolls.

<u>Mooney</u> – a measurement of rubber viscosity derived from use of
the Mooney viscometer, developed by Dr Melvin Mooney

<u>Odorant</u> – odorous substance used to disguise the characteristic
odour of vulcanisates or to give a specific odour

<u>Peptizer</u> – mastication aid, reclaiming agent, chemically
effective plasticizing agent with a powerful softening
effect on rubber, enabling reduction of the mixing time,
increased plasticity, and reduced viscosity of solutions.
Acts as an oxygen carrier and thus increases the oxidative
decomposition of the gel structure of rubber

<u>Plasticizer</u> – a material added to improve flexibility, particu-
larly at low temperatures

Ply – a single layer of rubber-coated textile or steel cord forming one element of a tyre casing

Plystock – a sheet of rubber-coated textile or steel cord from which a ply is cut

Polymerization regulator – material that controls the molecular weight of a polymer

Preservative – agent that prevents degradation

Reclaim – reclaimed rubber. Obtained from ground, vulcanized scrap from the production of natural and synthetic rubber articles, old rubber tyres, tubes and other such articles. Reclamation is achieved by replasticization (depolymerization), using heat and/or pressure and/or chemical agents. Used in compounding

Respirable dust – dust of a particle size small enough to be retained in the lungs; generally taken to be <8 μm in diameter

Retarder – a substance used to retard the speed of chemical reactions, i.e., to retard vulcanization and polymerization speeds and to prevent scorching during the mixing process

Scorch – premature start of vulcanization during mixing or shaping

Semi-bulk – a handling system in which raw materials are transferred from the original shipping container, to another container from which they are dispensed

Skiving – splitting or paring rubber to reduce it in thickness

Softener – material that softens rubber to facilitate its processing

Stabilizer – a compound added to prevent coagulation of rubber latex; an antioxidant used in emulsion polymerization to maintain the polymer in good condition during isolation, drying and storage of raw rubber

Tackifier – material used to increase the stickiness of compounds

Thermal black – carbon black produced by thermal decomposition of hydrocarbons in the absence of air

Tyre building – the process of building a tyre from its component parts before vulcanization

Vulcanite – (see Ebonite)

Vulcanization – the chemical reaction which brings about the formation of cross-links between polymer chains, giving a three-dimensional molecular structure. In this process, rubber is converted from a predominantly plastic to an elastic condition

Vulcanizing agents – all substances used to stabilize natural rubber or elastomers, usually with heating; some give vulcanisates particular properties, e.g., heat resistance

CHEMICALS USED OR PRODUCED IN THE RUBBER INDUSTRY

This appendix was prepared for IARC by SRI International under contract to the US National Cancer Institute. The reader should note, therefore, that in Tables 1 and 2, contrary to the usual practice of the IARC Monographs, neither the trade names nor the permissible levels have been verified by IARC from the original literature and that the presentation of the Chemical Abstracts Names differs in that (1) they have not been reversed; (2) 'sulfur' is spelled with a 'ph'; and (3) 'carbamic acid ester' is listed as 'carbamate'.

Introduction

Appendix 1 comprises four tables, in which chemicals either used or found as by-products in the rubber industry are identified. In Table 1 are listed those chemicals believed to have been used in the rubber industry in the US since 1975 and those used currently in western Europe. The chemicals are grouped according to structure and are listed alphabetically within each group. For each chemical, the Chemical Abstracts Service Registry Number (CAS No.), the structural formula, synonyms and trade names are given. Information is also provided on amounts of US production or imports, the class of use in rubber processing, the particular part of the rubber industry and the processes in which the chemical is used, reported levels of the chemical in the work place, and occupational standards that have been established in various countries. Monomers and elastomers are not included in Table 1, but are listed in Table 3. Also excluded are organic dyes and most plasticizers, which are believed to be associated primarily with the plastics and resins industry. Table 1 includes some compounds that were used in the rubber industry but have been withdrawn from use in certain countries.

Synonyms and trade names: The latest Chemical Abstracts Service Registry and IUPAC Systematic names are given, followed by the most common synonyms. Trade names for major products are listed separately.

US production: When no data on US production were available, amounts of US imports (indicated by the letter 'I') are given. When no data on US imports were available, estimates of production in western Europe (indicated by the letters 'WE') are given.

Use class: The way in which the chemical is used is indicated by means of the following code:

A   Accelerators, activators and vulcanizing agents

AN   Antioxidants, antiozonants and stabilizers

B   Bonding agents

BA   Blowing agents

C   Colourants

CLA   Conditioning and lubricating agents

F   Fillers

LM   Latex materials (including coagulants, stabilizers and preservatives)

M   Miscellaneous

P   Peptizers

PL   Plasticizers

PR   Polymerization regulators and materials

R   Retarders

S   Solvents

SO   Softeners

T   Tackifiers

Industries and processes: Industries are indicated by Roman numerals and processes by Arabic numbers, in accordance with the following outline:

I.   Tyres, tubes, remoulds, retreads
      1. Raw materials handling
      2. Weighing and mixing
      3. Milling, extruding, calendering
      4. Component building, assembling, rebuilding
      5. Press moulding, autoclaving, curing
      6. Inspecting, finishing, trimming, painting
      7. Storing and dispatching

II.   Other solid rubber goods, including rubber cables, belting and hoses, ebonite and vulcanite, rubber foot-wear, food processing equipment, aircraft de-icing equipment, automobile parts (seals, mounting, bushes), sports goods and toys, surgical and medical equipment (catheters, prostheses, etc)

      1. Raw materials handling
      2. Weighing and mixing
      3. Milling, extruding, calendering
      4. Component building, assembling
      5. Injection moulding, press moulding, autoclaving, curing, continuous vulcanization
      6. Inspecting, finishing, painting
      7. Storing and dispatching

III. Proofed rubber fabrics (including printers' blankets), adhesives and sealants

      1. Raw materials handling
      2. Weighing and mixing
      3. Spreading (impregnating, stretching and ironing)
      4. Curing
      5. Cutting
      6. Inspecting and finishing
      7. Storing and dispatching

IV.   Dipped latex products and foams

1.   Raw materials handling
2.   Weighing and mixing
3.   Frothing or dipping
4.   Curing
5.   Inspecting and finishing
6.   Storing and dispatching

Reported workplace levels (L): Examples are given of the highest
   airborne concentrations reported in the occupational environment in rubber processing when they exceeded the lowest
   occupational standard given in the next column. Each entry
   represents a separate study; sources for the data are indicated by footnotes. More detail is contained in Section V of
   this monograph.

Occupational standards (S): Recommended guidelines or governmental regulations which set occupational exposure limits
   for airborne substances in various countries are reported.
   They are given in a various ways: as ceiling (maximum
   allowable concentration) limits, time-weighted averages
   (TWA), or short-term exposure limits (STEL), which are
   ceiling values for a specified duration of time (30 min in
   the German Democratic Republic, 15 min in for the US),
   unless otherwise specified. Concentrations above ceiling
   limits but less than STEL are allowed for some chemicals;
   in such cases, the specified period of time during which
   this excursion is allowed is given following the peak value.
   For the US, Occupational Safety and Health Administration
   (OSHA) regulations are given, along with two types of
   recommended guidelines (National Institute for Occupational
   Safety and Health recommendations – USA-N – and American
   Conference of Governmental Industrial Hygienists recommendations – USA-A), because these recommendations frequently
   provide the basis for future OSHA regulations.

   The following is a list of the abbreviations used for the
names of countries, the year during which the standards were
issued and an indication of whether the standards are regulations
or guidelines:

Abbreviation	Country	Year	Status
A	Australia	1978	Guideline
BEL	Belgium	1978	Guideline
BUL	Bulgaria	1971	Regulation
CZ	Czechoslovakia	1976	Regulation
F	Finland	1975	Regulation
DDR	German Democratic Republic	1979	Regulation
BRD	Federal Republic of Germany	1979	Guideline
H	Hungary	1974	Regulation
I	Italy	1978	Guideline
J	Japan	1978	Guideline
N	The Netherlands	1978	Guideline
P	Poland	1976	Regulation
R	Romania	1975	Regulation
SWED	Sweden	1978	Guideline
S	Switzerland	1978	Regulation
USSR	USSR	1977	Regulation
USA	USA	1980	Regulation – Occupational Safety and Health Administration (OSHA)

Abbreviation	Country	Year	Status
USA-N	USA	1980	Guideline – National Institute for Occupationa Safety & Health (NIOSH)
USA-A	USA	1980	Guideline – American Conference of Governmenta Industrial Hygienists (ACGIH)
Y	Yugoslavia	1971	Regulation

Table 2 lists chemicals found as by-products in the rubber industry. As in Table 1, synonyms and trade names, Chemical Abstracts Service Registry Numbers, structural formulae, workplace levels and occupational standards are provided. The same codes as used in Table 1 identify the industry and process in which the by-product was identified and in which level were measured.

Table 3 comprises a list of monomers and elastomers used in the rubber industry; and Table 4 provides an indication of current production of elastomers.

Footnotes to Tables 1 and 2

a. US International Trade Commission (1977a,b); SRI International (1980a,b); SRI International estimates

b. International Labour Office (1980)

c. SRI International estimates

d. US Environmental Protection Agency (1980)

e. US Department of Commerce (1980b); e* (1980a)

f. US International Trade Commission (1980a); f* (1977b); f** (1978a); f*** (1979a)

g. SRI International estimates; includes t-octyl mercaptan and n-octyl mercaptan

h. SRI International estimates; includes all dodecyl mercaptans

i. Economic Research Service (1977)

J. Includes chrome orange

k. Excludes natural aluminium oxide

l. For countries other than the US, it is unclear whether this standard or guideline is a TWA or ceiling value

m. US International Trade Commission (1980b); m* (1977c); m** (1978b); m*** (1979b)

n. Natural and synthetic

o. US Department of the Interior (1980)

p. Recovered elemental

q. American Conference of Governmental Industrial Hygienists (1980)

r.   US Occupational Safety & Health Administration (1980)

s.   National Institute for Occupational Safety & Health (1980)

t.   National Institute for Occupational Safety & Health (1974)

u.   Van Ert et al. (1980)

v.   Butler & Taylor (1973)

w.   Borcherding et al. (1977)

x   Hollet & Schloemer (1978)

y.   Daniels (1980)

z.   Maier et al. (1974)

aa.   Gunter & Lucas (1975)

bb.   Levy (1975)

cc.   National Institute for Occupational Safety & Health (1976)

dd.   Pagnotto et al. (1979)

ee.   Burgess et al. (1977)

ff.   McGlothlin & Wilcox (1980)

gg.   Williams et al. (1980)

hh.   Noweir et al. (1972)

ii.   Rappaport & Fraser (1977)

jj.   Fajen et al. (1979)

kk.   Yeager et al. (1980)

ll.   Fajen (1980)

mm.   National Board of Occupational Safety & Health (1981)

nn.   Preussmann _et al._ (1981)

oo.   Preussmann _et al._ (1980)

TABLE 1

IDENTIFICATION, PRODUCTION, USE, WORKPLACE

OCCURRENCE AND STANDARDS FOR CHEMICALS

USED IN THE RUBBER INDUSTRY

Table 1. Table of contents by structural class

I. Organic Compounds
  A. Nitrogen Compounds
    1. Phenylenediamines

Name and CAS Reg. No.	Synonyms and Trade Names	Structural Formula	US Production -Thousand Kg (Year)	Use Class[a]	Indus-tries	Pro-cesses	Reported Workplace Levels(L)/Occupational Standards(S)[b,q,r,s]
Alkyl aryl-p-phenylenediamines --	Chem. Abstr.: -- IUPAC: -- Santoflex 134		450(1976)[c]	AN	I II IV	1-3 1-3 1-2	L:--/S: 5 mg/m^3 ceiling (USSR)
N,N'-Bis(1,4-dimethylpentyl)-p-phenylenediamine 3081-14-9	Chem. Abstr.: N,N'-bis(1,4-dimethyl-pentyl)-1,4-benzenediamine IUPAC: N,N'-bis(1,4-dimethyl-pentyl)-p-phenylenediamine N,N'-di(1,4-dimethylpentyl)-p-phenylenediamine Antioxidant 4030; Elastozone 33; Flexzone 4L; Santoflex 77; Tenamene 4; Tenemene: UOP 788		4.000(1976)[c]	AN	I II III IV	1-3 1-3 1-2 1-2	L:--/S: 5 mg/m^3 ceiling (USSR)
N,N'-Bis(1-ethyl-3-methylpentyl)-p-phenylenediamine 139-60-6	Chem. Abstr.: N,N'-bis(1-ethyl-3-methylpentyl)-1,4-benzenediamine IUPAC: N,N'-bis(1-ethyl-3-methyl-pentyl)-p-phenylenediamine Elastozone 31; Flexzone 8L; Santoflex 17; Tenamene 31; UOP 88		2,300(1976)[c]	AN	I II	1-2 1-2	L:--/S:--
N,N'-Bis(isopropyl)-p-phenylenediamine 4261-01-8	Chem. Abstr.: N,N'-bis(1-methylethyl)-1,4-benzenediamine IUPAC: N,N'-diisopropyl-p-phenylene-diamine		> 4.5 (1980)[c]	AN	--	--	L:--/S:--
N,N'-Bis(1-methylheptyl)-p-phenylenediamine 103-96-8	Chem. Abstr.: N,N'-bis(1-methyl-heptyl)-1,4-benzenediamine IUPAC: N,N'-bis(1-methylheptyl)-p-phenylenediamine N,N'-di(2-octyl)-p-phenylenediamine Antozite 1; Elastozone; Santoflex 217; Tenemene 30; UOP 288		2,300(1976)[c]	AN	I II III IV	1-3 1-3 1-2 1-2	L:--/S:--

Name and CAS Reg. No.	Synonyms and Trade Names	Structural Formula	US Production -Thousand Kg (Year)	Use Class [a]	Indus-tries	Pro-cesses	Reported Workplace Levels(L)/Occupational Standards(S) [b,q,r,s]
N,N'-Bis(1-methylpropyl)-o-phenylenediamine 13482-10-5	Chem. Abstr.: N,N'-bis(1-methylpropyl)-1,2-benzenediamine IUPAC: N,N'-di-sec-butyl-o-phenylene-diamine	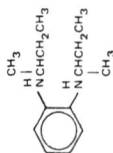	> 2.2(1980) [c]	AN	--	--	L:--/S:--
N,N'-Bis(1-methylpropyl)-p-phenylene-diamine 101-96-2	Chem. Abstr.: N,N'-bis(1-methylpropyl)-1,4-benzenediamine IUPAC: N,N'-di-sec-butyl-p-phenylene-diamine Antioxidant 22; Tenamene 2; Topanol M	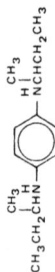	> 2.2(1980) [c]	AN	--	--	L:--/S:--
N-sec-Butyl-N'-phenyl-p-phenylenediamine 788-17-0	Chem. Abstr.: N-(1-methylpropyl)-N'-phenyl-1,4-benzenediamine IUPAC: N-sec-butyl-N'-phenyl-p-phenylenediamine Flexzone 5L	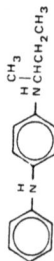	> 2.2(1980) [c]	AN	--	::	L:--/S:--
N-Cyclohexyl-N'-phenyl-p-phenylenediamine 101-87-1	Chem. Abstr.: N-cyclohexyl-N'-phenyl-1,4-benzenediamine IUPAC: N-cyclohexyl-N'-phenyl-p-phenylenediamine 4-(cyclohexylamino)diphenylamine Antioxidant 4010; Flexzone 6H; UOP 36		900(1976) [c]	AN	I 1-3, II 1-3, III 1-2, IV 1-2		L:--/S:--
Diaryl and alkylaryl p-phenylene-diamine, blended --	Chem. Abstr.: -- IUPAC: -- Flexzone 12L	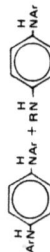	> 2.2(1960) [c]	AN	--	--	L:--/S:--
Diarylenediamines, mixed	Chem. Abstr.: -- IUPAC: --	Complex mixture	450(1976) [c]	AN	--	--	L:--/S:--

Name and CAS Reg. No.	Synonyms and Trade Names	Structural Formula	US Production -Thousand Kg (Year)	Use Class[a]	Indus-tries	Pro-cesses	Reported Workplace Levels(L)/Occupational Standards(S)[b,q,r,s]
Diaryl-p-phenylenediamine, mixed --	Chem. Abstr.: -- IUPAC: -- Wingstay 100; Wingstay 100 AZ; Wingstay 200		> 2.2(1980)[c]	AN	I II III	1-2 1-3 1-2	L:--/S:--
N,N'-Dicyclohexyl-p-phenylene-diamine 4175-38-6	Chem Abstr.: N,N'-dicyclohexyl-1,4-benzenediamine IUPAC: N,N'-dicyclohexyl-p-phenylenediamine N,N'-bis(cyclohexyl)-p-phenylenediamine UOP 26		2,300(1976)[c]	AN	I II III IV	1-3 1-3 1-2 1-2	L:--/S:--
N-(1,1-Dimethylamyl)-N'-phenyl-p-phenylenediamine 3081-01-4	Chem. Abstr.: N-(1,4-dimethylpentyl)-N'-phenyl-1,4-benzenediamine IUPAC: N-(1,4-dimethylpentyl)-N'-phenyl-p-phenylenediamine		>2.2(1980)[c]	AN	--	--	L:--/S:--
N-(1,3-Dimethylbutyl)-N'-phenyl-p-phenylenediamine 793-24-8	Chem. Abstr.: N-(1,3-dimethylbutyl)-N'-phenyl-1,4-benzenediamine IUPAC: N-(1,3-dimethylbutyl)-N'-phenyl-p-phenylenediamine Antioxidant 4020; Diafen 13; Flexzone 7L, 7F; Permanax 120; Santoflex 13; UOP 588; Vulkanox 4020; Wingstay 300		> 450(1977)[d]	AN	I II III IV	1-3 1-3 1-2 1-2	L:--/S: 5 mg/m^3 ceiling (USSR)
N,N'-Di-2-naphthyl-p-phenylenediamine 93-46-9	Chem. Abstr.: N,N'-di-2-naphthalenyl-1,4-benzene-diamine IUPAC: N,N'-di-2-naphthyl-p-phenylenediamine N,N'-bis(2-naphthyl)-p-phenylenediamine; DNPD Aceto DIPP; AgeRite White; Antigene F; Antioxidant DNP, 123; ASM-DNT; Diafen NN; Nonox CI; Santowhite CI; Tisperse MB-2X		>0.45(1979)[f]	AN	I II III IV	1-3 1-3 1-2 1-2	L:--/S:--

Name and CAS Reg. No.	Synonyms and Trade Names	Structural Formula	US Production -Thousand Kg (Year)	Use Class [a]	Indus-tries	Pro-cesses	Reported Workplace Levels(L)/Occupational Standards(S)[b,q,r,s]
N,N'-Diphenyl-p-phenylene-diamine 74-31-7	Chem. Abstr.: N,N'-diphenyl-1,4-benzenediamine IUPAC: N,N'-diphenyl-p-phenylene-diamine diphenyl-p-phenylenediamine AgeRite DPPD; Alkofane DIP; Diafen FF; DPPD; Flexamine G; JZF; Nonflex H; Nonox DPPD; Permanax 18; Stabilizer DPPD		> 45(1977)[d]	AN	I II III IV	1-3 1-3 1-2 1-2	L:--/S:--
N-Isopropyl-N'-phenyl-p-phenylenediamine 101-72-4	Chem. Abstr.: N-(1-methylethyl)-N'-phenyl-1,4-benzenediamine IUPAC: N-isopropyl-N'-phenyl-p-phenylenediamine p-isopropylaminodiphenylamine Antigen 36; Antioxidant 4010; Cyzone IP; Diafen FP; Flexone 3-C; Ipogrox; Nocrac 810 NA; Nonox ZA; Orflex PP; Ozonon 3C; Permanax IPPD; Santoflex IP; Santoflex 36		4,100(1976)[c]	AN	I II III IV	1-3 1-3 1-2 1-2	L:--/S: 2 mg/m^3 ceiling (USSR)
N-(1-Methylheptyl)-N'-phenyl-p-phenylenediamine 15233-47-3	Chem. Abstr.: N-(1-methylheptyl)-N'-phenyl-1,4-benzenediamine IUPAC: N-(1-methylheptyl)-N'-phenyl-p-phenylenediamine UOP 688		1,400(1976)[c]	AN	I II III IV	1-3 1-3 1-2 1-2	L:--/S:--
N-(1-Methylpentyl)-N'-phenyl-p-phenylenediamine 61792-45-8	Chem. Abstr.: N-(1-methylpentyl)-N'-phenyl-1,4-benzenediamine IUPAC: N-(1-methylpentyl)-N'-phenyl-p-phenylenediamine		>0.45(1979)[f]	AN	--	--	L:--/S:--

Name and CAS Reg. No.	Synonyms and Trade Names	Structural Formula	US Production -Thousand Kg (Year)	Use Class[a]	Indus-tries	Pro-cesses	Reported Workplace Levels(L)/Occupational Standards(S)[b,q,r,s]
N-Phenyl-p-phenylenediamine 101-54-2	Chem. Abstr.: N-phenyl-1,4-benzene-diamine IUPAC: N-phenyl-p-phenylenediamine p-aminodiphenylamine; N-phenyl-p-aminoaniline; semidin; p-semidine Diphenyl Black; Luxan Black R; Peltol BR, BRII; Variamine Blue RT		> 0.45(1977)[d]	AN	--	--	L:--/S:--
Toluenediamines 95-80-7 and 823-40-5	Chem. Abstr.: 4-methyl-1,3-benzene-diamine and 2-methyl-1,3-benzene-diamine IUPAC: toluene-2,4-diamine and toluene-2,6-diamine Eucanine GB; Fouramine J; Fourrine M, 94; Nako TMT; Pelagol J, Grey J; Pontamine Developer TN; Renal MD; Zoba GKE		58,500(1977)[d]	AN	--	--	L:--/S: 2-10 mg/m^3 ceiling (R, USSR) 2-5 mg/m^3 TWA (DDR USSR) 4 mg/m^3 STEL (DDR)

2. Diphenylamines

Name and CAS Reg. No.	Synonyms and Trade Names	Structural Formula	US Production -Thousand Kg (Year)	Use Class [a]	Indus- tries	Pro- cesses	Reported Workplace Levels(L)/Occupational Standards(S)[b,q,r,s]
4,4'-Bis(α,α-dimethylbenzyl)-diphenylamine 10081-67-1	Chem. Abstr.: 4-(1-methyl-1-phenyl-ethyl)-N-[4-(1-methyl-1-phenyl-ethyl)phenyl] benzenamine; IUPAC: 4,4'-bis(α,α-dimethylbenzyl)-diphenylamine; Permanax 49HV	[structural formula]	106(1978I) m***	A	I, II, III, IV	1-3, 1-3, 1-2, 1-2	L:--/S:--
4,4'-Dinonyldiphenylamine 24925-59-5	Chem. Abstr.: 4-nonyl-N-(4-nonylphenyl)-benzenamine; IUPAC: 4,4'-dinonyldiphenylamine	[structural formula]	>0.5(1980WE)[c]	AN	II	1-2	L:--/S:--
P,p-Dioctyldiphenylamine 101-67-7	Chem. Abstr.: 4-octyl-N-(4-octyl-phenyl)benzenamine; IUPAC: 4,4'-dioctyldiphenylamine bis(p-octylphenyl)amine; Vanlube 81	[structural formula]	>6.8(1980)[c]	AN	II	1-2	L:--/S:--
Diphenylamine, styrenated --	Chem. Abstr.: styrenated N-phenyl-benzenamine; IUPAC: styrenated diphenylamine	[structural formula]	>0.45(1979)[f]	AN	--	--	L:--/S:--
Diphenylamine, substituted --	Chem. Abstr.: substituted N-phenyl-benzenamine; IUPAC: substituted diphenylamine; Naugard 445	[structural formula]	>0.45(1979)[f]	AN	I, II, III, IV	1-3, 1-3, 1-2, 1-2	L:--/S:--
p-Hydroxydiphenylamine 122-37-2	Chem. Abstr.: 4-(phenylamino)phenol; IUPAC: p-anilinophenol; p-oxydiphenylamine; N-phenyl-p-aminophenol; VTI 1	[structural formula]	45(1976)[c]	AN	--	--	L:--/S:0.5 mg/m^3 ceiling (USSR)

Name and CAS Reg. No.	Synonyms and Trade Names	Structural Formula	US Production -Thousand Kg (Year)	Use Class [a]	Indus-tries	Pro-cesses	Reported Workplace Levels(L)/Occupational Standards(S) [b],q,r,s
4-Isopropoxy diphenylamine 101-73-5	Chem. Abstr.: 4-(1-methylethoxy)-N-phenylbenzenamine IUPAC: 4-isopropoxydiphenylamine p-hydroxydiphenylamine isopropyl ether Age Rite 150		>0.45(1977)[f] **	AN	II	1-2	L:--/S:--
N-Nitrosodiphenylamine 86-30-6	Chem. Abstr.: N-nitroso-N-phenyl-benzenamine IUPAC: N-nitrosodiphenylamine diphenylnitrosamine Curetard A; Delac J; Naugard TJB; Redax; Retarder J; Vulcatard A; Vulkalent A; Vultrol		284(1979)[f]	R	I, II, III, IV	1-3, 1-3, 1-2, 1-2	L: 13.1 $\mu g/m^3$ ff: 12.4 $\mu g/m^3$ ll S: --
Nonylated diethyldiphenylamine --	Chem. Abstr.: nonylated diethyl deriva-tive of N-phenylbenzenamine IUPAC: nonylated diethyl derivative of diphenylamine		>2.2(1980)[c]	AN	--	--	L:--/S:--
3. Other Aromatic Amines							
N,N'-Diphenylethylenediamine 150-61-8	Chem. Abstr.: N,N'-diphenyl-1,2-ethanediamine IUPAC: N,N'-diphenylethylenediamine 1,2-dianilinoethane; N,N'-ethylene-dianiline NODX; Stabilite		<450(1976)[c]	AN	--	--	L:--/S:--
N,N'-Diphenyl-1,3-propanediamine 104-69-8	Chem. Abstr.: N,N'-diphenyl-1,3-propanediamine IUPAC: N,N'-diphenyl-1,3-propanediamine N,N'-diphenyl-1,3-propylene-diamine Warcoat GPC		450(1976)[c]	AN	--	--	L:--/S:--

Name and CAS Reg. No.	Structural Formula	Synonyms and Trade Names	US Production -Thousand Kg (Year)	Use Class[a]	Indus-tries	Pro-cesses	Reported Workplace Levels(L)/Occupational Standards(S)[b,q,r,s]
N,N'-Di-o-tolylethylenediamine 94-92-8		Chem. Abstr.: N,N'-bis(2-methyl-phenyl)-1,2-ethanediamine IUPAC: N,N'-di-o-tolylethylene-diamine Stabilite ALBA	450(1976)[c]	AN	--	--	L:--/S:--
4,4'-Methylenebis(2-chloro-aniline) 101-14-4		Chem. Abstr.: 4,4'-methylenebis-(2-chlorobenzenamine) IUPAC: 4,4'-methylenebis(2-chloro-aniline) MOCA Diamet KH; Quodorole	>900 (1977)[d]	AN	--	--	L: 82 µg (wipe samples)aa S: 0.22 mg/m^3 Ceiling (BEL,N,S,I,); 0.02-0.22 mg/m^3 TWA (A,USA-A)
Nonyldiphenylamine mixture (mono-, di-, & tri-) --	R = C_9H_{19} x + y = 1, 2, or 3	Chem. Abstr.: -- IUPAC: -- Polylite	450(1976)[c]	AN	I II III IV	1-3 1-3 1-2 1-2	L:--/S:--
Octylated diphenylamine 70528-82-4	R = C_8H_{17} x + y = 1, 2, 3, or 4	Chem. Abstr.: Octylated N-phenylbenzen-amine IUPAC: octylated diphenylamine octyldiphenylamine Age Rite Stalite S; Akrochem Antioxidant S; Antioxidant OCD; Cyanox 8; Pennox A, ODP; Permanax CD; Wylox ADPF	3,825(1979)[f]	AN	I II III IV	1-3 1-3 1-2 1-2	L:--/S:--

Name and CAS Reg. No.	Synonyms and Trade Names	Structural Formula	US Production -Thousand Kg (Year)	Use Class [a]	Indus- tries	Pro- cesses	Reported Workplace Levels(L)/Occupational Standards(S)[b,q,r,s]
Octyldiphenylamine, alkylated --	Chem. Abstr.: alkylated octyl deriva- tive of N-phenylbenzenamine IUPAC: alkylated octyl derivative of diphenylamine AgeRite NEPA	Unknown	>0.45(1979)[f]	AN	I II III IV	1-3 1-3 1-2 1-2	L:--/S:--
Octyldiphenylamine mixtures (mono-, nonyl-, & di-) --	Chem. Abstr.: -- IUPAC: --	Unknown	3,600(1976)[c]	AN	--	--	L:--/S:--
p-(p-Toluenesulphonamido)diphenyl- amine 100-93-6	Chem. Abstr.: 4-methyl-N-[4- (phenylamino)phenyl] benzene- sulphonamide IUPAC: 4'-anilino-p-toluenesulphon- anilide p-(p-tolylsulphonylamido)diphenylamine Aranox	450(1976)[c]	AN	I II III IV	1-3 1-3 1-2 1-2	L:--/S:--
4,4'-Methylenedianiline 101-77-9	Chem. Abstr.: 4,4'-methylenebis - (benzenamine) IUPAC: 4,4'-methylenedianiline 4,4'-diaminodiphenylmethane; methylenebisaniline; p,p'-methylene- dianiline Epicure DDM; Epikure DDM; HT972; Tonox	>4,504(1977)[d]	AN	I II III IV	1-3 1-3 1-2 1-2	L:--/S:--

4. Aromatic Amine – Aldehyde (Ketone) Condensates

Name and CAS Reg. No.	Synonyms and Trade Names	Structural Formula	US Production –Thousand Kg (Year)	Use Class[a]	Indus- tries	Pro- cesses	Reported Workplace Levels(L)/Occupational Standards(S)[b,q,r,s]
Acetaldehyde-aniline condensate --	Chem. Abstr.: acetaldehyde reaction product with aniline IUPAC: acetaldehyde reaction product with aniline		> 0.45(1976)[f*]	A	--	--	L:--/S:--
Aldol-(mixed α- and β-)naphthyl-amine condensate --	Chem. Abstr.: 3-hydroxybutanal reaction product with 1- and 2-naphthyl-amines IUPAC: 3-hydroxybutyraldehyde reaction product with 1- and 2-naphthylamines Nonox S	Indefinite	(Used in the past but has been discontinued by some countries)				
Aldol-α-naphthylamine condensate --	Chem. Abstr.: 3-hydroxybutanal reaction product with 1-naphthylamine IUPAC: 3-hydroxybutyraldehyde reaction product with 1-naphthylamine	Indefinite 	> 1(1980WE)[c]	AN	--	--	L:--/S:--
Butyraldehyde-aniline condensate 68411-20-1	Chem. Abstr.: butanal reaction product with aniline IUPAC: butyraldehyde reaction product with aniline Accelerate 832; 808 Accelerator; Antox Special,Rubber Antioxidant; Beutene; Vanax 808; Vanox AT		> 0.9(1979)[f]	AN	I II III IV	1-3 1-3 1-2 1-2	L:--/S:--
n-Butyraldehyde-aniline condensate --	Chem. Abstr.: n-butanal reaction product with aniline IUPAC: n-butyraldehyde reaction product with aniline		> 0.9(1979)[f]	A	I II III IV	1-3 1-3 1-2 1-2	L:--/S:--

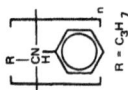

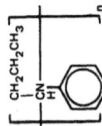

Name and CAS Reg. No.	Synonyms and Trade Names	Structural Formula	US Production -Thousand Kg (Year)	Use Class[a]	Indus-tries	Pro-cesses	Reported Workplace Levels(L)/Occupational Standards(S)[b,q,r,s]
Diarylamine-ketone-aldehyde condensate --	Chem. Abstr.: aldehydes reaction products with ketones and diaryl-amines IUPAC: aldehydes reaction products with ketones and diarylamines BXA	Indefinite	>0.5(1980WE)[c]	AN	I II III IV	1-3 1-3 1-2 1-2	L:--/S:--
Diarylamine-ketone condensate --	Chem. Abstr.: ketones reaction products with diarylamines IUPAC: ketones reaction products with diarylamines	Indefinite	>2.2(1980)[c]	AN	II	1-2	L:--/S:--
Diphenylamine-acetone condensate 9003-79-6	Chem. Abstr.: 2-propanone polymer with N-phenylbenzen-amine IUPAC: acetone polymer with diphenylamine Agerite Superflex; Agerite Superflex Solidroform; Aminox; BLE-25; Cyanoflex 50, 100; Permanax B, BL, BLN	Indefinite	>0.9(1979)[f]	AN	I II III IV	1-3 1-3 1-2 1-2	L:--/S:--
Heptaldehyde-aniline condensate --	Chem. Abstr.: heptanal reaction product with aniline IUPAC: heptanal reaction product with aniline Hepteen Base	$\left[\begin{array}{c}(CH_2)_5CH_3 \\ CN \\ H \end{array}\right]_n$ (phenyl group)	>0.45(1979)[f]	A	I II III IV	1-3 1-3 1-2 1-2	L:--/S:--
N-Phenyl-2-naphthylamine-acetone condensate --	Chem. Abstr.: 2-propanone reaction product with N-phenyl-2-naphthylamine IUPAC: acetone reaction product with N-phenyl-2-naphthylamine	Indefinite	>0.2(1980)[c]	AN	--	--	L:--/S:--

5. Quinolines

Name and CAS Reg. No.	Synonyms and Trade Names	Structural Formula	US Production -Thousand Kg (Year)	Use Class [a]	Indus-tries	Pro-cesses	Reported Workplace Levels(L)/Occupational Standards(S)[b,q,r,s]
1,2-Dihydro-6-dodecyl-2,2,4-tri-methylquinoline 89-28-1	Chem. Abstr.: 6-dodecyl-1,2-dihydro-2,2,4-trimethylquinoline; IUPAC: 6-dodecyl-1,2-dihydro-2,2,4-trimethylquinoline; Santoflex DD	$CH_3(CH_2)_{11}$ ... (structural formula)	1,800(1976)[c]	AN	I II III IV	1-3 1-3 1-2 1-2	L:--/S: 5 mg/m^3 ceiling (USSR)
1,2-Dihydro-6-ethoxy-2,2,4-tri-methylquinoline 91-53-2	Chem. Abstr.: 6-ethoxy-1,2-dihydro-2,2,4-trimethylquinoline; IUPAC: 6-ethoxy-1,2-dihydro-2,2,4-trimethylquinoline; ethoxyquin; Amea 100; Dave's Nitrigard; EMQ; EQ; Niflex; Nocrac AW; Permanax 103; Santoflex A, AW; Santoquin; Quinol ED	CH_3CH_2O ... (structural formula)	> 90(1977)[d]	AN	I II III IV	1-3 1-3 1-2 1-2	L:--/S: 5 mg/m^3 ceiling (USSR)
1,2-Dihydro-2,2,4-trimethyl-quinoline 147-47-7	Chem. Abstr.: 1,2-dihydro-2,2,4-trimethylquinoline; IUPAC: 1,2-dihydro-2,2,4-trimethylquinoline; acetone anil; Age Rite MA; Resin D; Akrochem Antioxidant DQ; Antioxidant HS; Cyanox 12 Antioxidant; Flectol H, Flakes; Naugard Q; Pennox HR; (polymerized products)	CH_3 ... (structural formula)	> 4.5(1977)[d]	AN	I II III IV	1-3 1-3 1-2 1-2	L:--/S:--

Name and CAS Reg. No.	Synonyms and Trade Names	Structural Formula	US Production -Thousand Kg (Year)	Use Class [a]	Indus- tries	Pro- cesses	Reported Workplace Levels(L)/Occupational Standards(S) [b,q,r,s]
Poly(2,2,4-trimethyl-1,2-di- hydroquinoline) 26780-96-1	Chem. Abstr.: 1,2-dihydro-2,2,4- trimethylquinoline, homopolymer IUPAC: 1,2-dihydro-2,2,4-trimethyl- quinoline, homopolymer acetoanil; trimethyldihydroquinoline polymer AgeRite Resin D, MA; Antigene ROF; Antioxidant HSL; Flectol H; Nocrac 224; Nonflex RD; Permanax 45; Polnoks R		340(1977I) [m,**]	AN	I II III IV	1-3 1-3 1-2 1-2	L:--/S: 1 mg/m^3 ceiling (USSR)

6. Arylguanidines

Name and CAS Reg. No.	Synonyms and Trade Names	Structural Formula	US Production -Thousand Kg (Year)	Use Class[a]	Indus-tries	Pro-cesses	Reported Workplace Levels(L)/Occupational Standards(S)[b,q,r,s]
Dicatechol borate, di-o-tolylguanidine salt 16971-82-7	Chem. Abstr.: hydrogen bis[1,2-benzenediolato(2-)-O,O']borate (1-) compound with N,N'-bis-(2-methylphenyl)guanidine (1:1) / IUPAC: hydrogen bis[pyrocatecholato(2-)]borate (1-) compound with 1,3-di-o-tolyl-guanidine (1:1) / Permalax; Permalux		>0.45(1979)[f]	A	I II III IV	1-3 1-3 1-2 1-2	L:--/S:--
1,3-Diphenylguanidine 102-06-7	Chem. Abstr.: N,N'-diphenyl-guanidine / IUPAC: 1,3-diphenylguanidine DPG / Accelerator D; Denax; DPG; Melaniline; Vulcacit D; Vulkozit		2,300(1976)[c]	A	I II III IV	1-3 1-3 1-2 1-2	L:--/S:--
1,3-Di-o-tolylguanidine 97-39-2	Chem. Abstr.: N,N'-bis(2-methylphenyl)guanidine / IUPAC: 1,3-di-o-tolylguanidine / DOTG; Eveite DOTG; Vulkacit DOTG		2,300(1972)[c]	A	I II III IV	1-3 1-3 1-2 1-2	L:--/S:--
o-Tolyl biguanidine 27550-75-0	Chem. Abstr.: N-(2-methylphenyl)-1,2-hydrazinedicarboximidamide / IUPAC: 1-o-tolylbiguanidine / 1-o-tolylbiguanide; 1-o-tolylbiguanidine; o-tolyl biguanidide		>2.5(1980WE)[c]	A	--	--	L:--/S:--

Name and CAS Reg. No.	Synonyms and Trade Names	Structural Formula	US Production -Thousand Kg (Year)	Use Class[a]	Indus-tries	Pro-cesses	Reported Workplace Levels(L)/Occupational Standards(S)[b,q,r,s]
1,2,3-Triphenylguanidine 101-01-9	Chem. Abstr.: N,N',N''-triphenyl-guanidine; IUPAC: 1,2,3-triphenylguanidine	(structure)	> 0.5(1980WE)[c]	A	--	--	L:--/S:--
7. Alkyl amines							
Di-n-butylamine 111-92-2	Chem. Abstr.: N-butyl-1-butanamine; IUPAC: dibutylamine	$CH_3(CH_2)_3$—NH—$(CH_2)_3CH_3$	2,345 (1979)[f]	A	II III	1-2 1-2	L:--/S:--
N,N-Diethylhydroxylamine 3710-84-7	Chem. Abstr.: N-ethyl-N-hydroxy-ethanamine; IUPAC: N,N-diethylhydroxylamine	CH_3CH_2—NOH—CH_3CH_2	> 0.45(1979)[f]	AN	--	--	L:--/S:--
N-Ethylcyclohexylamine 5459-93-8	Chem. Abstr.: N-ethylcyclohexanamine; IUPAC: N-ethylcyclohexylamine; Accelerator HX; Vulkacit HX	(structure) NCH_2CH_3	> 0.45(1979)[f]	A	I II III IV	1-3 1-3 1-2 1-2	L:--/S:--
Hexamethylenetetramine 100-97-0	Chem. Abstr.: 1,3,5,7-tetraazatri-cyclo [3.3.1.1(3,7)] decane; IUPAC: hexamethylenetetramine; aminoform; HMTA; Aceto HMT; Antihydral; Duirexol; Ekagam H; Formin; Herax UTS; Poly Slab; Poly Gel; Uramin; Uratune; Uritone; Urodeine; Urotropin; Xametrin	(structure)	53,550 (1979)[f]	A	I II	1-3 1-2	L:--/S:--
Hexamethyleneimine 111-49-9	Chem. Abstr.: hexahydro-1H-azepine; IUPAC: hexahydro-1H-azepine; azacycloheptane; 2-(1-hexamethylenimine); homopiperidine; perhydroazepine; G O	(structure)	> 1400(1977)[d]	A	--	--	L:--/S: 0.5 mg/m^3 Ceiling (USSR)

Name and CAS Reg. No.	Synonyms and Trade Names	Structural Formula	US Production -Thousand Kg (Year)	Use Class[a]	Indus-tries	Pro-cesses	Reported Workplace Levels(L)/Occupational Standards(S)[b,q,r,s]
N-(1-Methylheptyl)ethanolamine 26535-68-2	Chem. Abstr.: 2-[(1-methylheptyl)amino]-ethanol IUPAC: 2-[(1-methylheptyl)amino]-ethanol	$CH_3CH_2CH_2CH_2CH_2CH_2CHNHCH_2CH_2OH$ (with CH_3)	>2.2(1980)[c]	AN	--	--	L:--/S:--
Triethyltrimethylene triamine 7779-27-3	Chem. Abstr.: 1,3,5-triethylhexa-hydro-1,3,5-triazine IUPAC: 1,3,5-triethylhexahydro-s-triazine triethyl-trimethylenetriamine Vancide TH	CH_2CH_3, N—CH_2CH_3, CH_3CH_2—N	>0.45(1979)[f]	A	II III IV	1-2 1-2 1-2	L:--/S:--
8. Carbamates							
Bis(4-aminocyclohexyl)methane carbamate 15484-34-1	Chem. Abstr.: 4-amino-α-(4-aminocyclohexyl)cyclohexane-methanol, carbamate (ester) IUPAC: bis(4-aminocyclohexyl)methyl carbamate Diak No. 4	$[H_2N$—cyclohexyl—$CHOCNH_2 (=O)]_2$	>0.45(1979)[f***]	A	--	--	L:--/S:--
Dimethylethanolamine, toluene-2,4-diisocyanate adduct 57718-03-3	Chem. Abstr.: bis[2-(dimethyl-amino)ethyl](4-methyl-1,3-phenylene)bis[carbamate] IUPAC: bis[2-(dimethylamino)ethyl]-toluene-2,4-dicarbamate	$NCOCH_2CH_2N(CH_3)_2$, $NCOCH_2CH_2N(CH_3)_2$, CH_3	450(1976)[c]	A	--	--	L:--/S:--
Ethylenediamine carbamate 109-58-0	Chem. Abstr.: (2-aminoethyl)carbamic acid IUPAC: (2-aminoethyl)carbamic acid	$H_2NCH_2CH_2NCOH$ (=O)	>0.45(1979)[f]	A	--	--	L:--/S:--
Hexamethylenediamine carbamate 1017-89-5	Chem. Abstr.: carbamic acid, compound with 1,6-hexanediamine IUPAC: carbamic acid, compound with 1,6-hexanediamine	$H_2N(CH_2)_6NCOH$ (=O)	>4.5(1980)[c]	A	--	--	L:--/S:--

9. Miscellaneous

Name and CAS Reg. No.	Synonyms and Trade Names	Structural Formula	US Production -Thousand Kg (Year)	Use Class[a]	Indus- tries	Pro- cesses	Reported Workplace Levels(L)/Occupational Standards(S)[b,q,r,s]
4-Aminobiphenyl 92-67-1	Chem. Abstr.: (1,1'-biphenyl)-4-amine IUPAC: 4-biphenylamine p-aminobiphenyl; 4-phenylaniline; xenylamine; p-xenylamine		(Used in the past but has been discontinued by some countries)				
Aromatic polyamine, hindered --	Chem. Abstr.: hindered aromatic polyamine IUPAC: hindered aromatic polyamine	Indefinite	> 2.2(1980)[c]	AN	--	--	L:--/S:--
2,2'-Azobisisobutyronitrile 78-67-1	Chem. Abstr.: 2,2'-azobis(2-methyl-propanenitrile) IUPAC: 2,2'-azodiisobutyronitrile Aceto AZIB; Genitron; Pianofor AN; Porofor N; Poly-Zole AZDN; Vazo		> 450(1977)[d]	BA	--	--	L:--/S:--
1,1'-Azobisformamide 123-77-3	Chem. Abstr.: diazenedicarboxamide IUPAC: 1,1'-azobis(formamide) Azobiscarbonamide; Azocel 504, 506, 508, 525; Azobiscarboxamide; Celogen AZ; Delta (1,1')-biurea; Genitron; Kempore; Lucel ADA; Pinhole; Porofor 505; Unifoam		> 495(1977)[d]	BA	I II III IV	1-3 1-3 1-2 1-2	L:--/S:--
Azosulphamide 133-60-8	Chem. Abstr.: 6-(acetylamino)-3-((4-(aminosulphony)phenyl)azo)-4-hydroxy-2,7-naphthalene disulphonic acid, disodium salt IUPAC: 6-acetamido-4-hydroxy-3-[[p-sulphamoylphenyl)azo]-2,7-naphthalenedisulphonic acid, disodium salt Drometil; Leuconeoprontosil; Neoprontosil disodium salt; Prontosil S; Streptocid Rubrim; Streptozon S, II		0.05(1976I)[m*]	AN	--	--	L:--/S:--

Name and CAS Reg. No.	Synonyms and Trade Names	Structural Formula	US Production -Thousand Kg (Year)	Use Class [a]	Indus- tries	Pro- cesses	Reported Workplace Levels(L)/Occupational Standards(S)[b,q,r,s]
Benzidine 92-87-5	Chem. Abstr.: (1,1'-biphenyl)-4,4'-diamine; IUPAC: benzidine; p,p'-bianiline; 4,4'-bianiline; 4,4'-biphenyldiamine; CI Azoic Diazo Component 112; p,p'-diaminobiphenyl; 4,4'-diaminobiphenyl; Fast Corinth Base B	H_2N—(biphenyl)—NH_2	(Used in the past but has been discontinued by some countries)				
4,4'-Bis(sec-butylamino)-diphenyl-methane 5285-60-9	Chem. Abstr.: 4,4'-methylenebis-(N-(1-methylpropyl) benzenamine) IUPAC: 4,4'-methylenebis(N-sec-butylaniline)		> 2.2(1980)[c]	AN	--	--	L:--/S:--
Bis(cinnamylidene)hexamethylene-diamine 140-73-8	Chem. Abstr.: N,N'-Bis(3-phenyl-2-propenylidene)-1,6-hexanediamine IUPAC: N,N'-dicinnamylidene-1,6-hexanediamine Diak No. 3	$C_6H_5CH=CHCH=N(CH_2)_6N=CHCH=CH$	> 0.45(1979)[f]	A	III	1-2	L:--/S:--
n-Butyraldehyde-butylamine condensate 68411-19-8	Chem. Abstr.:-- IUPAC:--	$[CH_3CH_2CH_2C\!=\!NCH_2CH_2CH_2CH_3]_x$	>0.45(1979)[f]	A	--	--	L:--/S:--
Dibenzylamine 103-49-1	Chem. Abstr.: N-(phenylmethyl)-benzenemethanamine IUPAC: dibenzylamine N-benzylbenzylamine	CH_2NCH_2	>0.45(1979)[f]	A	II III	1-2 1-2	L:--/S:--
N,N'-Dimethyl-N,N'-dinitrosotere-phthalamide 133-55-1	Chem. Abstr.: N,N'-dimethyl-N,N'-dinitroso-1,4-benzenedicarboxamide IUPAC: N,N'-dimethyl-N,N'-dinitroso-terephthalamide BL 353; Nitrosan		270(1976)[c]	BA	--	--	L:--/S:--

Name and CAS Reg. No.	Synonyms and Trade Names	Structural Formula	US Production -Thousand Kg (Year)	Use Class [a]	Indus- tries	Pro- cesses	Reported Workplace Levels(L)/Occupational Standards(S)[b],[q],[r],[s]
Dimethylformamide 68-12-2	Chem. Abstr.: N,N-dimethylformamide IUPAC: N,N-dimethylformamide N,N-dimethylmethanamide; DMF; N-formyldimethylamine		4.5 (1979)[f]	S	I II III IV	1-3 1-3 1-2 1-2	L:--/S:-- 10-60 mg/m³ Ceiling (BUL, CZ,P,R,USSR,Y) 30-60 mg/m³ TWA (A,BEL,CZ,F,DDR, BRD,I,J,N,R, SWED,S,USA,USA-A) 60 mg/m³ STEL (USA-A, DOR)
N,N-Dimethyl-p-nitrosoaniline 138-89-6	Chem. Abstr.: N,N-dimethyl-4-nitroso-benzenamine IUPAC: N,N-dimethyl-p-nitrosoaniline p-(dimethylamino)nitrosobenzene; dimethyl(p-nitrosophenyl)amine; 4-nitrosodimethylaniline Accelerine		>45(1977)[d]	A	--	--	L:--/S:--
Dinitrosopentamethylenetetramine 101-25-7	Chem. Abstr.: 3,7-dinitroso-1,5,7-tetraazabicyclo(3.3.1)nonane IUPAC: 3,7-dinitroso-1,3,5,7-tetraazabicyclo(3.3.1)nonane 3,7-di-N-nitrosopentamethylene-tetramine DNPT; Opex 93, 141; Porofor DNO; Vulcacel BN, B-40, BN-94; Unicel ND, NDX, 100		> 0.45(1979)[f]	BA	I II III IV	1-3 1-3 1-2 1-2	L:--/S:--
3,7-Dioctylphenothiazine 6044-61-7	Chem. Abstr.: 3,7-dioctyl-10H-pheno-thiazine IUPAC: 3,7-dioctylphenothiazine		> 0.45(1976)[c]	M	--	--	L:--/S:--

Name and CAS Reg. No.	Synonyms and Trade Names	Structural Formula	US Production -Thousand Kg (Year)	Use Class [a]	Indus- tries	Pro- cesses	Reported Workplace Levels(L)/Occupational Standards(S)[b,q,r,s]
N-Ethylbenzylamine 14321-27-8	Chem. Abstr.: N-ethylbenzene-methanamine IUPAC: N-ethylbenzylamine benzylethylamine		> 0.5(1980WE)[c]	M	--	--	L:--/S:--
N-Ethyldibenzylamine 10479-25-1	Chem. Abstr.: N-ethyl-N-(phenylmethyl)-benzenemethanamine IUPAC: N-ethyldibenzylamine		> 0.5(1980WE)[c]	M	--	--	L:--/S:--
N-Methyl-N,4-dinitrosoaniline 99-80-9	Chem. Abstr.: N-methyl-N,4-di-nitrosobenzenamine IUPAC: N-methyl-N,p-dinitrosoaniline Elastopar; Heat Pre; Nitrosan K		(Used in the past but not believed to be currently used)				
4,4'-Methylenedicarbanilic acid, diphenyl ester 101-65-5	Chem. Abstr.: diphenyl(methylene-di-4-phenylene)bis[carbamate] IUPAC: diphenyl 4,4'-methylene-dicarbanilate diphenyl diphenylmethane-p,p'-di-carbamate; diphenyl N,N'-(methylene-bis(4-phenylene))dicarbamate; diphenyl(methylenedi-p-phenylene)di-carbamate Hylene MP		> 90(1977)[d]	B	I II III	1-3 1-3 1-2	L:--/S:--
N-(2-Methyl-2-nitropropyl)-4-nitrosoaniline 24458-48-8	Chem. Abstr.: N-(2-methyl-2-nitropropyl)-4-nitrosobenzenamine IUPAC: N-(2-methyl-2-nitropropyl)-p-nitrosoaniline Nitrol		450(1976)[c]	UN	--	--	L:--/S:--

Name and CAS Reg. No.	Synonyms and Trade Names	Structural Formula	US Production -Thousand Kg (Year)	Use Class [a]	Indus-tries	Pro-cesses	Reported Workplace Levels(L)/Occupational Standards(S) [b,q,r,s]
m-Phenylenebismaleimide 3006-93-7	Chem. Abstr.:1,1'-(1,3-phenylene)-bis[1H-pyrrole-2,5-dione] IUPAC: N,N'-m-phenylenedimaleimide 1,3-bismaleimidobenzene; 1,3-di-maleimidobenzene; m-phenylenedi-maleimide; HVA 2		>45(1977)[d]	A	II	1-2	L:--/S:--
Phenylhydrazine 100-63-0	Chem. Abstr.: phenylhydrazine IUPAC: phenylhydrazine hydrazinobenzene		289(1979I)[m]	BA	--	--	L:--/S: 22-25 mg/m^3 Ceiling (R,Y) 15-22 mg/m^3 TWA (A BEL,F,BRD,N,R,S, USA,USA-A) 45 ng/m^3 STEL (USA-A)
N-Phenyl-1-naphthylamine 90-30-2	Chem. Abstr.: N-phenyl-1-naphthalen-amine IUPAC: N-phenyl-1-naphthylamine phenyl-alpha-naphthylamine; Additin 30; Antioxidant PAN; Naugard PAN; Neozone; Nonox A, AN		>45(1977)[d]	AN	I II III IV	1-3 1-3 1-2 1-2	L:--/S:--
N-Phenyl-2-naphthylamine 135-88-6	Chem. Abstr.: N-phenyl-2-naphthalen-amine IUPAC: N-phenyl-2-naphthylamine 2-anilinonaphthalene; 2-naphthyl-phenylamine; 2-phenylaminonaphthalene; N-phenyl-β-naphthylamine; Aceto PBN; AgeRite Powder; Antioxidant PBN, 116; Neozone D; Nilox PENA; Nonox D, DN; Vulkanox PBN		709(1975)[f*]	AN	I II III	1-2 1-2 1-2	L:--/S:--

Name and CAS Reg. No.	Synonyms and Trade Names	Structural Formula	US Production -Thousand Kg (Year)	Use Class[a]	Indus-tries	Pro-cesses	Reported Workplace Levels(L)/Occupational Standards(S)[b,q,r,s]
Poly-p-dinitrosobenzene —	Chem. Abstr.: 1,4-dinitrosobenzene homopolymer IUPAC: p-dinitrosobenzene polymer		>0.45(1979)[f]	A	II	1-2	L:--/S:--
Pyridine 110-86-1	Chem. Abstr.: pyridine IUPAC: pyridine azabenzene; azine		>45(1977)[d]	S	--	--	L:--/S: 5-15 mg/m³ Ceiling (BUL, CZ, R, USSR, Y) 5-16 mg/m³ TWA (A, BEL, CZ, F, DDR, BRD, H, I, N, R, SWED, S, USA-A) 30-36 mg/m³ STEL (DDR, USA-A)
p-Toluenesulphonylhydrazide 1576-35-8	Chem. Abstr.: 4-methylbenzene-sulphonic acid, hydrazide IUPAC: p-toluenesulphonic acid, hydra-zide Celogen TSH; Tosylhydrazine		>2.2(1980)[c]	BA	I II III IV	1-3 1-3 1-2 1-2	L:--/S:--
Urea 57-13-6	Chem. Abstr.: urea IUPAC: urea carbamide BIK; Polymel Purca-, RIA, CS, NC; Ureaphil; Urevert; Varioform II		6,324,358 (1979)[e]	BA	I II III IV	1-3 1-3 1-2 1-2	L:--/S:--

B. Sulphur Compounds
1. Mercaptans

Name and CAS Reg. No.	Synonyms and Trade Names	Structural Formula	US Production -Thousand Kg (Year)	Use Class[a]	Indus-tries	Pro-cesses	Reported Workplace Levels(L)/Occupational Standards(S)[b,q,r,s]
Alkyl mercaptans, mixed --	Chem. Abstr.: -- IUPAC: --	RSH	>0.45(1979)[f]	PR	--	--	L:--/S:--
Amyl mercaptoacetate 6380-70-7	Chem. Abstr.: pentyl mercaptoacetate IUPAC: pentyl mercaptoacetate	$HSCH_2COC_5H_{11}$	>0.5(1980WE)[c]	A	--	--	L:--/S:--
Aryl mercaptans --	Chem. Abstr.: -- IUPAC: --	ArSH	45(1976)[c]	P	--	--	L:--/S:--
Cetyl-stearyl mercaptan 2917-26-2 and 2885-00-9	Chem. Abstr.: 1-hexadecanethiol and 1-octadecanethiol IUPAC: 1-hexadecanethiol and 1-octadecanethiol hexadecyl and octadecyl mercaptans	RSH $R = n-C_{16}H_{33}$ and $n-C_{18}H_{37}$	>0.5(1980WE)[c]	M	--	--	L:--/S:--
2,5-Dimercapto-1,3,4-thiadiazole 1072-71-5	Chem. Abstr.: 1,3,4-thiadiazolidine-2,5-dithione IUPAC: 1,3,4-thiadiazole-2,5-dithiol Bismuthiol I; PY 61H		>0.45(1979)[f]	A	--	--	L:--/S:--
Disodium 2,5-dimercapto-1,3,4-thiadiazole 55906-42-8	Chem. Abstr.: 1,3,4-thiadiazolidine-2,5-dithione, disodium salt IUPAC: disodium 1,3,4-thiadiazole-2,5-dithiolate		>2.2(1980)[c]	A	--	--	L:--/S:--
n-Dodecyl mercaptan 112-55-0	Chem. Abstr.: 1-dodecanethiol IUPAC: 1-dodecanethiol lauryl mercaptan; 1-mercaptododecane DDM 100	$CH_3(CH_2)_{11}SH$	7700(1976)[h]	PR	I II IV	1-3 1-3 1-2	L:--/S:--
tert-Dodecyl mercaptan 25103-58-6	Chem. Abstr.: tert-dodecanethiol IUPAC: tert-dodecanethiol tert-dodecylthiol 4-P Mercaptan; Sulfole 120	R_2CSH with R_1, R_3 $R_1 + R_2 + R_3 = C_{11}$	7700(1976)[h]	PR	I II IV	1-3 1-3 1-2	L:--/S: 5 mg/m^3 ceiling (USSR)

Name and CAS Reg. No.	Synonyms and Trade Names	Structural Formula	US Production -Thousand Kg (Year)	Use Class [a]	Indus-tries	Pro-cesses	Reported Workplace Levels(L)/Occupational Standards(S)[b,q,r,s]
Ethylene glycol bis(thioglycolate) 123-81-9	Chem. Abstr.: mercaptoacetic acid, 1,2-ethanediyl ester IUPAC: ethylene bis(mercapto-acetate) ethylene glycol dimercaptoacetate; glycol dimercaptoacetate	$$HSCH_2COCH_2CH_2OCCH_2SH$$ with O double bonds	> 0.45(1979)[f]	A	--	--	L:--/S:--
2-Ethylhexyl mercaptoacetate 7659-86-1	Chem. Abstr.: mercaptoacetic acid, 2-ethylhexyl ester IUPAC: 2-ethylhexylmercaptoacetate 2-ethylhexyl thioglycolate	$$HSCH_2COCH_2CHCH_2CH_2CH_2CH_3$$ with CH_2CH_3	> 2.2(1980)[c]	AN	--	--	L:--/S:--
tert-Hexadecyl mercaptan 25360-09-2	Chem. Abstr.: tert-hexadecanethiol IUPAC: tert-hexadecanethiol	$R_2 - C SH$ with R_1, R_3; $R_1 + R_2 + R_3 = C_{15}$	> 0.45(1979)[f]	PR	--	--	L:--/S:--
n-Hexyl mercaptan 111-31-9	Chem. Abstr.: 1-hexanethiol IUPAC: 1-hexanethiol hexyl mercaptan	$CH_3(CH_2)_5SH$	> 0.45(1979)[f**]	PR	--	--	L:--/S:--
2-Mercaptothiazoline 96-53-7	Chem. Abstr.: 2-thiazolidinethione IUPAC: 2-thiazoline-2-thiol Metabasal; Thyroidan	SH, N ring	> 1.5(1980WE)[c]	A	--	--	L:--/S:--
n-Octyl mercaptan 111-88-6	Chem. Abstr.: 1-octanethiol IUPAC: 1-octanethiol 1-mercaptooctane; octylthiol NOM	$CH_3(CH_2)_7SH$	900(1976)[g]	PR	--	--	L:--/S:--
tert-Octyl mercaptan 141-59-3	Chem. Abstr.: 2,4,4-trimethyl-2-pentanethiol IUPAC: 2,4,4-trimethyl-2-pentanethiol tert-octylthiol; 1,1,3,3-tetramethyl-1-butanethiol TOM	CH_3CCH_2CSH with CH_3 groups	900(1976)[g]	PR	I 1-3 II 1-3 IV 1-2		L:--/S:--

Name and CAS Reg. No.	Synonyms and Trade Names	Structural Formula	US Production -Thousand Kg (Year)	Use Class[a]	Indus-tries	Pro-cesses	Reported Workplace Levels(L)/Occupational Standards(S)[b,q,r,s]
Pentachlorobenzenethiol 133-49-3	Chem. Abstr.: pentachlorobenzenethiol; IUPAC: pentachlorobenzenethiol pentachlorothiophenol		>45(1977)[d]	P	I II	1-2 1-2	L:--/S:--
Pentachlorothiophenol, zinc salt 117-97-5	Chem. Abstr.: pentachlorobenzenethiol, zinc salt; IUPAC: zinc bis(pentachlorobenzene-thiolate) zinc pentachlorothiophenate; Endor; Renacit IV, VIII; Reptazin Zn; Saginol		230(1976)[c]	P	I II III IV	1-3 1-3 1-2 1-2	L:--/S:--
n-Tetradecyl mercaptan 2079-95-0	Chem. Abstr.: 1-tetradecanethiol; IUPAC: 1-tetradecanethiol myristyl mercaptan	$CH_3(CH_2)_{13}SH$	>4.5(1980)[c]	PR	--	--	L:--/S:--
p-Thiocresol 106-45-6	Chem. Abstr.: 4-methylbenzenethiol; IUPAC: p-toluenethiol 1-mercapto-4-methylbenzene; 4-toluenethiol; p-tolyl mercaptan		> 0.5(1980WE)[c]	PR	--	--	L:--/S:--
Tridecyl mercaptan 19484-26-5	Chem. Abstr.: 1-tridecanethiol; IUPAC: 1-tridecanethiol mixed primary tridecyl mercaptan PTM	$C_{12}H_{25}-CH_2SH$	> 2.2(1980)[c]	PR	--	--	L:--/S:--
Xylenethiol 25550-52-1	Chem. Abstr.: dimethylbenzenethiol; IUPAC: xylenethiol xylyl mercaptan		> 0.45 (1977)[d]	P	--	--	L:--/S:--

2. Thiocarbamates

Name and CAS Reg. No.	Synonyms and Trade Names	Structural Formula	US Production -Thousand Kg (Year)	Use Class [a]	Indus-tries	Pro-cesses	Reported Workplace Levels(L)/Occupational Standards(S)[b,q,r,s]
Activated dithiocarbamates --	Chem. Abstr.: -- IUPAC: -- Setsit 5,9,51,104	Indefinite	> 0.45(1976)[f]*	A	I II III IV	1-3 1-3 1-2 1-2	L:--/S:--
Carbon disulphide and 1,1'-methylenedipiperidine (reaction product) 75-15-0 and 880-09-1	Chem. Abstr.: 1,1'-methylenebis-(piperidine) reaction product with carbon disulphide IUPAC: 1,1'-methylenedipiperidine reaction product with carbon disulphide R-2 Crystals	Indefinite	>2.2(1980)[c]	A	--	--	L:--/S:--
Diamyldithiocarbamic acid, diamylammonium salt --	Chem. Abstr.: dipentylcarbamodithioic acid, compound with N-pentyl-1-penta-mine IUPAC: dipentyldithiocarbamic acid, compound with dipentylamine	C_5H_{11} $\backslash$ $NC-S^-$ $[C_5H_{11})_2NH_2^+$ / S / C_5H_{11} /	> 0.5(1980WE)[c]	A	--	--	L:--/S:--
Diamyldithiocarbamic acid, zinc salt 15337-18-5	Chem. Abstr.: bis(dipentylcarbamodithioato-S,S')zinc IUPAC: bis(dipentyldithiocarbamato)zinc dipentyldithiocarbamic acid, zinc salt; zinc dipentyldithiocarbamate Amyl Zimate; Vanlube AZ	$\left[\begin{array}{c} C_5H_{11} \\ C_5H_{11} \end{array} NC-S^- \right]_2 Zn^{++}$	> 04.5(1980)[c]	A	I II III IV	1-3 1-3 1-2 1-2	L:--/S:--
Dibenzyldithiocarbamic acid, sodium salt 55310-46-8	Chem. Abstr.: bis(phenylmethyl)carbamodithioic acid, sodium salt IUPAC: sodium dibenzyldithio-carbamate	(dibenzyl structure) NCS^-Na^+	> 4.5(1977)[d]	A	--	--	L:--/S:--

Name and CAS Reg. No.	Synonyms and Trade Names	Structural Formula	US Production -Thousand Kg (Year)	Use Class[a]	Indus-tries	Pro-cesses	Reported Workplace Levels(L)/Occupational Standards(S)[b,q,r,s]
Dibenzyldithiocarbamic acid, zinc salt 14726-36-4	Chem. Abstr.: bis[bis(phenylmethyl)-carbamodithioato-S,S']zinc IUPAC: bis(dibenzyldithiocarbamato)-zinc zinc dibenzyldithiocarbamate Arazate		> 4.5(1977)[d]	A	I II III IV	1-3 1-3 1-2 1-2	L:--/S:--
Dibutyldithiocarbamic acid, cadmium salt 14566-86-0	Chem. Abstr.: bis(dibutylcarbamodi-thioato-S,S')cadmium IUPAC: bis(dibutyldithiocarbamato)-cadmium cadmium dibutyldithiocarbamate		> 0.5(1980WE)[c]	A	--	--	L:--/S:--
Dibutyldithiocarbamic acid, N,N-dimethylcyclohexylamine salt 149-82-6	Chem. Abstr.: dibutylcarbamodithioic acid compound with N,N-dimethyl-cyclohexanamine (1:1) IUPAC: dibutyldithiocarbamic acid compound with N,N-dimethylcyclo-hexylamine (1:1) N,N-dimethylcyclohexylammonium dibutyldithiocarbamate RZ50B, -100		> 0.45(1977)[f]**	A	I II III IV	1-3 1-3 1-2 1-2	L:--/S:--
Di-n-butyldithiocarbamic acid, molybdenum salt 68412-26-0	Chem. Abstr.: bis(dibutylcarbamodi-thioato)di-μ-oxodioxodimolybdenum, sulphurized IUPAC: bis(dibutyldithiocarbamato)di-μ-oxodioxodimolybdenum, sulphurized Molyvan A		> 2.2(1980)[c]	A	--	--	L:--/S:--
Dibutyldithiocarbamic acid, nickel salt 13927-77-0	Chem. Abstr.: bis(dibutylcarbamodi-thioato-S,S')nickel IUPAC: bis(dibutyldithiocarbamato)-nickel nickel dibutyldithiocarbamate Rylex NBC		>45(1977)[d]	A,AN	II	1-2	L:--/S:--

Name and CAS Reg. No.	Synonyms and Trade Names	Structural Formula	US Production –Thousand Kg (Year)	Use Class [a]	Indus-tries	Pro-cesses	Reported Workplace Levels(L)/Occupational Standards(S) [b,q,r,s]
Dibutyldithiocarbamic acid, potassium salt 136-29-8	Chem. Abstr.: dibutyl carbamodithioic acid, potassium salt; IUPAC: potassium dibutyldithiocarbamate	$[CH_3(CH_2)_3]_2 N-C(=S)-S^-\ K^+$	> 2.2(1980) [c]	A	--	--	L:--/S:--
Dibutyldithiocarbamic acid, sodium salt 136-30-1	Chem. Abstr.: dibutylcarbamo-dithioic acid, sodium salt; IUPAC: sodium dibutyldithio-carbamate	$[CH_3(CH_2)_3]_2 N-C(=S)-S^-\ Na^+$	> 50.4(1977) [d]	A	IV	1-2	L:--/S:--
Dibutyldithiocarbamic acid, zinc salt 136-23-2	Butidone; Butyl Namate; Pennac SDB; Tepidone; Vulcacure NB-25 Chem. Abstr.: bis(dibutylcarbamo-dithioato-S,S')zinc; IUPAC: bis(dibutyldithiocarbamato)-zinc Aceto ZDBD; Butazate 50-D; Butazin; Butyl Zimate; Butyl Ziram; S Oxinol BZ; Vulcacure ZB; Vulkacit LDB	$\left[[CH_3(CH_2)_3]_2 N-C(=S)-S^- \right]_2 Zn^{++}$	>104(1977) [d]	A	I II III IV	1-3 1-3 1-2 1-2	L:--/S:--
Diethyldithiocarbamic acid, ammonium salt 21124-33-4	Chem. Abstr.: diethylcarbamodithioic acid, ammonium salt; IUPAC: ammonium diethyldithio-carbamate	$(CH_3CH_2)_2 N-C(=S)-S^-\ NH_4^+$	> 0.5(1980WE) [c]	A	--	--	L:--/S:--
Diethyldithiocarbamic acid, cadmium salt 14239-68-0	Chem. Abstr.: bis(diethylcarbamodithio-ato-S,S')cadmium; IUPAC: bis(diethyldithiocarbamato)-cadmium cadmium diethyldithiocarbamate Cadmate	$\left[(CH_3CH_2)_2 N-C(=S)-S^- \right]_2 Cd^{++}$	> 0.5(1980WE) [c]	A	I II III IV	1-3 1-3 1-2 1-2	L:--/S:--
Diethyldithiocarbamic acid, cadmium salt and bis(diethyl-thiocarbamoyl) disulphide mixture 14239-68-0 and 97-77-8	Chem. Abstr.: bis(diethylcarbamo-dithioato-S,S')cadmium and tetra-ethylthioperoxydicarbonic diamide-[((CH₂)₂N)C(S)]₂S₂]; IUPAC: bis(diethyldithiocarbamato)-cadmium and bis(diethylthiocarbamoyl) disulphide	$\left[(CH_3CH_2)_2 N-C(=S)-S^- \right]_2 Cd^{++}$ + $(CH_3CH_2)_2 NCSSCN(CH_2CH_3)_2$	>0.45(1979) [f]	A	--	--	L:--/S:--

Name and CAS Reg. No.	Synonyms and Trade Names	Structural Formula	US Production -Thousand Kg (Year)	Use Class [a]	Indus-tries	Pro-cesses	Reported Workplace Levels(L)/Occupational Standards(S)[b,q,r,s]
Diethyldithiocarbamic acid, nickel salt 14267-17-5	Chem. Abstr.: bis(diethylcarbamodi-thioato-S,S')nickel; IUPAC: bis(diethyldithiocarbamato)-nickel; nickel diethyldithiocarbamate	$[(CH_3CH_2)_2NCS_2]_2 Ni^{++}$	> 0.5(1980WE)[c]	A	--	--	L:--/S:--
Diethyldithiocarbamic acid, selenium salt 21559-14-8	Chem. Abstr.: tetrakis(diethylcar-bamodithioato-S,S')selenium; IUPAC: tetrakis(diethyldithiocar-bamato)selenium; selenium diethyldithiocarbamate; Ethyl Selenac	$[(CH_3CH_2)_2NCS_2]_4 Se^{++++}$	>0.45(1979)[f]	A	I II III IV	1-3 1-3 1-2 1-2	L:--/S:--
Diethyldithiocarbamic acid, sodium salt 148-18-5	Chem. Abstr.: diethylcarbamo-dithioic acid, sodium salt; IUPAC: sodium diethyldithio-carbamate; Thiocarb	$(CH_3CH_2)_2NCS_2^- \; Na^+$	> 5.8(1977)[d]	A	IV	1-2	L:--/S:--
Diethyldithiocarbamic acid, tellurium salt 20941-65-5	Chem. Abstr.: tetrakis(diethyl-carbamodithioato- S,S')tellurium; IUPAC: tetrakis(diethyldithiocar-bamato)tellurium; Ethyl Tellurac	$[(CH_3CH_2)_2NCS_2]_4 Te^{++++}$	>0.45(1979)[f]	A	I II	1-3 1-3	L:--/S:--
Diethyldithiocarbamic acid, zinc salt 14324-55-1	Chem. Abstr.: bis(diethylcarbamo-dithioato-S,S')zinc; IUPAC: bis(diethyldithiocarbamato)-zinc; zinc diethyldithiocarbamate; Etazin; Ethazate; Ethazate 50-D; Ethyl Cymate; Ethyl Zimate; Ethyl Ziram; Hermat ZDK; Vulcacure ZE; Vulkacit ZDK, LDA	$[(CH_3CH_2)_2NCS_2]_2 Zn^{++}$	775(1979)[f]	A	I II III IV	1-3 1-3 1-2 1-2	L:--/S:--
Diisobutyl dithiocarbamic acid, nickel salt 15317-78-9	Chem. Abstr.: bis[bis(2-methylpropyl)-carbamodithioato-S,S']nickel; IUPAC: bis(diisobutyldithio-carbamato)nickel; Isobutyl Niclate	$[((CH_3)_2CHCH_2)_2NCS_2]_2 Ni^{++}$	> 2.2(1980)[c]	A,AN	--	--	L:--/S:--

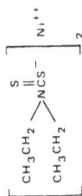

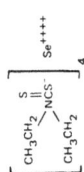

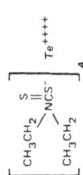

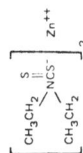

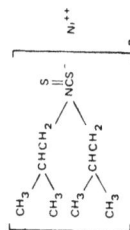

Name and CAS Reg. No.	Synonyms and Trade Names	Structural Formula	US Production -Thousand Kg (Year)	Use Class[a]	Indus-tries	Pro-cesses	Reported Workplace Levels(L)/Occupational Standards(S)[b,q,r,s]
Dimethyldithiocarbamic acid bismuth salt 21260-46-8	Chem. Abstr.: tris(dimethylcarbamo-dithioato-S,S')bismuth IUPAC: tris(dimethyldithiocarbamato)-bismuth bismuth dimethyldithiocarbamate Bismate	$\left[\begin{array}{c} CH_3 \\ CH_3 \end{array} N \overset{S}{\underset{NCS^-}{\|}} \right]_3 Bi^{+++}$	> 0.45(1979)[f]	A	I II III IV	1-3 1-3 1-2 1-2	L:--/S:--
Dimethyldithiocarbamic acid, cadmium salt 14949-60-1	Chem. Abstr.: cadmium bis(dimethyl-carbamodithioate) IUPAC: cadmium bis(dimethyldi-thiocarbamate) cadmium dimethyldithiocarbamate	$\left[\begin{array}{c} CH_3 \\ CH_3 \end{array} N \overset{S}{\underset{NCS^-}{\|}} \right]_2 Cd^{++}$	>1(1980WE)[c]	A	--	--	L:--/S:--
Dimethyldithiocarbamic acid, copper salt 137-29-1	Chem. Abstr.: bis(dimethylcarbamo-dithioato-S,S')copper IUPAC: bis(dimethyldithio-carbamato)copper copper dimethyldithiocarbamate Cumate; Hermat Cu; Wolfen	$\left[\begin{array}{c} CH_3 \\ CH_3 \end{array} N \overset{S}{\underset{NCS^-}{\|}} \right]_2 Cu^{++}$	>0.45(1979)[f]	A	I II IV	1-3 1-3 1-2	L:--/S:--
Dimethyldithiocarbamic acid, lead salt 19010-66-3	Chem. Abstr.: bis(dimethylcarbamo-dithioato-S,S')lead IUPAC: bis(dimethyldithio-carbamato)lead lead dimethyldithiocarbamate Ledate; Methyl Ledate	$\left[\begin{array}{c} CH_3 \\ CH_3 \end{array} N \overset{S}{\underset{NCS^-}{\|}} \right]_2 Pb^{++}$	>0.45(1979)[f]	A	I II III IV	1-3 1-3 1-2 1-2	L:--/S:--
Dimethyldithiocarbamic acid, dimethylammonium salt 2614-98-4	Chem. Abstr.: dimethylcarbamodi-thioic acid compound with N-methylmethananine (1:1) IUPAC: dimethyldithiocarbamic acid compound with dimethylamine (1:1) dimethylamine dimethyldithiocarbamate	$\begin{array}{c} CH_3 \\ CH_3 \end{array} N \overset{S}{\underset{NCS^-}{\|}} (CH_3)_2NH_2^+$	> 0.45(1978)[f***]	A	--	--	L:--/S:--

Name and CAS Reg. No.	Synonyms and Trade Names	Structural Formula	US Production -Thousand Kg (Year)	Use Class[a]	Indus-tries	Pro-cesses	Reported Workplace Levels(L)/Occupational Standards(S)[b,q,r,s]
Dimethyldithiocarbamic acid, potassium salt 128-03-0	Chem. Abstr.: dimethylcarbamodi-thioic acid, potassium salt; IUPAC: potassium dimethyldithio-carbamate; Vulnopol KM	CH_3 / N–C(=S)–NCS^- K^+	>45(1977)[d]	PR	I II III IV	1-3 1-3 1-2 1-2	L:--/S:--
Dimethyldithiocarbamic acid, selenium salt 144-34-3	Chem. Abstr.: tetrakis(dimethyl-carbamodithioato-S,S')selenium; IUPAC: tetrakis(dimethyldithio-carbamato)selenium; selenium dimethyldithiocarbamate; Methyl Selenac	$[CH_3$ / N–C(=S)–$NCS^-]_4$ Se^{++++}	>0.45(1979)[f]	A	I II III IV	1-3 1-3 1-2 1-2	L:--/S:--
Dimethyldithiocarbamic acid, sodium salt 128-04-1	Chem. Abstr.: dimethylcarbamodi-thioic acid, sodium salt; IUPAC: sodium dimethyldithio-carbamate; Aceto SDD 40; Alcobam NM; Diram; NSL; Sharstop 204; Sodam; Thiostop N; Volnopol NM; Wing Stop B	CH_3 / N–C(=S)–NCS^- Na^+	>1,530(1977)[d]	PR	I II III IV	1-3 1-3 1-2 1-2	L:--/S:--
Dimethyldithiocarbamic acid, sodium salt and sodium polysulphide 128-04-1 and 1344-08-7	Chem. Abstr.: sodium dimethyl-carbamodithioate and sodium poly-sulphide (Na_2S_x); IUPAC: sodium dimethyldithio-carbamate and sodium polysulphide	CH_3 / N–C(=S)–NCS^- Na^+ + Na_2S_x	>0.45(1979)[f]	A	--	--	L:--/S:--
Dimethyldithiocarbamic acid, zinc salt 137-30-4	Chem. Abstr.: bis(dimethylcarbamo-dithioato-S,S')zinc; IUPAC: bis(dimethyldithiocarbamato)-zinc; zinc bis(dimethyldithiocarbamate); Methasan; Methazate; Methyl Zimate; Methyl Ziram; Vulcacure ZM-45; Vulkacit L; Ziram	$[CH_3$ / N–C(=S)–$NCS^-]_2$ Zn^{++}	1,694(1979)[f]	A	I II III IV	1-3 1-3 1-2 1-2	L:--/S:--

Name and CAS Reg. No.	Synonyms and Trade Names	Structural Formula	US Production -Thousand Kg (Year)	Use Class[a]	Indus- tries	Pro- cesses	Reported Workplace Levels(L)/Occupational Standards(S)[b,q,r,s]
2,4-Dinitrophenyl dimethyldithiocarbamate 89-37-2	Chem. Abstr.: dimethylcarbamodithioic acid, 2,4-dinitrophenyl ester IUPAC: 2,4-dinitrophenyl dimethyldithiocarbamate		>0.45(1978)[f]***	A	--	--	L:--/S:--
Dipentyldithiocarbamic acid, lead salt 36501-84-5	Chem. Abstr.: bis(dipentylcarbamodithioato-S,S')lead IUPAC: bis(dipentyldithiocarbamato)lead diamyldithiocarbamic acid, lead salt; lead dipentyldithiocarbamate		>2.2(1980)[c]	A	--	--	L:--/S:--
Ethylenebis(dithiocarbamic acid), disodium salt 142-59-6	Chem. Abstr.: 1,2-ethanediylbis-carbamodithioic acid, disodium salt IUPAC: disodium ethylenebis(dithiocarbamate) Chem Bam; Dithane A40, D14; Nabam; Nafun IPO; Parzate		>0.9(1979)[f]	A	--	--	L:--/S:--
Ethylphenyldithiocarbamic acid, zinc salt 14634-93-6	Chem. Abstr.: bis(ethylphenylcarbamodithioato-S,S')zinc IUPAC: bis(N-ethyldithiocarbanilato) zinc ethylphenyldithiocarbamate Accelerator EFK; Hermat FEDK; Vulkacit P extra N		15(1979I)[m]	A	I II III IV	1-3 1-3 1-2 1-2	L:--/S:--
Monoethyl dithiocarbamic acid, sodium salt 13036-87-8	Chem. Abstr.: ethylcarbamodithioic acid, monosodium salt IUPAC: sodium ethyldithiocarbamate sodium ethyldithiocarbamate		0.5(1980WE)[c]	A	--	--	L:--/S:--
Nitro-pentamethylenedithiocarbamic acid, zinc salt --	Chem. Abstr.: bis(nitro-1-piperidine-carbodithioato-S,S') zinc IUPAC: bis(nitro-1-piperidinecarbo-dithioato) zinc		0.6(1976I)[m]*	A	--	--	L:--/S:--

Name and CAS Reg. No.	Synonyms and Trade Names	Structural Formula	US Production -Thousand Kg (Year)	Use Class [a]	Indus-tries	Pro-cesses	Reported Workplace Levels(L)/Occupational Standards(S)[b,q,r,s]
Pentamethylenedithiocarbamic acid, copper salt 15225-85-1	Chem. Abstr.: bis(1-piperidinecarbodithioato-S,S')copper; IUPAC: bis(1-piperidinecarbodithioato)-copper; copper pentamethylenedithiocarbamate; piperidinecarbodithioic acid, copper salt	$[\mathrm{N{-}CS^-}]_2\,Cu^{++}$	>0.5(1980WE)[c]	A	--	--	L:--/S:--
Pentamethylenedithiocarbamic acid, lead salt 41556-46-1	Chem. Abstr.: bis(1-piperidinecarbodithioato-S,S')lead; IUPAC: bis(1-piperidinecarbodithioato)-lead; lead pentamethylenedithiocarbamate; piperidinecarbodithioic acid, lead salt	$[\mathrm{N{-}CS^-}]_2\,Pb^{++}$	> 0.5(1980WE)[c]	A	--	--	L:--/S:--
Pentamethylenedithiocarbamic acid, zinc salt 13878-54-1	Chem. Abstr.: bis(1-piperidinecarbodithioato-S,S')zinc; IUPAC: bis(1-piperidinecarbodithioato)-zinc; zinc pentamethylenedithiocarbamate; Vulkacit ZP	$[\mathrm{N{-}CS^-}]_2\,Zn^{++}$	> 1.5(1980WE)[c]	A	IV	1-2	L:--/S:--
Piperidinecarbodithioic acid, piperidinium potassium salts 98-77-1 and --	Chem. Abstr.: 1-piperidinecarbodithioic acid compound with piperidine (1:1) and potassium 1-piperidine-carbodithioate; IUPAC: 1-piperidinecarbodithioic acid compound with piperidine (1:1) and potassium 1-piperidine-carbodithioate; PMP (accelerator)	$[\mathrm{N{-}CS^-}]_2 \cdot H_2N^+ \cdot K^+$	>0.45(1979)[f]	A	--	--	L:--/S:--

Name and CAS Reg. No.	Synonyms and Trade Names	Structural Formula	US Production -Thousand Kg (Year)	Use Class[a]	Indus- tries	Pro- cesses	Reported Workplace Levels(L)/Occupational Standards(S)[b,q,r,s]

3. Benzothiazoles
   a. Sulphenamides

N-t-Butyl-2-benzothiazole-sulphenamide 95-31-8	Chem. Abstr.: N-(1,1-dimethylethyl)-2-benzothiazolesulphenamide IUPAC: N-tert-butyl-2-benzo-thiazolesulphenamide TBBS Delac NS; Norceler NS; Pennac; Santocure NS; Vulkacit NZ		>45(1977)[d]	A	I II III IV	1-3 1-3 1-2 1-2	L:--/S:--
N-Cyclohexyl-2-benzothiazolyl-sulphenamide 95-33-0	Chem. Abstr.: N-cyclohexyl-2-benzothiazolesulphenamide IUPAC: N-cyclohexyl-2-benzo-thiazolesulphenamide Accelerator CZ; Conac A, S; Curax; Cydac; Delac S; Ekagam; Nocceler CZ; Pennac CBS; Rhodifax 16; Royal CBTS; Santocure; Sulfenax CB, CB 30, TSB; Vulkacite CZ; Vulcafor CBS		2,403(1979)[f]	A	I II III IV	1-3 1-3 1-2 1-2	L:--/S:--
N,N-Dicyclohexyl-2-benzothiazolyl-sulphenamide 4979-32-2	Chem. Abstr.: N,N-dicyclohexyl-2-benzothiazolesulphenamide IUPAC: N,N-dicyclohexyl-2-benzo-thiazolesulphenamide Vulkacit DZ, D2		85(1979)[m]	A	I II III IV	1-3 1-3 1-2 1-2	L:--/S:--

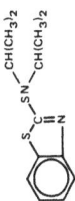

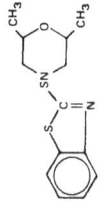

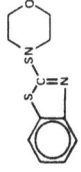

Name and CAS Reg. No.	Synonyms and Trade Names	Structural Formula	US Production -Thousand Kg (Year)	Use Class [a]	Indus-tries	Pro-cesses	Reported Workplace Levels(L)/Occupational Standards(S) b,q,r,s
N,N-Diisopropyl-2-benzothiazole-sulphenamide 95-29-4	Chem. Abstr.: N,N-bis(1-methylethyl)-2-benzothiazolesulphenamide IUPAC: N,N-diisopropyl-2-benzo-thiazolesulphenamide DIBS Dipac; Dipak		>0.45(1979) [f]	A	I II III IV	1-3 1-3 1-2 1-2	L:--/S:--
N-(2,6-Dimethylmorpholino)-2-benzo-thiazole sulphenamide 102-78-3	Chem. Abstr.: N-(2,6-dimethyl-4-morpho-linyl)-2-benzothiazolesulphenamide IUPAC: N-(2,6-dimethylmorpholino)-2-benzothiazolesulphenamide 2-(2,6-dimethyl-4-morpholinothio)-benzothiazole Santocure 26		> 0.45(1978) [f***]	A	--	--	L:--/S:--
N-Oxydiethylene-2-benzothiazole-sulphenamide 102-77-2	Chem. Abstr.: 4-(2-benzothiazolyl-thio)morpholine IUPAC: 2-(morpholinothio)benzo-thiazole 2-(4-morpholinylmercapto)benzo-thiazole Amax; NOBS Special; Nocceler MSA; Santocure MOR; Sulfenamide M; Sulfenax MODR; Vulkacit MOZ; Vulcafor BSM		> 9.9(1979) [f]	A	I II III IV	1-3 1-3 1-2 1-2	L:--/S:--

b. Miscellaneous

Name and CAS Reg. No.	Synonyms and Trade Names	Structural Formula	US Production -Thousand Kg (Year)	Use Class[a]	Indus-tries	Pro-cesses	Reported Workplace Levels(L)/Occupational Standards(S)[b,q,r,s]
2-Benzothiazyl-N,N-diethylthio-carbamoyl sulphide 95-30-7	Chem. Abstr.: diethylcarbamo-dithioic acid, 2-benzothiazolyl ester IUPAC: 2-benzothiazolyl diethyl-dithiocarbamate Ethylac		0.4(1979I)[m]	A	II	1-2	L:--/S:--
1 3-Bis(2-benzothiazolylmercapto-methyl)urea 95-35-2	Chem. Abstr.: N,N'-bis[(2-benzo-thiazolylthio)methyl]urea IUPAC: 1,3-bis[(2-benzothiazolylthio)-methyl]urea		> 0.45(1979)[f]	A	--	--	L:--/S:--
2,2'-Dithiobis(benzothiazole) 120-78-5	Chem. Abstr.: 2,2'-dithiobis-benzothiazole IUPAC: 2,2'-dithiobis(benzothiazole) mercaptobenzothiazole disulphide Accel TM; Altax; Ekagam GS; MBTS; Royal MBTS; Thiofide (MBTS); Vulkacit DM		7,454(1979)[f]	A	I II III IV	1-3 1-3 1-2 1-2	L:--/S:--

Name and CAS Reg. No.	Synonyms and Trade Names	Structural Formula	US Production -Thousand Kg (Year)	Use Class [a]	Indus- tries	Pro- cesses	Reported Workplace Levels(L)/Occupational Standards(S) [b,q,r,s]
2-Mercaptobenzothiazole 149-30-4	Chem. Abstr.: 2(3H)-benzothiazole-thione IUPAC: 2-benzothiazolethiol MBT Accelerator M; Captax; Ekagam C; Pennac MBT; Preumax MBT; Thiotax; Vulkacit M		>90(1977)[d]	A	I II III IV	1-3 1-3 1-2 1-2	L:--/S:--
2-Mercaptobenzothiazole, copper salt 4162-43-0	Chem. Abstr.: 2(3H)-benzothiazole-thione, copper(2+) salt IUPAC: copper(2+) bis(2-benzothiazole-thiolate) copper mercaptobenzothiazolate; copper 2-mercaptobenzothiazole	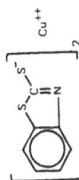	> 0.45(1979)[f]	A	--	--	L:--/S:--
2-Mercaptobenzothiazole, sodium salt 2492-26-4	Chem. Abstr.: 2(3H)-benzothiazole-thione, sodium salt IUPAC: sodium 2-benzothiazolethiolate sodium 2-mercaptobenzothiazole Duodex; Nacap		6,639(1979)[f]	A	--	--	L:--/S:--
2-Mercaptobenzothiazole, zinc chloride 149-30-4 and 7646-85-7	Chem. Abstr.: 2(3H)-benzothiazole-thione and zinc chloride IUPAC: 2-benzothiazolethiol and zinc chloride Caytur 4	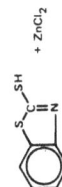	>0.45(1979)[f]	A	II III	1-3 1-2	L:--/S:--

Name and CAS Reg. No.	Synonyms and Trade Names	Structural Formula	US Production -Thousand Kg (Year)	Use Class[a]	Indus-tries	Pro-cesses	Reported Workplace Levels(L)/Occupational Standards(S)[b,q,r,s]
2-Mercaptobenzothiazole, zinc salt 155-04-4	Chem. Abstr.: 2(3H)-benzothiazole-thione, zinc salt IUPAC: zinc bis(2-benzothiazole-thiolate) zinc mercaptobenzothiazolate Pennac ZT; O-X-A-F; Vulkaat ZM; Zetax; ZMBT		927(1979)[f]	A	I II III IV	1-3 1-3 1-2 1-2	L:--/S:--
4-Morpholinyl-2-benzothiazyl disulphide 95-32-9	Chem. Abstr.: 2-(4-morpholinyl-dithio)benzothiazole IUPAC: 2-(morpholinodithio)-benzothiazole 2-benzothiazolylmorpholino disulphide Morfax; Vulcuren 2		>450(1977)[d]	A	I II III IV	1-3 1-3 1-2 1-2	L:--/S:--

4. Xanthates

Name and CAS Reg. No.	Synonyms and Trade Names	Structural Formula	US Production -Thousand Kg (Year)	Use Class[a]	Indus-tries	Pro-cesses	Reported Workplace Levels(L)/Occupational Standards(S)[b,q,r,s]
Di-n-butylxantho disulphide 105-77-1	Chem. Abstr.: dibutyl thioperoxydi-carbonate [((HO)C(S))₂S2] IUPAC: O,O-dibutyl dithiobis[thioformate] dibutyl dixanthogen; dibutylxanthogen CPB	$\left[CH_3(CH_2)_3OC\overset{S}{\parallel}S \right]_2$	≥4.5(1977)[d]	A	I II III IV	1-3 1-3 1-2 1-2	L:--/S:--
Diisopropylxantho disulphide 105-65-7	Chem. Abstr.: bis(1-methylethyl) thioperoxy-dicarbononate [((HO)C(S))₂S2] IUPAC: O,O-diisopropyl dithiobis [thioformate] bis(2-propyl) dixanthogen; diisopropyl-xanthogen disulphide Diproxid	$\left[(CH_3)_2CHOC\overset{S}{\parallel}S \right]_2$	>0.45(1979)[f]	A	--	--	L:--/S:--
Zinc diisopropyl xanthate 42590-53-4	Chem. Abstr.: zinc bis[O-(1-methyl-ethyl)carbonodithioate] IUPAC: zinc bis(O-isopropyl dithio-carbamate)	$\left[(CH_3)_2CHOC\overset{S}{\parallel}S^- \right]_2 Zn^{++}$	> 0.45(1979)[f]	A	--	--	L:--/S:--

Name and CAS Reg. No.	Synonyms and Trade Names	Structural Formula	US Production -Thousand Kg (Year)	Use Class a	Indus- tries	Pro- cesses	Reported Workplace Levels(L)/Occupational Standards(S) b,q,r,s
5. Sulphides and Disulphides a. Thioethers							
Alkylphenolsulphides --	Chem. Abstr.: -- IUPAC: --	Unknown	2.7(1979)^m	A	--	--	L:--/S:--
p-t-Amylphenol sulphide 98-26-0	Chem. Abstr.: 2,2'-thiobis[4-(1,1-dimethylpropyl)phenol] IUPAC: 2,2'-thiobis[4-tert-pentylphenol]		900(1976)^c	T	--	--	L:--/S:--
4,4'Thiobis(6-t-butyl-m-cresol) 96-69-5	Chem. Abstr.: 4,4'-thiobis[2-(1,1-dimethylethyl)]-5-methylphenol IUPAC: 4,4'-thiobis(6-tert-butyl-m-cresol) 4,4'-thiobis(2-tert-butyl-5-methyl phenol) Disperol MB-61; Santonox; Santowhite Crystals; Thioalkofen; Thioalkophene; Yoshinox S,SR		1,800(1972)^c	AN	II III IV	1-2 1-2 1-2	L:--/S: 10 mg/m^3 TWA (A,BEL,N,USA-A) 20 mg/m^3 STEL (USA-A)

Name and CAS Reg. No.	Synonyms and Trade Names	Structural Formula	US Production -Thousand Kg (Year)	Use Class [a]	Indus- tries	Pro- cesses	Reported Workplace Levels(L)/Occupational Standards(S)[b,q,r,s]
Thiobisphenol 2664-63-3	Chem. Abstr.: 4,4'-thiobis[phenol] IUPAC: 4,4'-thiodiphenol p,p'-dihydroxydiphenyl sulphide; bis(4-hydroxyphenyl)sulphide		> 2.2(1980)[c]	AN	--	--	L:--/S:--
Thiobisphenol, alkylated ---	Chem. Abstr.: -- IUPAC: --	Indefinite	>0.45(1979)[f]	AN	--	--	L:--/S:--

b. Thiurams

Name and CAS Reg. No.	Synonyms and Trade Names	Structural Formula	US Production -Thousand Kg (Year)	Use Class [a]	Indus-tries	Pro-cesses	Reported Workplace Levels(L)/Occupational Standards(S)[b,q,r,s]
Bis(diethyldithiocarbamoyl) disulphide 97-77-8	Chem. Abstr.: tetraethylthioperoxy-dicarbonic diamide [((H$_2$N)C(S))$_2$S$_2$] IUPAC: bis(diethylthiocarbamoyl) disulphide tetraethylthiuram disulphide Accelerator Thiuram Cyuram DS; Ethyl Tuads; Etiurac; Tuex	$$\left[\begin{array}{c}CH_3CH_2 \\ CH_3CH_2\end{array}N\!-\!\underset{\;\;\parallel}{C}\!-\!NCS\atop S\right]_2$$	> 45(1977)[d]	A	I II III IV	1-3 1-3 1-2 1-2	L:--/S:--
Bis(diethyldithiocarbamoyl) disulphide and Bis(dimethylthiocarbamoyl) disulphide 97-77-8 and 137-26-8	Chem. Abstr.: tetraethylthioperoxy-dicarbonic diamide [((H N)C(S))$_2$S$_2$] and tetramethylthioperoxydi-carbonic diamide [((H$_2$N)C(S))$_2$S$_2$] IUPAC: bis(diethylthiocarbamoyl) disulphide and bis(dimethylthio-carbamoyl) disulphide bis(mixed alkylthiocarbamoyl) disulphides; tetraalkylthiuram di-sulphides, mixed; methyl and ethyl thiurams, mixed Pennac TM	$$\left[\begin{array}{c}CH_3CH_2 \\ CH_3CH_2\end{array}N\!-\!\underset{\;\;\parallel}{C}\!-\!NCS\atop S\right]_2 + \left[\begin{array}{c}CH_3 \\ CH_3\end{array}N\!-\!\underset{\;\;\parallel}{C}\!-\!NCS\atop S\right]_2$$	> 0.45(1979)[f]	A	--	--	L:--/S:--

Name and CAS Reg. No.	Synonyms and Trade Names	Structural Formula	US Production -Thousand Kg (Year)	Use Class [a]	Industries	Processes	Reported Workplace Levels(L)/Occupational Standards(S)[b,q,r,s]
Bis(dimethylthiocarbamoyl) disulphide 137-26-8	Chem. Abstr.: tetramethylthioperoxy-dicarbonic diamide $[(H_2NJC(S))_2S_2]$ IUPAC: bis(dimethylthiocarbamoyl) disulphide tetramethylthiuram disulphide Accelerator Thiuram; Methyl Thiram; Methyl Tuads; Metiurac; Royal TMTD; Thiram B, 75, 80; Thiurad; Thiuram D, M; TMTD; TMTDS; Vulcafor TMTD; Vulkacit Thiuram		> 0.9(1979)[f]	A	I II III IV	1-3 1-3 1-2 1-2	L:--/S: 0.05-5mg/m³ ceiling (P, USSR, Y) 1-5 mg/m³ TWA (A, BEL, F, DDR, BRD, I, N, R, S, USA, USA-A) 5-10 mg/m³ STEL (DDR, USA-A)
Bis(dimethylthiocarbamoyl)sulphide 97-74-5	Chem. Abstr.: tetramethylthiodicarbonic diamide $[(H_2NJC(S))_2S]$ IUPAC: bis(dimethylthiocarbamoyl) sulphide tetramethylthiuram monosulphide tetramethylthiuram sulphide Akrochem TMTM; Cyuram MS; Methyl Tuads; Monex; Mono-Thiurad; Pennac MS; Thiuram MM; Urads; Vulkacit Thiuram MS		> 0.9(1979)[f]	A	I II III IV	1-3 1-3 1-2 1-2	L:--/S: 5mg/m³ (USA)
Bis(dimethylthiocarbamoyl) tetra-sulphide 97-91-6	Chem. Abstr.: bis((dimethylamino)-thioxomethyl) tetrasulphide IUPAC: bis(dimethylthiocarbamoyl) tetrasulphide tetramethylthiuram tetrasulphide		>0.45(1979)[f]	A	--	--	L:--/S: 5mg/m³ (USA)

Name and CAS Reg. No.	Synonyms and Trade Names	Structural Formula	US Production -Thousand Kg (Year)	Use Class [a]	Indus- tries	Pro- cesses	Reported Workplace Levels(L)/Occupational Standards(S)[b,q,r,s]
Bis(isopropyloctadecylthio-carbamoyl)disulphide 35318-10-6	Chem. Abstr.: N,N'-bis(1-methylethyl)-N,N'-dioctadecylthioperoxydi-carbonic diamide [((H2N)C(S))2S2] IUPAC: bis(isopropyloctadecylthio-carbamoyl) disulphide N,N'-Dioctadecyl-N,N'diisopropyl-thiuram disulphide	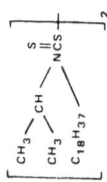	>0.45(1979)[f]	A	--	--	L:--/S:--
Bis(methylphenylthiocarbamoyl)di-sulphide 10591-84-1	Chem. Abstr.: N,N'-dimethyl-N,N'-diphenylthioperoxydicarbonic diamide $[((H_2N)C(S))_2S_2]$ IUPAC: bis(methylphenylthio-carbamoyl) disulphide dimethyldiphenylthiuram disulphide Vulkacit J	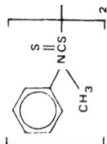	5.6(1979I)[m]	A	II	1-2	L:--/S:--
Bis(morpholinothiocarbamoyl) disulphide 51480-09-2	Chem. Abstr.: 4,4'-(dithiodicarbono-thioyl)bis(morpholine) IUPAC: bis(morpholinothiocarbonyl) disulphide	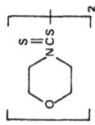	>0.45(1979)[f]	A	--	--	L:--/S:--
Dicyclopentamethylenethiuram disulphide 94-37-1	Chem. Abstr.: 1,1'-(dithiodicarbonothioyl)-bis(piperidine) IUPAC: bis(piperidinothiocarbonyl) disulphide dipentamethylene thiuram disulphide		> 0.5(1980WE)[c]	A	--	--	L:--/S:--

Name and CAS Reg. No.	Synonyms and Trade Names	Structural Formula	US Production -Thousand Kg (Year)	Use Class [a]	Indus- tries	Pro- cesses	Reported Workplace Levels(L)/Occupational Standards(S) [b,q,r,s]
Di-N,N'-pentamethylenethiuram hexasulphide 971-15-3	Chem. Abstr: 1,1'-(hexathiodicarbono-thioyl)bis(piperidine) IUPAC: bis(piperidinothiocarbonyl) hexasulphide Akrochem DPTT; Sulfads; Tetrone A		>2.2(1980) [c]	A	I II III IV	1-3 1-3 1-2 1-2	L:--/S:--
Dipentamethylenethiuram mono-sulphide 725-32-6	Chem. Abstr.: 1-piperidinecarbodithioic acid, anhydrosulphide IUPAC: bis(piperidinothiocarbonyl) sulphide dipentamethylenethiuram sulphide		> 0.5(1980WE) [c]	A	IV	1-2	L:--/S:--
Di-N,N'-pentamethylenethiuram tetrasulphide 120-54-7	Chem. Abstr.: 1,1'-(tetrathiodi-carbonothioyl)bis(piperidine) IUPAC: bis(piperidinothiocarbonyl) tetrasulphide dipentamethylenethiuram tetrasulphide Noksera TRA; Tetrone A; Thiuram MT; Worceler TRA		>0.9(1979) [f]	A	I II III IV	1-3 1-3 1-2 1-2	L:--/S:--
Tetrabutylthiuram disulphide 1634-02-2	Chem. Abstr.: tetrabutylthioperoxy-dicarbonic diamide [((H₂N)C(S))₂S₂] IUPAC: bis(dibutylthiocarbamoyl) disulphide 1,1'-dithiobis(N,N-dibutylmethane-thioamide)		>2.2(1980) [c]	A	--	--	L:--/S:--

Name and CAS Reg. No.	Synonyms and Trade Names	Structural Formula	US Production -Thousand Kg (Year)	Use Class a	Indus-tries	Pro-cesses	Reported Workplace Levels(L)/Occupational Standards(S)b,q,r,s

c. Miscellaneous

Name and CAS Reg. No.	Synonyms and Trade Names	Structural Formula	US Production -Thousand Kg (Year)	Use Class a	Indus-tries	Pro-cesses	Reported Workplace Levels(L)/Occupational Standards(S)b,q,r,s
Aryl disulphides, mixed --	Chem. Abstr.: -- IUPAC: --	Ar—SS—Ar	> 2.2(1980)c	P	--	--	L:--/S:--
Carbon bisulphide 75-15-0	Chem. Abstr.: carbon disulphide IUPAC: carbon disulphide	S=C=S	> 117,000 (1977)d	S,A	I II III	1-3 1-3 1-2	L:--/S: 10-150 mg/m³ Ceiling (BUL,P,R, USSR,Y,USA) 3-60 mg/m³ TWA (A, BEL, CZ,F,DDR,BRD, H,I,J,N,R,SWED,S, USA,USA-N,USA-A) 30-100 mg/m³ STEL (DDR,USA-N) 300 mg/m³ 30 min. peak (USA)
Morpholine disulphide 103-34-4	Chem. Abstr.: 4,4'-dithiobismorpholine IUPAC: 4,4'-dithiodimorpholine Accel R; Sulfasan R; Vulnoc	[structure]	0.5(1980WE)c	A	I II III IV	1-3 1-3 1-2 1-2	L:--/S:--

Name and CAS Reg. No.	Synonyms and Trade Names	Structural Formula	US Production -Thousand Kg (Year)	Use Class [a]	Indus- tries	Pro- cesses	Reported Workplace Levels(L)/Occupational Standards(S)[b,q,r,s]
2',2'''-Dithiobis(benzanilide) 135-57-9	Chem. Abstr.: N,N'-(dithiodi-2,1-phenylene)bis-benzamide IUPAC: 2',2'''-dithiobis(benzanilide) o-(benzoylamino)phenyl disulphide; bis(2-benzamidophenyl)disulphide; o,o'-dibenzamidophenyl disulphide Peptazin BAFD; Peptisant 10; Pepton 22	*(structural formula)*	450(1976)[c]	P	I II	1-2 1-2	L:--/S:--
Dixylyl disulphides, mixed 27080-90-6	Chem. Abstr.: bis(dimethylphenyl) disulphide IUPAC: Dixylyl disulphide tetramethyldiphenyl disulphide	*(structural formula)*	>45(1977)[d]	P	--	--	L:--/S:--

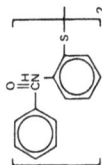

6. Thioureas

Name and CAS Reg. No.	Synonyms and Trade Names	Structural Formula	US Production -Thousand Kg (Year)	Use Class[a]	Indus-tries	Pro-cesses	Reported Workplace Levels(L)/Occupational Standards(S)[b,q,r,s]
Dialkylthiourea --	Chem. Abstr.: dialkylthiourea IUPAC: dialkylthiourea Pennzone L	$\overset{S}{\underset{H\ \ H}{RNCNR}}$	> 2.2(1980)[c]	AN,A	I II III IV	1-3 1-3 1-2 1-2	L:--/S:--
1,3-Di-n-butyl-2-thiourea 109-46-6	Chem. Abstr.: N,N'-dibutyl-thiourea IUPAC: 1,3-dibutyl-2-thiourea Pennzone B	$CH_3(CH_2)_3\overset{S}{\underset{H\ \ H}{NCN}}(CH_2)_3CH_3$	900(1976)[c]	A	I II III IV	1-3 1-3 1-2 1-2	L:--/S:--
1,3-Diethyl-2-thiourea 105-55-5	Chem. Abstr.: N,N'-diethyl-thiourea IUPAC: 1,3-diethyl-2-thiourea Pennzone E	$CH_3CH_2\overset{S}{\underset{H\ \ H}{NCN}}CH_2CH_3$	> 0.9(1979)[f]	A	I II III IV	1-3 1-3 1-2 1-2	L:--/S:--
1,3-Diphenyl-2-thiourea 102-08-9	Chem. Abstr.: N,N'-diphenyl-thiourea IUPAC: thiocarbanilide diphenylthiourea Rhenocure CA; Stabilisator C; Vulkacit CA	(diphenyl thiourea structure)	>45(1977)[d]	A	II	1-2	L:--/S:--

Name and CAS Reg. No.	Synonyms and Trade Names	Structural Formula	US Production -Thousand Kg (Year)	Use Class [a]	Indus- tries	Pro- cesses	Reported Workplace Levels(L)/Occupational Standards(S)[b,q,r,s]
Di-o-tolylthiourea 137-97-3	Chem. Abstr.: N,N'-bis(2-methyl-phenyl)thiourea IUPAC: 2,2'-dimethylthiocarbanilide 1,3-di-l-tolyl-2-thiourea		> 0.45(1980)[f]	A	--	--	L:--/S:--
3-Ethyl-l,l-dimethyl-2-thiourea 15361-86-1	Chem. Abstr.: N'-ethyl-N,N-dimethylthiourea IUPAC: 3-ethyl-l,l-dimethyl-2-thiourea l-ethyl-3,3-dimethylthiourea		>450(1976)[c]	A	--	--	L:--/S:--
1,3-Ethylene-2-thiourea 96-45-7	Chem. Abstr.: 2-imidazolidine-thione IUPAC: 2-imidazolidinethione 4,5-dihydro-2-mercaptoimidazole; imidazoline-2(3)-thione; ETU Akrochem ETU; ETU-2; NA-22, 220, 227; Pennac CRA; Sodium-22 neoprene accelerator; Vulkacit NPVIC; Warecure C		>45(1977)[d]	A	II III	1-3 1-2	L:--/S:--
Tetramethylthiourea 2782-91-4	Chem. Abstr.: tetramethylthiourea IUPAC: 1,1,3,3-tetramethyl-2-thiourea Basthioryl		> 0.45(1977)[f**]	A	--	--	L:--/S:--

Name and CAS Reg. No.	Synonyms and Trade Names	Structural Formula	US Production -Thousand Kg (Year)	Use Class [a]	Indus- tries	Pro- cesses	Reported Workplace Levels(L)/Occupational Standards(S) [b,q,r,s]
N,N,N'-Tributyl thiourea 2422-88-0	Chem. Abstr.: tributylthiourea IUPAC: 1,1,3-tributyl-2-thiourea 1,1,3-tributylthiourea TBTU	$CH_3(CH_2)_3$ $CH_3(CH_2)_3$ N—$\overset{S}{\overset{\|}{C}}$—N(CH$_2$)$_3CH_3$	> 0.5(1980WE)[c]	A	--	--	L:--/S:--
1,1,3-Trimethyl-2-thiourea 2489-77-2	Chem. Abstr.: trimethylthiourea IUPAC: 1,1,3-trimethyl-2-thiourea Thiate EF-2	CH_3 CH_3 N—$\overset{S}{\overset{\|}{C}}$—NCH$_3$	> 0.45(1979)[f]	A	II III	1-3 1-2	L:--/S:--

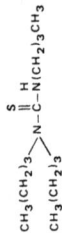

Name and CAS Reg. No.	Synonyms and Trade Names	Structural Formula	US Production -Thousand Kg (Year)	Use Class[a]	Indus- tries	Pro- cesses	Reported Workplace Levels(L)/Occupational Standards(S)[b,q,r,s]

7. Miscellaneous

Name and CAS Reg. No.	Synonyms and Trade Names	Structural Formula	US Production -Thousand Kg (Year)	Use Class[a]	Indus- tries	Pro- cesses	Reported Workplace Levels(L)/Occupational Standards(S)[b,q,r,s]
Alkyl sulphonates --	Chem. Abstr.: -- IUPAC: --	Indefinite	--	LM	IV	1-3	L:--/S:--
Benzenesulphonyl hydrazide 80-17-1	Chem. Abstr.: benzenesulphonic acid, hydrazide IUPAC: benzenesulphonic acid, hydrazide phenylsulphohydrazide Celogen BSH; Genitron BSH; Nitropore OBSH; Porofor BSH		56(1979)[m]	BA	I II III IV	1-3 1-3 1-2 1-2	L:--/S:--
2-Benzimidazolethiol, zinc salt 3030-80-6	Chem. Abstr.: 1,3-dihydro-2H-ben- zimidazole-2-thione, zinc salt IUPAC: zinc bis(2-benzimidazole- thiolate) 2-mercaptobenzimidazole, zinc salt; zinc mercaptobenzimidazolate Antioxidant ZMB		> 0.45(1977)[d]	AN	II IV	1-2 1-2	L:--/S:--
N-(Cyclohexylthio)phthalimide 17796-82-6	Chem. Abstr.: 2-(cyclohexylthio)-1H- isoindole-1,3(2H)-dione IUPAC: N-(cyclohexylthio) phthalimide Santogard PVI		> 0.45(1979)[f]	R	I II	1-2 1-2	L:--/S:--

Name and CAS Reg. No.	Synonyms and Trade Names	Structural Formula	US Production -Thousand Kg (Year)	Use Class [a]	Indus- tries	Pro- cesses	Reported Workplace Levels(L)/Occupational Standards(S)[b,q,r,s]
2-Mercaptobenzimidazole 583-39-1	Chem. Abstr.: 1,3-dihydro-2H-benzimidazole-2-thione IUPAC: 2-benzimidazolethiol o-phenylenethiourea; 2-thio-benzimidazole; Antigene MB; Antioxidant MB; ASM-MB; Permanax 21; Vulkanox MB		>4.5(1977)[d]	AN	I II IV	1-3 1-3 1-2	L:--/S:--
2-Mercaptotoluimidazole 53998-10-6	Chem. Abstr.: 1,3-dihydro-4(or 5)-methyl-2H-benzimidazole-2-thione IUPAC: 4 (or 5)-methyl-2-benzimidazolethiol methyl-2-benzimidazolethiol Vanox MTI		>2.2(1980)[c]	A,AN	I II III IV	1-3 1-3 1-2 1-2	L:--/S:--
2-Mercaptotoluimidazole, zinc salt 61617-00-3	Chem. Abstr.: 1,3-dihydro-4(or 5)-methyl-2H-benzimidazole-2-thione, zinc salt (2:1) IUPAC: zinc bis [4(or 5)-methyl-2-benzimidazolethiolate] Vanox ZMTI		>2.2(1980)[c]	A,AN	I II III IV	1-3 1-3 1-2 1-2	L:--/S:--
p,p'-Oxybis(benzenesulphonyl-hydrazide) 80-51-3	Chem. Abstr.: 4,4'-oxybis[benzene-sulphonic acid], dihydrazide IUPAC: 4,4'-oxydibenzenesulphonic acid, dihydrazide p,p'-oxybis(benzenesulphonyl hydrazide) Celogen OT; Celnike S; Genitron OB; Serogen		>0.45(1979)[f]	BA	I II III IV	1-3 1-3 1-2 1-2	L:--/S:--
N-Oxydiethylenethiocarbamoyl-N'-oxydiethylenesulphenamide 13752-51-7	Chem. Abstr.: 4-[(4-morpholinylthio)-thioxomethyl]morpholine IUPAC: 4,4'-[thio(thiocarbonyl)]di-morpholine N,N'-bis(oxydiethylene) thiocarbamoyl-sulphenamide Care Rite 18		>2.2(1980)[c]	AN	--	--	L:--/S:--

Name and CAS Reg. No.	Synonyms and Trade Names	Structural Formula	US Production -Thousand Kg (Year)	Use Class [a]	Indus-tries	Pro-cesses	Reported Workplace Levels(L)/Occupational Standards(S)[b,q,r,s]
Sodium alkyl sulphates --	Chem. Abstr.:-- IUPAC:--	ROSO^-Na^+	$> 0.45 (1979)^f$	CLA	I II III IV	1,5 1,5 1,5 1,4	L:--/S:--
p-Toluenesulphonic acid, zinc salt 13438-45-4	Chem. Abstr.: 4-methylbenzenesulphonic acid, zinc salt IUPAC: zinc p-toluenesulphonate	$\left[\text{CH}_3\!\!-\!\!\bigcirc\!\!-\!\!\text{SO}_3^- \right]_2 \text{Zn}^{++}$	$> 0.45 (1977)^{f**}$	A	--	--	L:--/S:--
p-Toluenesulphonylsemicarbazide 10396-10-8	Chem. Abstr.: 4-methylbenzenesulphonic acid, 2-(aminocarbonyl)hydrazide IUPAC: 1-(p-tolylsulphonyl)-semicarbazide Celogen RA	$\text{CH}_3\!\!-\!\!\bigcirc\!\!-\!\!\underset{O}{\overset{O}{S}}\!\!-\!\!\text{NNCNH}_2$	$\geqslant 0.45 (1979)^f$	BA	I II III	1-3 1-3 1-2	L:--/S:--

C. Oxygen Compounds
1. Phenols
a. Carbon-bridged phenols

Name and CAS Reg. No.	Synonyms and Trade Names	Structural Formula	US Production -Thousand Kg (Year)	Use Class [a]	Indus- tries	Pro- cesses	Reported Workplace Levels(L)/Occupational Standards(S)[b,q,r,s]
Bisphenol, hindered --	Chem. Abstr.: hindered bisphenol IUPAC: hindered bisphenol Naugawhite	Indefinite	>1.4(1979)[f]	AN	I II III IV	1-3 1-3 1-2 1-2	L:--/S:--
4,4'-Butylidenebis(6-t-butyl)-m-cresol 85-60-9	Chem. Abstr.: 4,4'-butylidenebis[2-(1,1-dimethylethyl)-5-methylphenol] IUPAC: 4,4'-butylidenebis(6-tert-butyl-m-cresol) Arulex PBA '5; Santowhite Powder; SWP; Sumilit BBM; Sumilizer BBM	[structural formula]	>0.45(1979)[f]	AN	--	--	L:--/S:--
4-Chloro-2,6-bis(2,4-dihydroxybenzyl)phenol 31265-39-1	Chem. Abstr.: 4,4'-[(5-chloro-2-hydroxv-1,3-phenylene)bis(methylene]bis(1,3-benzenediol) IUPAC: 4,4'-[(5-chloro-2-hydroxy-m-phenylene)dimethylene]diresorcinol	[structural formula]	>0.45(1979)[f]	M	--	--	L:--/S:--
2,2'-Methylenebis(6-t-butyl)-p-cresol 119-47-1	Chem. Abstr.: 2,2'-methylenebis[6-(1,1-dimethylethyl)-4-methyl-phenol] IUPAC: 2,2'-methylenebis[6-tert-butyl-p-cresol] Antioxidant 1, 2246, BKF; Advastab 405; Antage W 400; Bisalkofen BP; Caiso 2246; CAO 5, 14; Catolin 14; Chemanox 21; Lederle 2246; NG 2246; Nocrac N56; Plastanox 2246	[structural formula]	>45(1977)[d]	AN	I II III IV	1-3 1-3 1-2 1-2	L:--/S:--

Name and CAS Reg. No.	Synonyms and Trade Names	Structural Formula	US Production -Thousand Kg (Year)	Use Class[a]	Indus-tries	Pro-cesses	Reported Workplace Levels(L)/Occupational Standards(S)[b,q,r,s]
2,2'-Methylenebis(6-t-butyl)-4-ethylphenol 88-24-4	Chem. Abstr.: 2,2'-methylenebis[6-(1,1-dimethylethyl)-4-ethylphenol] IUPAC: 2,2'-methylenebis[6-tert-butyl-4-ethylphenol] Antioxidant 425; Anti-Oxidant MBP-5P; Chemanox 22; Plastanox 425; Yoshinox 425		>0.45(1979)[f]	AN	I II III IV	1-3 1-3 1-2 1-2	L:--/S:--
4,4'-Methylenebis(2,6-di-tert-butyl-phenol) 118-82-1	Chem. Abstr.: 4,4'-methylenebis[2,6-bis(1,1-dimethylethyl)phenol] IUPAC: 4,4'-methylenebis(2,6-di-tert-butylphenol) Antioxidant E702; Bimox M; Ethyl 702; Ionox 220		>0.45(1979)[f]	AN	--	--	L:--/S:--
4,4'-Methylenebis(2,6-dimethyl-phenol) 5384-21-4	Chem. Abstr.: 4,4'-methylenebis(2,6-dimethylphenol) IUPAC: 4,4'-methylenedi-2,6-xylenol bis(4-hydroxy-3,5-dimethylphenyl)methane		>0.5(1980WE)[c]	AN	--	--	L:--/S:--
2,2'-Methylenebis-6-(1-methyl-cyclohexyl)-p-cresol 77-62-3	Chem. Abstr.: 2,2'-methylenebis-[4-methyl-6-(1-methylcyclohexyl)-phenol] IUPAC: 2,2'-methylenebis[6-(1-methylcyclohexyl)-p-cresol] Bisalkofen MTSP; Ionox WSP; Nonox WSP; Permanax WSP		>0.9(1979)[f]	AN	--	--	L:--/S:--
2,2'-Methylenebis(4-methyl-6-nonylphenol) 7786-17-6	Chem. Abstr.: 2,2'-methylenebis(4-methyl-6-nonylphenol) IUPAC: 2,2'-methylenebis(6-nonyl-p-cresol) 2,2'-methylenebis(6-nonyl-4-methyl-phenol) Naugawhite		>2.2(1980)[c]	AN	I II III IV	1-3 1-3 1-2 1-2	LS:--/S:--

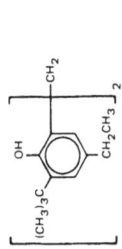

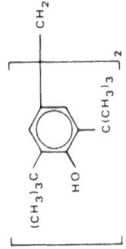

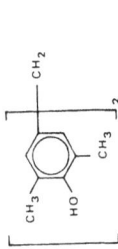

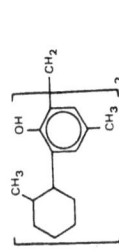

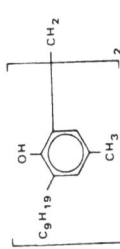

Name and CAS Reg. No.	Synonyms and Trade Names	Structural Formula	US Production -Thousand Kg (Year)	Use Class [a]	Indus-tries	Pro-cesses	Reported Workplace Levels(L)/Occupational Standards(S)[b,q,r,s]
Phenol, polymeric, hindered --	Chem. Abstr.: -- IUPAC: --	Indefinite	> 2.2(1980)[c]	AN	--	--	L:--/S:--
Polyphenol, alkylated --	Chem. Abstr.: alkylated polyphenol IUPAC: alkylated polyphenol	Indefinite	2,500(1976)[c]	AN	--	--	L:--/S:--
1,1,3-Tris(2-methyl-4-hydroxy-5-t-butylphenyl)butane 1843-03-4	Chem. Abstr.: 4,4',4"-(1-methyl-1-propanyl-3-ylidene)tris[2-(1,1-dimethylethyl)-5-methylphenol] IUPAC: 4,4',4"-(1-methyl-1-propanyl-3-ylidene)tris[6-tert-butyl-m-cresol)] Topanol CA, KA; Trisalkofen BMB		> 0.45(1979)[f]	AN	--	--	L:--/S:--
1,3,5-Trimethyl-2,4,6-tris-(3,5-di-tert-butyl-4-hydroxy-benzyl)benzene 1709-70-2	Chem. Abstr.: 4,4',4"-[(2,4,6-trimethyl-1,3,5-benzenetriyl)tris(methylene)]-tris[2,6-bis(1,1-dimethylethyl)phenol] IUPAC: α,α',α"-(2,4,6-trimethyl-s-phenenyl)-tris(2,6-di-tert-butyl-p-cresol) Agidol 40; Antioxidant 40, 330; Ethyl 330; Ethyl Antioxidant 330; Ionox 330; Irganox 330	 where R = --CH$_2$--	33(1979)[m]	AN	--	--	L:--/S:--
Tris(3,5-di-t-butyl-4-hydroxy-benzyl)isocyanurate 27676-62-6	Chem. Abstr.: 1,3,5-tris[[3,5-bis-(1,1-dimethylethyl)-4-hydroxyphenyl]-methyl]-1,3,5-triazine-2,4,6(1H,3H,5H)-trione IUPAC: 1,3,5-tris(3,5-di-tert-butyl-4-hydroxybenzyl)-s-triazine-2,4,6-(1H,3H,5H)-trione	 R = --CH$_2$--	> 0.45(1977)[f**]	AN	--	--	L:--/S:--

b. Alkylated phenols

Name and CAS Reg. No.	Synonyms and Trade Names	Structural Formula	US Production -Thousand Kg (Year)	Use Class[a]	Indus- tries	Pro- cesses	Reported Workplace Levels(L)/Occupational Standards(S)[b,q,r,s]
o-Cresol, alkylated --	Chem. Abstr.: alkylated 2-methylphenol IUPAC: alkylated o-cresol		>0.45(1979)[f]	AN	--	--	L:--/S:--
p-Cresol, alkylated --	Chem. Abstr.: alkylated 4-methylphenol IUPAC: alkylated p-cresol		>2.2(1980)[c]	AN	--	--	L:--/S:--
2,6-Di-tert-butyl-p-cresol 128-37-0	Chem. Abstr.: 2,6-bis(1,1-dimethyl-ethyl)-4-methylphenol IUPAC: 2,6-di-tert-butyl-p-cresol BHT; butylated hydroxytoluene AO 4K; CAD 1,3; Dalpac; DBPC; Deenax; Impruvol; Ionol; Naugard BHT; Nonox TBC; Parabar 441; Sustane BHT; Stavox; Tenamene 3; Tenox BHT; Topanol OC, O; Vanulic PC, PCX; Vianol		10,350 (1978)[c]	AN	I II III IV	1-3 1-3 1-2 1-2	L:--/S: 10 mg/m^3 TWA (A, BEL, N, S, USA-A) 20 mg/m^3 STEL (USA-A)
2,4-Di(α-methylbenzyl) phenol 2769-94-0	Chem. Abstr.: 2,4-bis(1-phenylethyl)phenol IUPAC: 2,4-bis(α-methylbenzyl)phenol 2,4-bis(phenylethylidene)phenol		>0.5(1980WE)[c]	AN	--	--	L:--/S:--

Name and CAS Reg. No.	Synonyms and Trade Names	Structural Formula	US Production -Thousand Kg (Year)	Use Class[a]	Indus- tries	Pro- cesses	Reported Workplace Levels(L)/Occupational Standards(S)[b,q,r,s]
Phenol, alkylated --	Chem. Abstr.: alkylated phenol IUPAC: alkylated phenol Antioxidant KSM; Cyanox 251 antioxidant; Nevastain 21, A, B; Stabilite 454, 455; Wingstay T		3210(1977)[f]	AN	I II III IV		1-3 1-3 1-2 1-2 L:--/S:--
Phenol, hindered --	Chem. Abstr.: hindered phenol IUPAC: hindered phenol Antioxidant 431; Irganox 1035; Mastermix Stabilizer B 1017 MB; Stabilite 49-466, 467, 470; Antioxidant 431	Indefinite	> 0.9(1979)[f]	AN	I II III IV		1-3 1-3 1-2 1-2 L:--/S:--
Phenol, styrenated 61788-44-1	Chem. Abstr.: styrenated phenol IUPAC: styrenated phenol Stabilite 49-456, 464-SP; Wingstay S, V		383(1979)[f]	AN	I II III IV		1-3 1-3 1-2 1-2 L:--/S:--

Name and CAS Reg. No.	Synonyms and Trade Names	Structural Formula	US Production -Thousand Kg (Year)	Use Class[a]	Indus-tries	Pro-cesses	Reported Workplace Levels(L)/Occupational Standards(S)[b,q,r,s]
c. Aminophenols							
N-Butyroyl-p-aminophenol 101-91-7	Chem. Abstr.: N-(4-hydroxyphenyl)-butanamide IUPAC: 4'-hydroxybutyranilide p-butyramidophenol; N-butyryl-p-aminophenol; p-(butyroylamino)phenol; 4-butyramidophenol Suconox-4	$C_3H_7C\underset{O}{\overset{\parallel}{}}\overset{H}{\underset{}{N}}$ —⟨ ⟩— OH	>2.2(1980)[c]	AN	--	--	L:--/S:--
N-Lauroyl-p-aminophenol 103-98-0	Chem. Abstr.: N-(4-hydroxyphenyl)-dodecanamide IUPAC: 4'-hydroxydodecananilide N-lauroyl-4-aminophenol Suconox-12; Suconox-112	$C_{11}H_{23}C\overset{O}{\overset{\parallel}{}}N$ —⟨ ⟩— OH	>2.2(1980)[c]	AN	--	--	L:--/S:--
N-Stearoyl-p-aminophenol 103-99-1	Chem. Abstr.: N-(4-hydroxyphenyl)-octadecanamide IUPAC: 4'-hydroxyoctadecananilide Suconox 18	$C_{17}H_{35}C\overset{O}{\overset{\parallel}{}}N$ —⟨ ⟩— OH	45(1976)[c]	AN	--	--	L:--/S:--

d. Hydroquinones

Name and CAS Reg. No.	Synonyms and Trade Names	Structural Formula	US Production -Thousand Kg (Year)	Use Class [a]	Indus-tries	Pro-cesses	Reported Workplace Levels(L)/Occupational Standards(S)[b,q,r,s]
p-Benzyloxyphenol 103-16-2	Chem. Abstr.: 4-(phenylmethoxy)phenol IUPAC: p-(benzyloxy)phenol hydroquinone benzyl ether; mono-benzyl ether hydroquinone AgeRite Alba; Benzoquin; Carmifal; Depigman; Dermochinona; Leucodinine; Monobenzon; Pigmex; Superlite		>2.2(1980)[c]	AN	--	--	L:--/S:--
2,5-Di-sec-butyl decylhydroquinone 61791-96-6	Chem. Abstr.: 3-decyl-2,5-bis(1-methylpropyl)-1,4-benzenediol IUPAC: 2,5-di-sec-butyl-3-decylhydro-quinone		>0.45(1979)[f]	AN	--	--	L:--/S:--
2,5-Di(1,1-dimethylpropyl)hydro-quinone 79-74-3	Chem. Abstr.: 2,5-bis(1,1-dimethyl-propyl)-1,4-benzenediol IUPAC: 2,5-di-tert-pentyl-hydroquinone Santovan A		>2.2(1980)[c]	AN	I II III IV	1-3 1-3 1-2 1-2	L:--/S:--
Hydroquinone 123-31-9	Chem. Abstr.: 1,4-benzenediol IUPAC: hydroquinone benzohydroquinone; 1,4-dihydroxy-benzene Arctuvin; Diak 5; Eldopaque; Eldoquin; HE 5; Phiaquin; Tecquinol; Tenox HQ		>4,995(1977)[d]	AN	--	--	L:--/S: 2 mg/m3 ceiling (P,R,Y,USA-N) 0.5-2 mg/m3 TWA (A,BEL,F,BRD,N,R,S,SWED,USA) 4 mg/m3 STEL (USA-A)

Name and CAS Reg. No.	Synonyms and Trade Names	Structural Formula	US Production -Thousand Kg (Year)	Use Class [a]	Indus- tries	Pro- cesses	Reported Workplace Levels(L)/Occupational Standards(S)[b,q,r,s]
Resorcinol 108-46-3	Chem. Abstr.: 1,3-benzenediol IUPAC: resorcinol m-hydroquinone; m-hydroxyphenol Developer C, R, RS; Fouramine RS; Fourrine 79, EW; Nako TGG; Pelagol Grey RS, RS		> 0.9(1979)[f]	BA	I II III IV	4 1-4 1-3 1-2	L: -- S: 45 mg/m^3 TWA (BEL,N,S,USA-A) 90 mg/m^3 STEL (USA-A)
e. Miscellaneous							
Phenyl-β-naphthol --	Chem. Abstr.: phenyl-2-naphthalenol IUPAC: phenyl-2-naphthol		≥0.5(1980WE)[c]	AN	--	--	L:--/S:--

Name and CAS Reg. No.	Structural Formula	US Production -Thousand Kg (Year)	Use Class[a]	Indus- tries	Pro- cesses	Reported Workplace Levels(L)/Occupational Standards(S)[b,q,r,s]
2. Quinones						
p-Benzoquinonedioxime 105-11-3		> 0.45(1980)[c]	A	I II III IV	1-3 1-3 1-2 1-2	L:--/S:--
Chem. Abstr.: 2,5-cyclohexadiene-1,4-dione, dioxime IUPAC: p-benzoquinone dioxime Actor Q; PQD						
Dibenzoyl-p-quinone dioxime 120-52-5		> 4.5(1980)[c]	A	I II III IV	1-3 1-3 1-2 1-2	L:--/S:--
Chem. Abstr.: 2,5-cyclohexadiene-1,4-dione, bis(0-benzoyloxime) IUPAC: p-benzoquinone, bis(0-benzoyl-oxime) dibenzoyl-p-benzoquinone dioxime; p-quinone dioxime dibenzoate; p-quinone dioxime dibenzoate; 1,4-bis(benzoyloxyimino)cyclohexa-2,5-diene Dibenzo GMF; Dilbenzo PQD; Vulnoc DGM						

3. Carboxylic Acids and Salts

Name and CAS Reg. No.	Synonyms and Trade Names	Structural Formula	US Production -Thousand Kg (Year)	Use Class [a]	Indus- tries	Pro- cesses	Reported Workplace Levels(L)/Occupational Standards(S)[b,q,r,s]
Acetic acid 64-19-7	Chem. Abstr.: acetic acid IUPAC: acetic acid ethanoic acid; ethylic acid; glacial acetic acid; methanecarboxylic acid; vinegar acid	$CH_3C\overset{O}{\underset{}{}}OH$	1,482,359 (1979)[f]	LM	IV	1-2	L:--/S: 5-50 mg/m^3 Ceiling (BUL, CZ, 15-25 mg/m^3 TWA (A,BEL,CZ,F, DDR,BRD,I,J,N, R,SWED,S,USA, USA-A) 20-37 mg/m^3 STEL (DDR, USA-A)
Ammonium acetate 631-61-8	Chem. Abstr.: acetic acid, ammonium salt IUPAC: ammonium acetate	$CH_3C\overset{O}{\underset{}{}}O^- \; NH_4^+$	>76.8 (1979)[f]	LM	IV	1-2	L:--/S:--
Benzoic acid 65-85-0	Chem. Abstr.: benzoic acid IUPAC: benzoic acid Retarder BAX, BA	C_6H_5COOH	34,669 (1979)[f]	SO	I II III IV	1-3 1-3 1-2 1-2	L:--/S:--
Calcium stearate 1592-23-0	Chem. Abstr.: octadecanoic acid, calcium salt IUPAC: calcium stearate Aquacal; Calstan; Flexichem CS; Nopcote C104; Stavinor 30; Witco G 339S	$[CH_3(CH_2)_{16}COO^-]_2 Ca^{++}$	23,904 (1979)[f]	F	I II III IV	1-3 1-3 1-2 1-2	L:--/S:--
Di-n-butylammonium oleate 7620-75-9	Chem. Abstr.: [Z]-9-octadecenoic acid compound with N-butyl-1-butanamine (1:1) IUPAC: oleic acid compound with dibutylamine (1:1)	$CH_3(CH_2)_7CH=CH(CH_2)_7COO^- \; H_2N^+(CH_2CH_2CH_3)_2$	>0.45 (1979)[f**]	A	--	--	L:--/S:--

Name and CAS Reg. No.	Synonyms and Trade Names	Structural Formula	US Production -Thousand Kg (Year)	Use Class [a]	Indus- tries	Pro- cesses	Reported Workplace Levels(L)/Occupational Standards(S) [b,q,r,s]
Dimethylammonium hydrogen isophthalate 71172-17-3	Chem. Abstr.: 1,3-benzenedicarboxylic acid, compound with N-methylmethan-amine (1:1) IUPAC: isophthalic acid, compound with dimethylamine (1:1) Vanax CPA		> 2.2(1980) [c]	AN,A	--	--	L:--/S:--
Lauric acid 143-07-7	Chem. Abstr.: dodecanoic acid IUPAC: lauric acid dodecylic acid; laurostearic acid ABL; Aliphat No. 4; Neo-Fat 12, 12-43; Ninol AA62 extra; Univol U-314	$CH_3(CH_2)_{10}COOH$	> 1,080(1977) [d]	SO	I II III IV	1-3 1-3 1-2 1-2	L:--/S:--
Methacrylic acid, zinc salt 13189-00-9	Chem. Abstr.: 2-methyl-2-propenoic acid, zinc salt IUPAC: zinc methacrylate		--	A	--	--	L:--/S:--
Oxalic acid 144-62-7	Chem. Abstr.: ethanedioic acid IUPAC: oxalic acid Aktisal; Aquisal		> 4,550(1977) [d]	BA	--	--	L:--/S: 1 mg/m^3 TWA (A, BEL, F, N, S, USA, USA-A) 2 mg/m^3 STEL (USA-A)
Ricinoleic acid 141-22-0	Chem. Abstr.: [R-(Z)]-12-hydroxy-9-octadecenoic acid IUPAC: ricinoleic acid ricinic acid	$CH_3(CH_2)_5CHCH_2CH=CH(CH_2)_7COOH.$ with OH	>455(1977) [d]	SO	--	--	L:--/S:--

Name and CAS Reg. No.	Structural Formula	Synonyms and Trade Names	US Production -Thousand Kg (Year)	Use Class [a]	Indus- tries	Pro- cesses	Reported Workplace Levels(L)/Occupational Standards(S)[b,q,r,s]
Salicylic acid 69-72-7		Chem. Abstr.: 2-hydroxybenzoic acid IUPAC: salicylic acid Psoriacid-S-Stift; Retarder W; Rutranex; Salonil	18,111[f] (1979)	R	II	1-2	L:--/S:--
Stearic acid 57-11-4	$CH_3(CH_2)_{16}COOH$	Chem. Abstr.: octadecanoic acid IUPAC: stearic acid 1-heptadecanecarboxylic acid Emery 400; Hydrofol Acid 150; Hystrene S-97, T-70, 80, 5016; Kam 1000, 2000, 3000; Neo-Fat 18; Stearex Beads; Vanicol	13,504 (1977)[d]	A, SO	I II III IV	1-3 1-3 1-2 1-2	L:--/S:--
Wood rosin 8050-09-7	Complex mixture	Chem. Abstr.: wood rosin IUPAC: wood rosin FF Wood Rosin; N Wood Rosin; Penbro; Rosin; W G Wood Rosin; W W Wood Rosin	26,000(1976)[c]	SO	I II III IV	1-3 1-3 1-2 1-2	L:--/S:--
Zinc laurate 2452-01-9	$\left[CH_3(CH_2)_{10}COO^-\right]_2 Zn^{++}$	Chem. Abstr.: dodecanoic acid, zinc salt IUPAC: zinc laurate zinc dilaurate	> 0.45(1979)[f]	A	--	--	L: 3.44 mg/m^3 (as zinc)[bb] S: --
Zinc stearate 557-05-1	$\left[CH_3(CH_2)_{16}COO^-\right]_2 Zn^{++}$	Chem. Abstr.: octadecanoic acid, zinc salt IUPAC: zinc stearate Dermarone; Metasap Zinc Stearate H; Stravinor ZN-E; Synpro stearate; Talculin Z; Wet:Zinc; Witco Zinc Stearate 11, 42; Zincote; Zinc Stearate ZS-50/50; LS7; PM Wettable	10,688(1979)[f]	A,CLA	I II III IV	1-3 1-3 1-2 1-2	L:--/S:--

Name and CAS Reg. No.	Synonyms and Trade Names	Structural Formula	US Production -Thousand Kg (Year)	Use Class [a]	Indus- tries	Pro- cesses	Reported Workplace Levels(L)/Occupational Standards(S)[b,q,r,s]
4. Anhydrides and Esters							
Castor oil 8001-79-4	Chem. Abstr.: castor oil; IUPAC: castor oil; phorbyol	Complex mixture	454(1975)[l]	SO	--	--	L:--/S:--
Cottonseed oil 8001-29-4	Chem. Abstr.: cottonseed oil; IUPAC: cottonseed oil	Complex mixture	>450(1977)[d]	SO	I; II; III; IV	1-3; 1-3; 1-2; 1-2	L:--/S:--
Dibutyl phthalate 84-74-2	Chem. Abstr.: 1,2-benzenedicarboxylic acid, dibutyl ester; IUPAC: dibutyl phthalate; butyl phthalate; DBP; Celluflex DBP; Elaol; Ergoplast FDB; Genoplast B; Hexaplas M/B; Palatinol C; Polycizer DBP; PX 104; Staflex DBP; Unimoll DB; Witcizer 300	[structure: $C{-}O{-}(CH_2)_3CH_3$ benzene diester]	7,789 (1979)[f] (includes di-isobutyl phthalate)	PL	II	1-2	L:--/S: 0.5-10 mg/m^3 Ceiling (BUL, CZ, USSR,Y) 5 mg/m^3 TWA (A, BEL,F,I,N,USA, USA-A) 10 mg/m^3 STEL (USA-A)
Di-2-ethylhexyl adipate 103-23-1	Chem. Abstr.: bis(2-ethylhexyl) hexanedioate; IUPAC: bis(2-ethylhexyl) adipate; DEHA; dioctyl adipate; DOA; Adipol 2EH; Bisoflex DOA; Effomoll DOA; Ergoplast AddO; Flexol A26; Kodaflex DOA; Monoplex DOA; Plastomoll DOA; Sicol 250; Truflex DOA; Vestinol OA; Wickenol 158; Witamol 320	[structure: $CH_2COCH_2CHICH_2)_3CH_3$ adipate ester]	21,186 (1979)[f]	PL	II	1-2	L:--/S:--
Di-2-ethylhexyl phthalate 117-81-7	Chem. Abstr.: bis(2-ethylhexyl)-1,2-benzenedicarboxylate; IUPAC: bis(2-ethylhexyl) phthalate; DEHP; dioctyl phthalate; DOP; Bisoflex 81, DOP; Compound 889; DAF 68; Ergoplast FDO; Eviplast 80, 81; Fleximel; Flexol DOP; Good-Rite GP 264; Kodaflex DOP; Octoil; Palatinol AH; Pittsburgh PX-138; Reomol D 79P; Sicol 150; Staflex DOP; Truflex DOP; Vestinol AH; Vinicizer 80; Witicizer 312	[structure: $COCH_2CHICH_2)_3CH_3$ benzene diester]	136,457 (1979)[f]	PL	II	1-2	L:--/S:--

Name and CAS Reg. No.	Synonyms and Trade Names	Structural Formula	US Production -Thousand Kg (Year)	Use Class [a]	Industries	Processes	Reported Workplace Levels(L)/Occupational Standards(S)b,q,r,s
Epoxidized soybean oil 8013-07-8	Chem. Abstr.: epoxidized soybean oil; IUPAC: epoxidized soybean oil; Drapex 104; Epoxizer P206; Epoxol 7-4; G-61; G-62; Paraplex G-60; Plastol 10	Complex mixture	32,346 [f] (1979)	SO	II IV	1-3 1-2	L:--/S:--
Ethyl acetate 141-78-6	Chem. Abstr.: ethyl acetate; IUPAC: ethyl acetate	$CH_3COCH_2CH_3$ (=O)	118,070 (1979) [f]	S	I II III	1-3 1-4 1-3	L:--/S: 200-2000 mg/m^3 Ceiling(BUL,H, CZ,P,USSR,R,Y) 200-1400 mg/m^3 TWA (A,CZ,DDR,R,I, SWED,A,BEL,F,BRD, J,N,S,USA,USA-A) 1500 mg/m^3 STEL (DDR)
Lanolin 8006-54-0	Chem. Abstr.: lanolin; IUPAC: lanolin; Agnolin; Alopurin; Cosmelan; Lanain; Lanalin; Lanesin; Lanichol; Laniol; Lanum	Complex mixture	>1179(1977) [d]	SO	--	--	L:--/S:--
Phthalic anhydride 85-44-9	Chem. Abstr.: 1,3-isobenzofurandione; IUPAC: phthalic anhydride; 1,2-benzenedicarboxylic anhydride; ESEN; Phthalandione; Retarder AK, ESEN, PD; TGL 6525; Vulcalent B/C	(benzene ring fused anhydride)	455,786 [f] (1979)	R	I II III IV	1-3 1-3 1-2 1-2	L:--/S: 1-15 mg/m^3 Ceiling (P,USSR,R, Y,CZ) 5-12 mg/m^3 TWA (A,F, SWED,S,CZ,DDR,BRD, I,R,BEL,N,USA, USA-A) 24-30 mg/m^3 STEL (USA-A,DDR)
Vulcanized vegetable oils --	Chem. Abstr.: vulcanized vegetable oils; IUPAC: vulcanized vegetable oils; Factice	Indefinite	--	SO	I II III IV	1-3 1-3 1-2 1-2	L:--/S:--

5. Peroxides

Name and CAS Reg. No.	Synonyms and Trade Names	Structural Formula	US Production -Thousand Kg (Year)	Use Class [a]	Indus-tries	Pro-cesses	Reported Workplace Levels(L)/Occupational Standards(S) [b,q,r,s]
Benzoyl peroxide 94-36-0	Chem. Abstr.: dibenzoyl peroxide IUPAC: benzoyl peroxide Benoxyl; Cadox BS; Lucidol , B50, G20, 50P; Luperco AST; Nayper BO; Oxylite; Panoxyl; Persadox	$\left[\text{benzene}-\text{CO}-\text{O}\right]_2$	3,992 [f] (1979)	A	II	1-2	L:--/S: 0.05 mg/m^3 Ceiling (BUL) 5 mg/m^3 TWA (A, BEL F, BRD,N,I,S,USA, USA-N, USA-A)
α,α'-Bis(tert-butylperoxyisopropyl)-benzene 25155-25-3	Chem. Abstr.: [phenylenebis(1-methyl-ethylene)]bis(1,1-dimethylethyl) peroxide IUPAC: (phenylenediisopropylidene)-bis(tert-butyl peroxide) Vul-Cup 40 KE	$(CH_3)_3COOC\begin{smallmatrix}CH_3\\CH_3\end{smallmatrix}-\text{benzene}-\begin{smallmatrix}CH_3\\CH_3\end{smallmatrix}CHOOC(CH_3)_3$	> 0.5 (1980WE) [c]	A	--	--	L:--/S:--
Bis(2,4-dichlorobenzoyl) peroxide 133-14-2	Chem. Abstr.: bis(2,4-dichlorobenzoyl) peroxide IUPAC: bis(2,4-dichlorobenzoyl) peroxide Cadox TS, TS 40, TS 50; Luperco CST; Siloprenvernetzea CL40	$\left[\text{Cl}_2\text{-benzene}-\text{CO}\right]_2$	> 0.9(1979) [f]	A	II III	1-3 1-3	L:--/S:--
tert-Butyl peroxide 110-05-4	Chem. Abstr.: bis(1,1-dimethylethyl) peroxide IUPAC: tert-butyl peroxide di-tert-butyl peroxide; DTBP Cadox TBP; Trigonox B	$\left[(CH_3)_3CO\right]_2$	>11(1979) [f]	A	--	--	L:--/S:--
tert-Butyl peroxybenzoate 614-45-9	Chem. Abstr.: 1,1-dimethylethyl benzene-carboperoxoate IUPAC: tert-butyl peroxybenzoate tert-butyl perbenzoate Chaloxyd TBPB; Esperox 10; Kayabutyl B; Luperox P; Perbutyl Z	$\text{benzene}-\overset{O}{\underset{}{C}}OOC(CH_3)_3$	1,610 [f] (1979)	A	--	--	L:--/S:--

Name and CAS Reg. No.	Synonyms and Trade Names	Structural Formula	US Production -Thousand Kg (Year)	Use Class [a]	Indus- tries	Pro- cesses	Reported Workplace Levels(L)/Occupational Standards(S)[b,q,r,s]
1,1-Di-tert-butylperoxy-3,3,5-trimethylcyclohexane 6731-36-8	Chem. Abstr.: (3,3,5-trimethylcyclohexylidene)bis[(1,1-dimethylethyl)peroxide] IUPAC: (3,3,5-trimethylcyclohexylidene)bis(tert-butyl peroxide) Luperco 231XI; Lupersol 231; Trigonox 29B50, 29B75, 29/40	(structural formula: trimethylcyclohexane with OOC(CH$_3$)$_3$ groups)	17(1979I)[m]	PR	I II III IV	1-3 1-3 1-2 1-2	L:--/S:--
Dicumyl peroxide 80-43-3	Chem. Abstr.: bis(1-methyl-1-phenylethyl) peroxide IUPAC: bis(α,α-dimethylbenzyl) peroxide; cumyl peroxide; α,α-dimethylbenzyl peroxide Di-Cup; Kayacumyl D; Luperco 500-40C, 500-4OKE; Luperox 500; Percumyl D, D40; Perkadox B	(structural formula: [C$_6$H$_5$–C(CH$_3$)(CH$_3$)–O]$_2$)	> 0.45(1979)[f]	A	I II III IV	1-3 1-3 1-2 1-2	L:--/S:--
2,5-Dimethyl-2,5-di(tert-butylperoxy)hexane 78-63-7	Chem. Abstr.: (1,1,4,4-tetramethyl-1,4-butanediyl)bis(1,1-dimethylethyl)peroxide IUPAC: (1,1,4,4-tetramethyltetramethylene)bis(tert-butyl peroxide) Kayahexa AD; Luperco 101; Lupersol 101; Perhexa 2.58, 3M 40; Triganox XQ8; Varox 50	(structural formula: CH$_3$COOC(CH$_3$)$_2$–C(CH$_2$)$_2$–COOCCH$_3$ with CH$_3$ groups)	>2.3 (1979)[f]	A	I II III IV	1-3 1-3 1-2 1-2	L:--/S:--

6. Aldehydes and Ketones

Name and CAS Reg. No.	Synonyms and Trade Names	Structural Formula	US Production -Thousand Kg (Year)	Use Class [a]	Indus-tries	Pro-cesses	Reported Workplace Levels(L)/Occupational Standards(S)[b,q,r,s]
Acetone 67-64-1	Chem. Abstr.: 2-propanone IUPAC: acetone dimethyl ketone	CH_3CCH_3 (=O)	1,184,652 (1979)[i]	S	I II III IV	1-3 1-4 1-3 1-3	L:--/S;--200-4000 mg/m^3 Ceiling (P, USSR,Y,R,CZ) 200-2400 mg/m^3 TWA (H,A,J,CZ,DDR,I, R,S,BEL,F,BRD,N, SWED,USA,USA-A) 2000-3000 mg/m^3 STEL (USA-A,DDR)
Cyclohexanone 108-94-1	Chem. Abstr.: cyclohexanone IUPAC: cyclohexanone Anone; Hexanon; Hytrol D; Nadone; Pimelic ketone; Pimelin ketone; Sextone	(cyclohexanone ring, =O)	395,098 (1979)[f]	S	II III	1,2,4 1-3	L:--/S; 10-400 mg/m^3 Ceiling (BUL,CZ,P,R,Y, USSR) 100-200 mg/m^3 TWA (A, BEL,CZ,F,I,BRD,J, R,N,S,SWED,USA, USA-A)
Formaldehyde 50-00-0	Chem. Abstr.: formaldehyde IUPAC: formaldehyde formalin BFV; Fannoform; Formol; Fyde; Ivalon; Lysoform; Morbicid; Superlysofam	HCHO	2,687,000 (1979)[f]	BA,LM	I II III IV	4 1-4 1-4 1-3	L:--/S: 0.5-7.5 mg/m^3 Ceiling (A,BEL,BUL, CZ,F,J,H,N,P,R,Y, SWED,USSR,USA, USA-A) 1-4.5 mg/m^3 TWA (DDR,BRD,H) 1.2 mg/m^3 30 min.STEL (USA-N) 2 mg/m^3 STEL (DDR) 15 mg/m^3 Peak 30 min. (USA)

Name and CAS Reg. No.	Synonyms and Trade Names	Structural Formula	US Production -Thousand Kg (Year)	Use Class[a]	Indus-tries	Pro-cesses	Reported Workplace Levels(L)/Occupational Standards(S)[b,q,r,s]
Methyl ethyl ketone 78-93-3	Chem. Abstr.: 2-butanone IUPAC: 2-butanone MEK	$CH_3CCH_2CH_3$ (O)	292,527[f] (1979)	S	I II III	1-3 1-4 1-3	L:--/S: 200 mg/m^3 Ceiling (BUL,P,USSR,R,Y) 200-590 mg/m^3 TWA (A,BEL,F,BRD,J,H, DDR,N,I,S,SWED, USA,USA-A) 600-885 mg/m^3 STEL (DDR,USA-A)
Methyl isobutyl ketone 108-10-1	Chem. Abstr.: 4-methyl-2-pentanone IUPAC: 4-methyl-2-pentanone hexone; MIBK	$CH_3CCH_2CH-CH_3$ (O) (CH_3)	85,512[f] (1979)	S	III	1-2	L: -- S: 200-410 mg/m^3 ceiling (P, R, Y) 200-410 mg/m^3 TWA (A,BEL,F,BRD,I,J, N,R,S,SWED,USA, USA-A) 510 mg/m^3 STEL (USA-A)

7. Alcohols

Name and CAS Reg. No.	Synonyms and Trade Names	Structural Formula	US Production -Thousand Kg (Year)	Use Class[a]	Indus-tries	Pro-cesses	Reported Workplace Levels(L)/Occupational Standards(S)[b,q,r,s]
Alkyl alcohols, mixed --	Chem. Abstr.: -- IUPAC: --	ROH	>0.45(1978)[f**]	CLA	I II III IV	1-3 1-3 1-2 1-2	L:--/S:--
Butyl alcohol 71-36-3	Chem. Abstr.: 1-butanol IUPAC: butyl alcohol n-butanol CCS 203; Hemostyp	$CH_3CH_2CH_2CH_2OH$	344,924 (1979)[f]	S	II III	1,2,4 1-3	L:--/S: 10-200 mg/m^3 Ceiling (CZ,P,R,USSR,Y, A,BEL,USA-A) 10-300 mg/m^3 TWA (F,BRD,N,S,H, I,J,CZ,USA,R,SWED)
Ethyl alcohol 64-17-5	Chem. Abstr.: ethanol IUPAC: ethyl alcohol anhydrous alcohol; alcohol; methyl-carbinol Jaysol; SD Alcohol 23-Hydrogen; Tecsol	CH_3CH_2OH	633,809 (1979)[f]	S	I II III IV	1-3 1-4 1-3 1-3	LS:--/S: 200-1900 mg/m^3 Ceiling (BUL, P,R,CZ,USSR,Y) 1000-1900 mg/m^3 TWA (A,BEL,CZ,DDR,H, I,F,BRD,N,R,SWED S,USA,USA-A) 3000 mg/m^3 STEL (DDR)
Glycerine 56-81-5	Chem. Abstr.: 1,2,3-propanetriol IUPAC: glycerol glycerin; glycyl alcohol Glyrol; Glysanin; Osmoglyn	CH_2OH $\mid$ $CHOH$ $\mid$ CH_2OH	67,448 (1979)[f]	SO	I II III IV	1-3 1-3 1-2 1-2	L:--/S: 10 mg/m^3 TWA (USA-A)

Name and CAS Reg. No.	Synonyms and Trade Names	Structural Formula	US Production -Thousand Kg (Year)	Use Class[a]	Indus- tries	Pro- cesses	Reported Workplace Levels(L)/Occupational Standards(S)[b,q,r,s]
Isopropyl alcohol 67-63-0	Chem. Abstr.: 2-propanol IUPAC: isopropyl alcohol isopropanol Alcojel; Alcosolve 2; Avantin; Combi-Schutz; Hartosol; Imsol A; Isohol; Lutosol; Petrohol; PRO; Propol; Takinaocol	$\mathrm{CH_3}$ $\quad\diagdown$ $\quad\quad\mathrm{CHOH}$ $\mathrm{CH_3}\diagup$	855,169 (1979)[f]	S	I II III	1-3 1-4 1-3	L:--/S: 980-2450 mg/m^3 Ceiling (Y,CZ) 200-980 mg/m^3 TWA (A,BEL,F,DDR,BRD,CZ, J,N,R,S,USA,SWED, USA-N,USA-A) 600-1986 mg/m^3 STEL (USA-A,USA-N,DDR)
Methyl alcohol 67-56-1	Chem. Abstr.: methanol IUPAC: methanol Carbinol; Wood alcohol	$\mathrm{CH_3OH}$	3,315,332 (1979)[f]	S	II III	1,2,4 1-3	L:--/S: 5-500 mg/m^3 Ceiling (BUL, R,CZ,P, USSR,Y) 50-260 mg/m^3 TWA (A,BEL,CZ,DDR,F, BRD,H,J,N,SWED, S,I,USA,USA-N, USA-A) 300-1048 mg/m^3 STEL (USA-A, USA-N, DDR)
Polyethylene glycol 25322-68-3	Chem. Abstr.: α-hydro-ω-hydroxy- poly(oxy-1,2-ethanediyl) IUPAC: polyethylene glycols 1,2 ethanediol homopolymer; ethylene glycol homopolymer; oxirane polymer; PEG Alcox E30, E160; Aquaffin; Bradsyn PEG; Carbowax; Chemiox E20; E1000; Emkapol 150, 200, 4200; ENT 1000; Gafanol E200, E300; Laprol 402; Lineartop P; Lutrol 9; Macrogol 400, 6000; Merpol OJ; Modopeg 4000; Nosilen; Nycoline; Oxide Wax A, An; PEO 10, 16, 18, 100; Plastigen PR 8086; Pluriol; Polikol; Polyglycol; Polyox; Polywax 600; Postanol; Solbase; Superox; Swasconol D-60, D-80; Terisan Z 75; Ucar 4C; Viterra 2 Hydrogel; WSR 35, 205 301, N-10, N-750, N-3000, N-Coag	$\mathrm{H(OCH_2CH_2)_nOH}$	40,692 (1979)[f]	M	I II	1-5 1-5	L:--/S:--

8. Miscellaneous

Name and CAS Reg. No.	Synonyms and Trade Names	Structural Formula	US Production -Thousand Kg (Year)	Use Class a	Indus-tries	Pro-cesses	Reported Workplace Levels(L)/Occupational Standards(S)b,q,r,s
Benzofurane derivative --	Chem. Abstr.: -- IUPAC: -- Antiozonant AFD	Indefinite	1.2(1979)m	AN	I II III IV	1-3 1-3 1-2 1-2	L:--/S:--
1,4-Dioxane 123-91-1	Chem. Abstr.: 1,4-dioxane IUPAC: p-dioxane diethylene dioxide; diethylene ether; dioxan; p-dioxan; dioxane	$OCH_2CH_2OCH_2CH_2$	6.8 (1979)f	S	--	--	L:--/S: 1-360 mg/m^3 Ceiling (BUL,P,R,USSR, Y) 90-360 mg/m^3 TWA (A, BEL,F,DDR,BRD,I,N, R,SWED,S,USA,USA-A) 3.6-600 mg/m^3 30 min. STEL (USA-N,DDR)
1,6-Hexanediol bis [3-(3,5-di-tert-butyl-4-hydroxyphenyl)propionate] 35074-77-2	Chem. Abstr.: 1,6-hexanediyl bis-[3,5-bis(1,1-dimethylethyl)-4-hydroxybenzenepropanoate] IUPAC: hexamethylene bis(3,5-di tert-butyl-4-hydroxyhydro-cinnamate) Irganox 259		6.5(1979)m	A	--	--	L:--/S:--

Name and CAS Reg. No.	Synonyms and Trade Names	Structural Formula	US Production -Thousand Kg (Year)	Use Class[a]	Indus-tries	Pro-cesses	Reported Workplace Levels(L)/Occupational Standards(S)[b,q,r,s]
Tetrahydrofuran 109-99-9	Chem. Abstr.: tetrahydrofuran IUPAC: tetrahydrofuran diethylene oxide; THF Oxolane		54,133 (1979)[c]	S	III	1-3	L:--/S: 100-590 mg/m^3 Ceiling (BUL,USSR, R,Y) 100-600 mg/m^3 TWA (A,BEL,F,R,DDR,I, SWED,BRD,N,S,USA, USA-A) 600-735 mg/m^3 STEL (USA-A,DDR)
Sodium pentachlorophenate 131-52-2	Chem. Abstr.: sodium pentachloro-phenate IUPAC: sodium pentachlorophenate sodium PCP; sodium pentachloro-phenol Dowicide G; Mystox D; PCP-Sodium; PKhFN	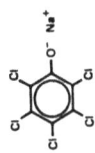	>2.3(1979)[f]	LM	IV	1-2	L:--/S:--

D. Phosphorus Compounds
1. Phosphites

Name and CAS Reg. No.	Synonyms and Trade Names	Structural Formula	US Production -Thousand Kg (Year)	Use Class[a]	Indus-tries	Pro-cesses	Reported Workplace Levels(L)/Occupational Standards(S)[b,q,r,s]
Alkylaryl phosphites, mixed --	Chem. Abstr.: -- / IUPAC: -- / AgeRite; Geltrol; Wytox 320	Indefinite	> 0.9(1979)[f]	AN	I, II, III, IV	1-3, 1-3, 1-2, 1-2	L:--/S:--
Di(nonylphenyl) phosphite --	Chem. Abstr.: -- / IUPAC: --	Indefinite	> 0.5(1980WE)[c]	AN	--	--	L:--/S:--
Diphenyl decyl phosphite 3287-06-7	Chem. Abstr.: decyl diphenyl phosphite / IUPAC: decyl diphenyl phosphite	(structure: phenyl-O-P(O)(OC$_{10}$H$_{21}$)-O-phenyl)	> 0.5(1980WE)[c]	AN	--	--	LS:--/S:--
Nonylphenyl phosphites, mixed --	Chem. Abstr.: -- / IUPAC: --	Indefinite	>1.8(1979)[f]	AN	I, II, III, IV	1-3, 1-3, 1-2, 1-2	L:--/S:--
Polymeric phosphites --	Chem. Abstr.: polymeric phosphites / IUPAC: polymeric phosphites / Wytox 345	Indefinite	> 0.9(1979)[f]	AN	I, II, IV	1-3, 1-3, 1-2	L:--/S:--
Polyphenolic phosphite, polyalkylated --	Chem. Abstr.: -- / IUPAC: -- / Vanox 13	Indefinite	> 0.9(1979)[f]	AN	I, II, III, IV	1-3, 1-3, 1-2, 1-2	L:--/S:--

Name and CAS Reg. No.	Synonyms and Trade Names	Structural Formula	US Production -Thousand Kg (Year)	Use Class[d]	Indus-tries	Pro-cesses	Reported Workplace Levels(L)/Occupational Standards(S)[b],q,r,s
Triaryl phosphites --	Chem. Abstr.: triaryl phosphites IUPAC: triaryl phosphites	$(ArO)_3 P$	>0.45(1979)[f]	AN	--	--	L:--/S:--
Trisnonylphenyl phosphite 26523-78-4	Chem. Abstr.: tris(nonylphenyl) phosphite IUPAC: Nonylphenol phosphite (3:1) Polygard; Stave TNPP; Weston 399, TNPP; Wytox 312	Indefinite	> 912(1977)[d]	AN	I II III IV	1-3 1-3 1-2 1-2	L:--/S:--

2. Phosphates and Phosphonates

Name and CAS Reg. No.	Synonyms and Trade Names	Structural Formula	US Production -Thousand Kg (Year)	Use Class[a]	Indus-tries	Pro-cesses	Reported Workplace Levels(L)/Occupational Standards(S)[b,q,r,s]
3,5-Di-tert-butyl-4-hydroxy-benzyl phosphonic acid, mono-ethyl ester, nickel salt 30947-30-9	Chem. Abstr.: ((3,5-bis(1,1-dimethyl-ethyl)-4-hydroxyphenyl)methyl)-phosphonic acid, monoethyl ester, nickel(2+) salt (2:1) IUPAC: nickel(2+) bis[ethyl(3,5-di-tert-butyl-4-hydroxybenzyl)-phosphonate] Irgastab 2002		50(1979I)[m]	M	--	--	L:--/S:--
Diethyldithiophosphoric acid 298-06-6	Chem. Abstr.: phosphorodithioic acid, O,O-diethyl ester IUPAC: diethyl hydrogen phosphorodithioate O,O'-diethyldithiophosphate; O,O'-diethyl hydrogen dithiophosphate; O,O'-diethyl phosphorodithioate		> 0.5(1980)[c]	A	--	--	L:--/S:--
Mono- and dialkyl phosphates, mixed --	Chem. Abstr.: -- IUPAC: --		> 0.45(1976)[f*]	CLA	--	--	L:--/S:--
Mono- and dialkyl phosphate, ammonium salts, mixed --	Chem. Abstr.: -- IUPAC: --		>0.45(1979)[f]	CLA	--	--	L:--/S:--

Name and CAS Reg. No.	Synonyms and Trade Names	Structural Formula	US Production -Thousand Kg (Year)	Use Class[a]	Indus-tries	Pro-cesses	Reported Workplace Levels(L)/Occupational Standards(S)[b,q,r,s]
Tris(2,3-dibromopropyl) phosphate 126-72-7	Chem. Abstr.: 2,3-dibromo-1-propanol phosphate (3:1) IUPAC: tris(2,3-dibromopropyl) phosphate TDPP: tris Anfram 3PB; Apex 462-5; Bromkal P67-6HP; ES 685; Firemaster LV-T 23P, T 23P; Flacavon R; Flammex AP, LV-T 23P, T23P; Forol HB32; Phoscon PE60; 3 PBR; T 238; Zetoflex ZN	$\begin{array}{l}BrCH_2CHBrCH_2O \\ BrCH_2CHBrCH_2O{-}P{=}O \\ BrCH_2CHBrCH_2O\end{array}$	2.3 (1977)[f**]	M	IV	1-5	L:--/S:--

E. Halogen Compounds

Name and CAS Reg. No.	Synonyms and Trade Names	Structural Formula	US Production -Thousand Kg (Year)	Use Class [a]	Indus- tries	Pro- cesses	Reported Workplace Levels(L)/Occupational Standards(S)[b,q,r,s]
Carbon tetrachloride 56-23-5	Chem. Abstr.: tetrachloromethane IUPAC: carbon tetrachloride carbona; carbon chloride; carbon tet; perchloromethane Benzinoform; Fasciolin; Flukoids; Neca-torina; R 10; Tetrafinol; Tetraform; Tetrasol; Univerm; Vermoestricid	CCl_4	321,507[f] (1979)	S	I II III	1-3 1-4 1-3	L:--/S: 1-163 mg/m^3 Ceiling (BUL,CZ,P, R,USA,USSR,Y) 5.6-65 mg/m^3 TWA (A,BEL,CZ,F,DDR,I, BRD,H,J,N,R,SWED, S,USA) 100-130 mg/m^3 STEL (DDR,USA-A) 12.6 mg/m^3 STEL 1 hour (USA-N) 1300 mg/m^3 5 min./ 4 hour peak (USA)
Chloroform 67-66-3	Chem. Abstr.: trichloromethane IUPAC: chloroform R-20	$CHCl_3$	160,218[f] (1979)	S	--	--	L:--/S: 50-250 mg/m^3 Ceiling (BUL,CZ, P,DDR,R,USA,Y) 10-240 mg/m^3 TWA (A, BEL,CZ,F,H,BRD,I, DDR,J,N,R,SWED,S, USA,USA-A) 225 mg/m^3 STEL (USA-A) 9.8 mg/m^3 STEL 1 hour (USA-N)

Name and CAS Reg. No.	Synonyms and Trade Names	Structural Formula	US Production -Thousand Kg (Year)	Use Class[a]	Indus-tries	Pro-cesses	Reported Workplace Levels(L)/Occupational Standards(S)[b,q,r,s]
Chlorotoluenes 95-49-8, 108-41-8 and 106-43-4	Chem. Abstr.: 1-chloro-2-methylbenzene, 1-chloro-3-methylbenzene and 1-chloro-4-methylbenzene; IUPAC: o-chlorotoluene, m-chlorotoluene and p-chlorotoluene		>0.9(1979)[f] (o-isomer) >0.45 (1979)[f] (p-isomer)	S	--	--	L:--/S: 0.5-395 mg/m³ Ceiling (R,USSR,Y) 5-250 mg/m³ TWA (BEL, N,R,A,USA,USA-A) 375 mg/m³ STEL (USA-A)
o-Dichlorobenzene 95-50-1	Chem. Abstr.: 1,2-dichlorobenzene; IUPAC: o-dichlorobenzene; Chloroben; Dilatin DB; Dowtherm E		25,701 (1979)[f]	S	--	--	L:--/S: 20-300 mg/m³ Ceiling (BEL,BUL,F, N,P,R,USSR,USA, USA-A,Y) 20-300 mg/m³ TWA (A, DDR,BRD.H,I,J,R,S, SWED) 300 mg/m³ STEL (DDR)
Ethylene dichloride 107-06-2	Chem. Abstr.: 1,2-dichloroethane; IUPAC: 1,2-dichloroethane; EDC; Brocide; Dichlor-Mulsion; Dutch Liquid	ClCH₂CH₂Cl	5,307,358 (1979)[f]	S	I II III	1-3 1-3 1-2	L: >1366 mg/m³[bb]; 140 mg/m³[cc] 10-400 mg/m³ Ceiling (CZ,P,R,USSR,Y,USA) 4-200 mg/m³ TWA (A, BEL,CZ,F,DDR,BRD,I,J, N,R,SWED,S,USA,USA-A, USA-N) 8-150 mg/m³ STEL (USA, USA-A,USA-N,DDR) 800 mg/m³ 5 min./3 hour peak (USA)
Fluorinated hydrocarbons --	Chem. Abstr.: --; IUPAC: --	Indefinite	396,560 (1979)[f]	M	I II	1-5 1-5	L:--/S:--

Name and CAS Reg. No.	Synonyms and Trade Names	Structural Formula	US Production -Thousand Kg (Year)	Use Class	Indus- tries	Pro- cesses	Reported Workplace Levels(L)/Occupational Standards(S)[b,q,r,s]
Methylene chloride 75-09-2	Chem. Abstr.: dichloromethane IUPAC: dichloromethane methylene dichloride Aerothene MM; Narkotel; R30; Solaesthin; Solmethine	CH_2Cl_2	284,962 (1979)[f]	S	I II III	1-3 1-4 1-3	L:--/S: 50-700 mg/m³ Ceiling (CZ,Y, P,R,USSR,USA,USA-N) 200-1740 mg/m³ TWA (A,BEL,CZ,F,DDR,I, BRD,J,N,R,SWED,S, USA,USA-N,USA-A) 870-1500 mg/m³ STEL (DDR,USA-A) 7200 mg/m³ 5 min./ 2 hours peak (USA)
Monochlorobenzene 108-90-7	Chem. Abstr.: chlorobenzene IUPAC: chlorobenzene MCB; phenyl chloride		145,531 (1979)[f]	S	I II III	1-3 1-3 1-2	L:--/S: 50-300 mg/m³ Ceiling (BUL,CZ, P,R,USSR,Y) 50-850 mg/m³ TWA (A. BEL,CZ,F,DDR,BRD, N,I,J,N,R,S,USA, USA-A) 150 mg/m³ STEL (DDR)
Perchloroethylene 127-18-4	Chem. Abstr.: tetrachloroethene IUPAC: tetrachloroethylene perc; perchlor; 1,1,2,2-tetrachloro-ethylene Ankilostin; Antisal; Dee-Solv; Di'Akene; Dow-per; ENT 1860; Fedal-Un; Nema; Perclene; PerSec; Tetlen; Tetracap; Tetralino; Tetravec; Tetroguer; Tetraleno; Tetropil	$Cl_2C=CCl_2$	347,863 (1979)[f]	S	I II III	1-3 1-4 1-3	L:--/S: 10-670 mg/m³ Ceiling (BUL,CZ,P, R,USSR,Y,USA) 50-670 mg/m³ TWA (A,BEL,CZ,F,DDR, BRD,H,I,J,N,R,SWED, S,USA-N,USA-A,USA) 670-1000 mg/m³ STEL (DDR,USA-A,USA-N) 2010 mg/m³ 5 min./2 hours peak (USA)

Name and CAS Reg. No.	Synonyms and Trade Names	Structural Formula	US Production -Thousand Kg (Year)	Use Class[a]	Indus-tries	Pro-cesses	Reported Workplace Levels(L)/Occupational Standards(S)[b,q,r,s]
Propylene dichloride 78-87-5	Chem. Abstr.: 1,2-dichloropropane IUPAC: 1,2-dichloropropane propylene chloride	$ClCH_2CHCH_3$	31,420 (1979)[f]	S	I II III IV	1-3 1-3 1-2 1-2	L:-/S: 10-350 mg/m^3 Ceiling (BUL,P,R, USSR,Y) 50-350 mg/m^3 TWA (A, BEL,F,DDR,BRD,N,R, S,USA,USA-A) 150-510 mg/m^3 STEL (DDR, USA-A)
1,1,1-Trichloroethane 71-55-6	Chem. Abstr.: 1,1,1-trichloroethane IUPAC: 1,1,1-trichloroethane methyl chloroform Aerothene TT; Chlorothene NU, VG; Chlorten; Inhibisol	CH_3CCl_3	322,351 (1979)[f]	S	II III	1,2,4 1-3	L: 716.6 mg/m^{3u} S: 20-2000 mg/m^3 Ceiling (CZ,R, USSR,Y) 380-1900 mg/m^3 TWA (A,BEL,CZ,F,DDR, BRD,I,J,N,R,SWED, USA,USA-A) 1900-2450 mg/m^3 STEL (DDR,USA-A, USA-N)
Trichloroethylene 79-01-6	Chem. Abstr.: trichloroethene IUPAC: trichloroethylene TCE; Tri Algylen; Anamenth; Chlorilen; Chlorylen; Densinfluat; Fluate; Germalgene; Narcogen; Narkosoid; Threthylene; Trethylene; Trichloran; Trichloren; Triclene; Trilene; Trimar; Westrosol	$Cl_2C=CHCl$	143,744 (1979)[f]	S	I II III	1-3 1-3 1-3	L:-/S: 10-1050 mg/m^3 Ceiling (BUL,CZ,P,R,USSR, Y,USA) 50-535 mg/m^3 TWA (A,BEL,CZ,F,DDR, BRD,H,I,J,N,R, SWED,S,USA,USA-A, USA-N) 800-1000 mg/m^3 STEL (DDR,USA-A) 1605 mg/m^3 5 min./ 2 hours peak (USA)

F. Hydrocarbons

L: 5.5 mg/m³ (C_5-C_8; alkanes (C_3-C_8)[x]

Name and CAS Reg. No.	Structural Formula	US Production -Thousand Kg (Year)	Use Class[a]	Indus-tries	Pro-cesses	Reported Workplace Levels(L)/Occupational Standards(S)[b,q,r,s]
Benzene 71-43-2	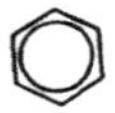 (benzene ring)	5,309,007 (1979)[f]	S	I II III	1-3 1-3 1-2	L: 38.4 mg/m³[u] ; 4.5 mg/m³[v] ; 6 mg/m³[w] (1935-1937) 780 mg/m³ (1935-1937)[t]; 375 mg/m³ (1961)[t]; 420 mg/m³ (1977)[t]; 137 mg/m³; 129 mg/m³[dd]; 8.4 mg/m³[ee] S: 5-80 mg/m³ Ceiling (CZ,I,J,P,S, USSR,Y,USA) 15-50 mg/m³ TWA (A,BEL,CZ,F,H, N,SWED,USA,USA-A) 75-100 mg/m³ STEL (DDR,USA-A) 3.2 mg/m³ STEL 1 hour (USA-N) 150 mg/m³ 10 min. peak (USA)
Coal tar oils 65996-82-9	Complex mixture	> 1,140,000 (1977)[d]	SO	--	--	L:--/S:--
Cyclohexane 110-82-7	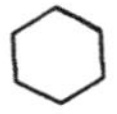 (cyclohexane ring)	1,091,376 (1979)[f]	S	I II III	1-3 1-3 1-2	L:--/S: 80-1050 mg/m³ Ceiling (BUL,P,R, USSR,Y) 514-1050 mg/m³ TWA (A,BEL,F,BRD,I,J. N,R,S,USA,USA-A) 1300 mg/m³ STEL (USA-A)

Chem. Abstr.: benzene
IUPAC: benzene
benzol; coal naphtha

Chem. Abstr.:--
IUPAC:--
chemical oil (coal); tar acid oil (coal)

Chem. Abstr.: cyclohexane
IUPAC: cyclohexane
hexahydrobenzene

Name and CAS Reg. No.	Synonyms and Trade Names	Structural Formula	US Production -Thousand Kg (Year)	Use Class[a]	Indus-tries	Pro-cesses	Reported Workplace Levels(L)/Occupational Standards(S)[b],[q],[r],[s]
Dipentene 138-86-3	Chem. Abstr.: 1-methyl-4-(1-methyl-ethenyl)cyclohexene IUPAC: p-mentha-1,8-diene limonene Cajeputen; Cinene; Dipenten; Eulimen; Kautschin; Nesol		>11.3(1980)[c]	S	--	--	L:--/S:--
heptane 42-82-5	Chem. Abstr.: heptane IUPAC: heptane dipropylmethane; n-heptane Skellysolve C	$CH_3(CH_2)_5CH_3$	>4.5(1979)[f]	S	I II III	1-4 1-4 1-2	L: 552 mg/m^3 [u] S: 200-2000 mg/m^3 ceiling (P,R,Y) 1200-2000 mg/m^3 TWA (A,BEL,F,BRD, I, N,R,S,USA,USA-A) 450 mg/m^3 STEL (USA-A)
xane 0-54-3	Chem. Abstr.: hexane IUPAC: hexane n-hexane Skellysolve B	$CH_3(CH_2)_4CH_3$	174,417 (1979)[f]	S	I II III	2-5 1-4 1-2	L: 1382 mg/m^3 [u] S: 400-1800 mg/m^3 ceiling (P,R,Y) 350-1800 mg/m^3 TWA (A,BEL,F,BRD,I,J, N,R,S,USA,USA-A) 450 mg/m^3 STEL (USA-A)
Isooctane 540-84-1	Chem. Abstr.: 2,2,4-trimethylpentane IUPAC: isooctane isobutyltrimethylmethane	$(CH_3)_3CCH_2CH(CH_3)_2$	45(1977)[d]	S	--	--	L:--/S: 700 mg/m^3 Ceiling (R) 500 mg/m^3 TWA (R)
Mineral Oil 8012-95-1	Chem. Abstr.:-- IUPAC:-- paraffin oil Flexon 845; Irrawax 361; Paraffin oil: Petrolatum, liquid; Primol D; Shellflex 371N; Sunpar 150; Ultrol 7; Uvasol	Complex mixture (may contain polycyclic aromatic hydrocarbons-- see Section VI)	--	SO	I II III IV	1-3 1-3 1-2 1-2	L:--/S: 5 mg/m^3 Ceiling (USSR) 3-5 mg/m^3 TWA (DDR,I,J)

Name and CAS Reg. No.	Synonyms and Trade Names	Structural Formula	US Production -Thousand Kg (Year)	Use Class[a]	Indus-tries	Pro-cesses	Reported Workplace Levels(L)/Occupational Standards(S)[b,q,r,s]
Mineral Rubber 64742-93-4	Chem. Abstr.:-- IUPAC:-- blown asphalt; condensed asphalt; hard hydrocarbon; oxidized asphalt M.R. No. 38 Mineral Rubber	Complex mixture	--	SO,F	--	--	L:--/S:--
Naphtha 8030-30-6	Chem. Abstr.: naphtha IUPAC: naphtha benzin; petroleum benzin; petroleum ether; petroleum naphtha Hi-Sol 10, 15; Rubber Solvent; Shell Sol B, B-8, BT67 EC	Complex mixture	3,855 (1979)[f]	S	I II III IV	1-4 1-4 1-2 1-2	L:--/S: 300-500 mg/m^3 Ceiling (P,Y) 200-400 mg/m^3 TWA (F,I,USA) Benzene soluble PAH, 0.2 mg/m^3 (A,BEL, USA-A)
Octane 111-65-9	Chem. Abstr.: octane IUPAC: octane n-octane	$CH_3(CH_2)_6CH_3$	> 2.2(1979)[f]	S	I	2,4	L:--/ S: 200-2350 mg/m^3 Ceiling (P,R,Y) 1450-2350 mg/m^3 TWA (A,BEL,F,BRD,I,N, R,SWED,S,USA,USA-A) 1800 mg/m^3 STEL(USA-A)
Pentane 109-66-0	Chem. Abstr.: pentane IUPAC: pentane n-pentane Skellysolve A	$CH_3(CH_2)_3CH_3$	32,285[f] (1979)	S	I	2,4	L: 576 mg/m^3[u] S: 100-2400 Ceiling mg/m^3(P,R,Y) 1500-2950 mg/m^3 TWA (A,BEL,F,BRD,I, N,R,S,SWED,USA,USA-A) 2250 mg/m^3STEL (USA-A)
Petrolatum 8009-03-8	Chem. Abstr.: petrolatum IUPAC: petrolatum Chresm White; Extra Amber; Pennsoline Soft Yellow; Penreco white; Perfecta; Petroleum jelly, Protopet; Snow White; Ultima White; White Protopet;	Complex mixture	>947,955[d] (1977)	SO,CLA	I II III IV	1-3 1-3 1-2 1-2	L:--/S:--

Name and CAS Reg. No.	Synonyms and Trade Names	Structural Formula	US Production -Thousand Kg (Year)	Use Class[a]	Indus-tries	Pro-cesses	Reported Workplace Levels(L)/Occupational Standards(S)[b,q,r,s]
Pitch 61789-60-4	Chem. Abstr.: pitch IUPAC: pitch pitch of tar Emery 786; Tolpit 35	Complex mixture	54,140 (1977)[d]	SO,A	I II III IV	1-3 1-3 1-2 1-2	L:--/S: 0.2 mg/m^3 Ceiling (Y) 0.1-0.2 mg/m^3 TWA (A, BEL, I, N, S, USA, USA-A, USA-N)
Toluene 108-88-3	Chem. Abstr.: methylbenzene IUPAC: toluene toluol Antisal la	CH_3-benzene	3,246,658 (1979)[f]	S	I II III	1-4 1-4 1-3	L: 188 mg/m^3 [u] ; 214 mg/m^3 [v] ; 988 mg/m^3 [z] S: 50-1300 mg/m^3 Ceiling (BUL,CZ, R.P.USA,USSR,Y) 50-750 mg/m^3 TWA (A,BEL,CZ,F,DDR, BRD,H,I,J,N,R, SWED,S,USA,USA-N, USA-A) 560-800 mg/m^3 STEL (USA-A,DDR) 750 mg/m^3 STEL 10 min. (USA-N) 1875 mg/m^3 10. min. peak (USA)
Xylene 1330-20-7	Chem. Abstr.: dimethylbenzene IUPAC: xylene xylol Dilan	CH_3-benzene-CH_3	3,320,098 (1979)[f]	S	I II III	1-4 1-4 1-3	L: 57 mg/m^3 [u] S: 50-1000 mg/m^3 Ceiling (BUL,CZ,R,Y) 50-870 mg/m^3 TWA (A,BEL,CZ,F,DDR, BRD,H,I,J,N,SWED, S,USA-A,USA-N) 600-655 mg/m^3 STEL (DDR,USA-A) 868 mg/m^3 STEL 10 min. (USA-N)

Name and CAS Reg. No.	Synonyms and Trade Names	Structural Formula	US Production -Thousand Kg (Year)	Use Class [a]	Indus- tries	Pro- cesses	Reported Workplace Levels(L)/Occupational Standards(S) [b,q,r,s]
p-Xylene 106-42-3	Chem. Abstr.: 1,4-dimethylbenzene IUPAC: p-xylene p-xylol		2,092,404 (1979)[f]	S	I II III	1-4 1-4 1-3	L: 57 mg/m^3[u] S: 50-1000 mg/m^3 Ceiling (BUL,CZ,R,Y) 50-870 mg/m^3 TWA (A,BEL,CZ,F,DDR, BRD,H,I,J,N,SWED, S,USA,USA-A,USA-N) 600-655 mg/m^3 STEL (DDR,USA-A) 868 mg/m^3 STEL 10 min. (USA-N)

G. Miscellaneous Organic Compounds

Name and CAS Reg. No.	Synonyms and Trade Names	Structural Formula	US Production -Thousand Kg (Year)	Use Class [a]	Indus- tries	Pro- cesses	Reported Workplace Levels(L)/Occupational Standards(S)[b,q,r,s]
Bitumen 8052-42-4	Chem. Abstr.: bitumen IUPAC: bitumen asphalt; asphaltum; Judean pitch; mineral pitch	Complex mixture	> 6,116,625 (1977)[d]	SO	--	--	L:--/S: **2**.5-5 mg/m^3 TWA (BEL, I, N, R, S, USA, USA-A) 10 mg/m^3 STEL (USA-A, USA-N)
6-tert-Butyl-m-cresol -- sulphur dichloride condensate --	Chem. Abstr. 2-(1,1-dimethylethyl)-5-methyl-phenol, reaction product with sulphur chloride (SCl$_2$) IUPAC: 6-tert-butyl-m-cresol,reaction product with sulphur chloride (SCl$_2$) Santowhite MK	Unknown	> 2.2(1980)[c]	AN	I II III IV	1-3 1-3 1-2 1-2	L:--/S:--
Casein 9000-71-9	Chem. Abstr.: casein IUPAC: casein Protaflex; Protoflex	Indefinite	55,434 (1979I)[e*]	LM	--	--	L:--/S:--
Cotton Fiber --	Chem. Abstr.: cotton fiber IUPAC: cotton fiber	Indefinite	--	F	I II III IV	1-3 1-3 1-2 1-2	L:--/S: 2-6 mg/m^3 Ceiling (CZ,DDR, USSR) 5 mg/m^3 (Y)[1]
Coumarone-indene resins 63393-89-5	Chem. Abstr.:-- IUPAC:-- Cumar; Cumrone; Natro-Rez 50-D; Nevillac; Nevindene; Piccoumaron; Piccovar	Complex mixture	> 900(1977)[d]	T, SO	I II III IV	1-3 1-3 1-2 1-2	L:--/S:--

Name and CAS Reg. No.	Synonyms and Trade Names	Structural Formula	US Production -Thousand Kg (Year)	Use Class[a]	Indus- tries	Pro- cesses	Reported Workplace Levels(L)/Occupational Standards(S)[b,q,r,s]
Phenol-formaldehyde resins 9003-35-4	Chem. Abstr.: phenol, polymer with formaldehyde IUPAC: phenol, polymer with formaldehyde formaldehyde-phenol resin Akrochem P-37, 49; PA-52; SP-G601- 6001, 6700, 6710	Indefinite	800,370[f] (1979)	SO	I II III IV	1-3 1-3 1-2 1-2	L:--/S:--
Pine Tar 8011-48-1	Chem. Abstr.: pine tar IUPAC: pine tar Aktar; Tarene; Tartac	Complex mixture	--	SO	I II III IV	1-3 1-3 1-2 1-2	
Silicones --	Chem. Abstr.: silicones IUPAC: silicones silicone fluids	Indefinite	98,835[f] (1979)	M	--	--	L:--/S:--

Name and CAS Reg. No.	Synonyms and Trade Names	Structural Formula	US Production -Thousand Kg (Year)	Use Class [a]	Indus-tries	Pro-cesses	Reported Workplace Levels(L)/Occupational Standards(S)[b,q,r,s]
Vinyltris(2-methoxyethoxy) silane 1067-53-4	Chem. Abstr.: 6-ethenyl-6-(2-methoxy-ethoxy)-2,5,7,10-tetraoxa-6-silaun-decane IUPAC: tris(2-methoxyethoxy)vinylsilane A 172; GF 58; NUCA 172	$CH_2 = CHSi(OCH_2CH_2OCH_3)_3$	> 0.5(1980WE)[c]	M	--	--	L:--/S:--
Wax base, Ozone Protector 80 --	Chem. Abstr.: Ozone protective wax base 80 IUPAC: Ozone protective wax base 80	Indefinite	> 0.45(1976)[c]	AN	--	--	L:--/S:--
Waxes and paraffinic products --	Chem. Abstr.: -- IUPAC: --	Complex mixture	>0.9(1978)[f++]	SO	--	--	L:--/S:--
Wood flour --	Chem. Abstr.: wood flour IUPAC: wood flour	Complex mixture	--	F	I II III IV	1-3 1-3 1-2 1-2	L:--/S: 10 mg/m^3 (DDR)

II. Inorganic Compounds

Name and CAS Reg. No.	Synonyms and Trade Names	Structural Formula	US Production -Thousand Kg (Year)	Use Class [a]	Indus-tries	Pro-cesses	Reported Workplace Levels(L)/Occupational Standards(S)[b,q,r,s]
Aluminium hydrate 21645-51-2	Chem. Abstr.: aluminium hydroxide [Al(OH)$_3$]; IUPAC: aluminium hydroxide; alumina hydrate; aluminic acid — Alcoa C30BF, C330, 333; Alugel; Alumigel; Alusal; Amberol ST 140F; Baco AF260; Calmogastrin; Hychol 705; Hydrafil; Hydral 710; Higilite H 31 S, H 42; Martinal A, AlS, F-a; Reheis F 1000; Solem SB-632	Al(OH)$_3$	>5,012(1977)[d]	AN	I, II, III, IV	1-3, 1-3, 1-2, 1-2	L:--/S:--
Aluminium oxide 1344-28-1	Chem. Abstr.: aluminium oxide [Al$_2$O$_3$]; IUPAC: aluminium oxide; alumina; aluminium trioxide; alumite — Al; Alcoa F-1; Almite; Alon C; Aloxite; Aluminite 37; Alumogel Al; Alundum 600; Cab-O-Grip; Catapal S; Compalox; Conopal; Dispal M, Alumina; Dotment 324, 358; Exolon XW60; Faserton; Fasertonerde; Hypalox II; KA161; KHP 2; Ketjen B; LA 6; Lucalox; Ludox CL; Martoxin; Microgrit WCA; Neobead C; Poraminar	Al$_2$O$_3$	5,739,478 (1979)[e,k]	F	--	--	L:--/S: 2 mg/m^3 Ceiling (USSR) 20 mg/m^3 (S)[1]
Aluminium silicate 14504-95-1	Chem. Abstr.: silicic acid [H$_2$SiO$_3$], aluminium salt (3:2); IUPAC: aluminium silicate [Al$_2$(SiO$_3$)$_3$] — Afton; Allen R; Apex; Barden R; Kaolloid; Optiwhite; Snobrite;	Al$_2$(SiO$_3$)$_3$	> 4.4(1980)[c]	F	I, II, III, IV	1-3, 1-3, 1-2, 1-2	L:--/S:--
Ammonia 7664-41-7	Chem. Abstr.: ammonia; IUPAC: ammonia; ammonia gas; spirit of hartshorn — Nitro-Sil; R 717	NH$_3$	16,859,673 (1979)[e]	A,LM	II, IV	4, 1-3	L:--/S: 20-80 mg/m^3 Ceiling (CZ,P,R, USSR,Y) 18-4Q mg/m^3 TWA (A,BEL,CZ,F,DDR, BRD,H,I,J,N,R, SWED,S,USA,USA-A) 25-27 mg/m^3 STEL (USA-A,DDR) 35 mg/m^3 STEL 5 min. (USA-N)

Name and CAS Reg. No.	Synonyms and Trade Names	Structural Formula	US Production -Thousand Kg (Year)	Use Class [a]	Indus-tries	Pro-cesses	Reported Workplace Levels(L)/Occupational Standards(S)[b,q,r,s]
Ammonium bicarbonate 1066-33-7	Chem. Abstr.: ammonium hydrogen carbonate IUPAC: ammonium hydrogen carbonate monoammonium carbonate	NH_4HCO_3	>229,635 (1977)[d]	F	--	--	L:--/S:--
Ammonium nitrate 6484-52-2	Chem. Abstr.: ammonium nitrate IUPAC: ammonium nitrate AN Varioform I	NH_4NO_3	6,788,553 (1979)[e]	M	--	--	L:--/S:--
Ammonium sulphate 7783-20-2	Chem. Abstr.: diammonium sulphate IUPAC: diammonium sulphate Dolamin	$(NH_4)_2SO_4$	2,556,722 (1979)[e]	LM	IV	1-2	L:--/S:--
Antimony trioxide 1309-64-4	Chem. Abstr.: antimony oxide $[Sb_2O_3]$ IUPAC: diantimony trioxide or antimony oxide (Sb_2O_3) antimony white; flowers of antimony Antox; Chemetron Fire Shield; Exitelite; Thermoguard B, S; Timonox	Sb_2O_3	>2700(1977)[d]	AN	I II III IV	1-3 1-3 1-2 1-2	L:--/S:--

Name and CAS Reg. No.	Synonyms and Trade Names	Structural Formula	US Production -Thousand Kg (Year)	Use Class[a]	Indus-tries	Pro-cesses	Reported Workplace Levels(L)/Occupational Standards(S)[b,q,r,s]
Asbestos 1332-21-4	Chem. Abstr.: asbestos IUPAC: asbestos Caldria Asbestos	Complex mixture	87(1980)[o]	F	--	--	L: >100,000 fibers> 5 µm long/cm³ y S: 2-8 mg/m³ Ceiling (CZ,USSR,Y) 1-4 mg/m³ (P)[1] 200 particles/cm³ (H) 1-5 fibers >5 µm long/cm³ (F,SWED)[1] 0.1-2 fibers >5 µm long/cm³ TWA (USA-A,USA-I) 10 fibers >5 µm long/cm³ Ceiling (USA) 0.5 fibers >5 µm long/cm³ STEL (USA-N)
Barium sulphate 7727-43-7	Chem. Abstr.: barium sulphate IUPAC: barium sulphate Baryte; Blanc fixe; C.I. Pigment White 21; permanent white Actybaryte; Bakontal; Barco B; Baridol; Bariwite; Baritop; Barosperse; Barotrast; Citobaryum; Enamel White; Eweiss; E-Z-Paque; Finemeal; Lactobaryt; Liquibarine; Micropaque; Neobar; Solbar; Supramikre; Unibaryt	BaSO₄	>54,593 (1977)[d]	F	I II III IV	1-3 1-3 1-2 1-2	L:--/S:--
Bentonite 1302-78-9	Chem. Abstr.: bentonite IUPAC: bentonite Albagel premium USP 4444; Tixoton; Volcaly Bentonite BC	Al₂O₃·4SiO₂·H₂O (Major component)	>450(1977)[d]	F	--	--	L:--/S:--

Name and CAS Reg. No.	Synonyms and Trade Names	Structural Formula	US Production -Thousand Kg (Year)	Use Class [a]	Indus-tries	Pro-cesses	Reported Workplace Levels(L)/Occupational Standards(S)[b,q,r,s]
Cadmium Yellow 1306-23-6	Chem. Abstr.: cadmium sulphide IUPAC: cadmium sulphide Cadmium Golden 366; Cadmium Lemon Yellow 527; Cadmium Primrose 819; Cadmium Yellow 000, 892, 10G, Deep, Golden, Lemon, Primrose, OZ dark, Primrose 47-4100; Cadmopur Golden Yellow N; Cadmopur Yellow; Capsebon; C.P. Golden Yellow 55; Ferro Lemon Yellow, Orange Yellow, Yellow	CdS	>149(1977)[d]	C	I II III IV	1-3 1-3 1-2 1-2	L:--/S:--
Calcium carbonate 471-34-1	Chem. Abstr.: calcium carbonate IUPAC: calcium carbonate chalk whiting; marble flour; Paris white; Pigment White 18 40-200; Allied Whiting; Amical; Atomite; Calcene; Calofort; Calopake; Calwhite; Camel-CARB,-TEX,-WITE; CC 100, 101, 109; CCC G, H, Q-White; Dirkalite; Dryca-Flo; Durmite; Gama-Sperse; Hakuenka CC; Hydrocarb; Kotamite; Laminar; OMYA; Omyalene; Omyalite; Polcarb; Purecal; Smithko Kalkarb; Socal; Solemite; Stan-white; Sturcal; Vicron; Witcarb	$CaCO_3$	193,199 (100% CaCO3) (1979)[e]	F	I II III IV	1-3 1-3 1-2 1-2	L:--/S: 10-20 mg/m^3 (F,I,S,USA-A)[1]
Calcium chloride 10043-52-4	Chem. Abstr.: calcium chloride [CaCl2] IUPAC: calcium chloride calcium dichloride Calcosan; Liquidow; Uramine MC	$CaCl_2$	1,080 (1975)[e]	LM	IV	1-2	L:--/S:--
Calcium nitrate 10124-37-5	Chem. Abstr.: nitric acid, calcium salt IUPAC: calcium dinitrate Norway saltpeter Synfat 1006	$Ca(NO_3)_2$	111,639 (1979)[e*]	LM	IV	1-2	L:--/S:--

Name and CAS Reg. No.	Synonyms and Trade Names	Structural Formula	US Production -Thousand Kg (Year)	Use Class [a]	Indus- tries	Pro- cesses	Reported Workplace Levels(L)/Occupational Standards(S)[b],[q],[r],[s]
Calcium oxide 1305-78-8	Chem. Abstr.: calcium oxide IUPAC: calcium oxide burnt lime; calcia; calcium monoxide; calx Caloxol W3; Calxyl; Desical; Rhenosorb C, F	CaO	7,891,695 (1977)[d]	A	II	1-2	L:--/S: 2-5 mg/m^3 Ceiling (P,R,Y) 2-5 mg/m^3 TWA (A, BEL, F, BRD, I, N, R, SWED, S, USA)
Calcium silicate 10034-77-2	Chem. Abstr.: silicic acid [H$_4$SiO$_4$], calcium salt (1:2) IUPAC: calcium silicate (Ca$_2$SiO$_4$) bicalcium silicate; dicalcium silicate; C2S	Ca$_2$SiO$_4$	0.9(1977)[d]	F	--	--	L:--/S: 10 mg/m^3 TWA (USA-A)
Calcium sulphate 7778-18-9	Chem. Abstr.: calcium sulphate IUPAC: calcium sulphate Crysalba; Drierite; Gibs; Thiolite	CaSO$_4$	>3,060,190 (1977)[d]	M	--	--	L:--/S: 20 mg/m^3(S)[1]
Carbon black 1333-86-4	Chem. Abstr.: carbon black IUPAC: carbon black C.I. Pigment Black 7; Channel Black; Columbia carbon; Corax P; Delussa Black FW; Furnex N 765; Philblack N550, 765; Printex 60; Regol 99; Spheron 6; Statex N550; Sterling N765, SO 1; TM-30; Witcoblak No. 100	C (may contain polycyclic aromatic hydrocarbons-- see Section VI)	>657,078 (1977)[d]	F	I II III IV	1-3 1-3 1-2 1-2	L:--/S: 3-20 mg/m^3 TWA (A, BEL, F, I, N, S, USA, SWED, USA-A, USA-N) 7 mg/m^3 STEL (USA-A) 0.1 mg/m^3 TWA in presence of polycyclic aromatic amines (USA-N)
Chrome Yellow 1344-37-2	Chem. Abstr.: C.I. Pigment Yellow 34 IUPAC: C.I. Pigment Yellow 34 Chromastral Green; Chrome Orange; Chrome Yellow Lemon; Chrome Yellow Middle; Chrome Yellow Primrose; Krolor Yellow; Lemon Chrome; Pure Lemon Chrome; Pure Middle Chrome; Pure Primrose Chrome; Supra Lemon Chrome; Vynamon Yellow	Indefinite	31,026(1979)[e,f]	C	II III	1-3 1-2	L:--/S:--

Name and CAS Reg. No.	Synonyms and Trade Names	Structural Formula	US Production -Thousand Kg (Year)	Use Class [a]	Indus- tries	Pro- cesses	Reported Workplace Levels(L)/Occupational Standards(S)[b,q,r,s]
Chromium oxide (Cr$_2$O$_3$) 1308-38-9	Chem. Abstr.: chromium oxide [Cr$_2$O$_3$] IUPAC: dichromium trioxide or chromium oxide (Cr$_2$O$_3$) chromia; C.I. Pigment Green 17 Casalis Green; Chrome Green; Chrome Oxide Green; GN-M; Green Chrome Oxide; Green Cinnabar; Levanox Green GA	Cr$_2$O$_3$	>590(1977)[d]	C	I II III IV	1-3 1-3 1-2 1-2	L:--/S: 0.01 mg/m^3 Ceiling (USSR) 0.1 mg/m^3 TWA (BEL, BUL, BRD)
Clay 1302-87-C	Chem. Abstr.: clay IUPAC: clay	Complex mixture	--	F	I II III IV	1-3 1-3 1-2 1-2	L:--/S: 1 2-4 mg/m^3 (USSR)
Graphite 7782-42-5	Chem. Abstr.: graphite IUPAC: graphite black lead; C.I. Pigment Black 10; mineral carbon AG 1500; Aquadag; Asbury 505; ATJ-S graphite; DC2; Electrographite; Fortafil 5Y; Grafoil; Hitco HMG 50; Korobon; Plumbago; Pyro-Carb 406; Seast SO; Stove Black; Thornel 40; Ucar 38	C	>51,760 (1977)[d]	F	I II III IV	1-3 1-3 1-2 1-2	L:--/S: 530 ppcm^3 Ceiling (Y) 530 ppcm^3 (BEL,USA, F)[1] 6 mg/m^3 Ceiling (CZ) 5 mg/m^3 TWA (SWED)
Ground glass --	Chem. Abstr.: -- IUPAC: -- Imsil; Processed mineral fiber	Complex mixture	--	F	--	--	L:--/S:--
Hydrazine 302-01-2	Chem. Abstr.: hydrazine IUPAC: hydrazine Levoxine; Oxytreat 35	H$_2$NNH$_2$	>905(1977)[d]	BA	--	--	L:--/S;--0.1-1.3 mg/m^3 Ceiling (BUL,N,S,USSR,Y) 0.1-1.3 mg/m^3 TWA (A,BEL,F,DDR,BRD,I, N,R,SWED,S,USA, USA-A) 0.2 mg/m^3 STEL (DDR) 0.04 mg/m^3 120 min. STEL (USA-N)

Name and CAS Reg. No.	Synonyms and Trade Names	Structural Formula	US Production -Thousand Kg (Year)	Use Class [a]	Indus-tries	Pro-cesses	Reported Workplace Levels(L)/Occupational Standards(S) [b,q,r,s]
Hydrogen peroxide 7722-84-1	Chem. Abstr.: hydrogen peroxide; IUPAC: hydrogen peroxide; Albone DS; Inhibine; Perhydrol; Peroxaan; Superoxol; T-Stuff	HOOH	101,598 (1979)[e]	LM,M	IV	1-2	L:--/S: 1-1.4 mg/m^3 Ceiling (BUL, I,N,S,USA-A,Y) 1.4-1.5 mg/m^3 TWA (A,BEL,F,BRD,I,N, S,USA-A) 3 mg/m^3 STEL (USA-A)
Iron oxide 1309-37-1	Chem. Abstr.: iron oxide [Fe$_2$O$_3$]; IUPAC: diiron trioxide or iron oxide (Fe$_2$O$_3$); bauxite residue; colloidal ferric oxide; Pigment Red 101; red iron oxide; rouge; turkey red; Bayer S11; Caput Mortuum; Cerven H; Colcothar; Colliron; Crocus; Deanox; Feiac; Ferrugo; Krokus; Mapico Red R220-3; Pigdex 100; Prussian Red; Redoxaid; Rubigo	Fe$_2$O$_3$	> 289,278 [d] (1977)	C	I II III IV	1-3 1-3 1-2 1-2	L:--/S: 4-6 mg/m^3 (USSR) 3.5 mg/m^3 TWA (SWED)
Lead chromate 7758-97-6	Chem. Abstr.: chromic acid [H$_2$CrO$_4$], lead(2+) salt (1:1); IUPAC: lead chromate; C.I. 7600; crocite; Pigment Green 15; plumbous chromate; Canary Chrome Yellow 40-2250; Chrome Green; Chrome Green UC61; Chrome Green UC74; Chrome Green UC76; Chrome Lemon; Chrome Yellow 5G; Chrome Yellow GF; Chrome Yellow LF; Chrome Yellow Light 1066; Chrome Yellow Light 1075; Chrome Yellow Medium 1074; Chrome Yellow Medium 1085; Chrome Yellow Medium 1295; Chrome Yellow Medium 1298; Chrome Yellow Primrose 1010; Chrome Yellow Primrose 1015; Cologne Yellow; Dainichi Chrome Yellow G; Leipzig Yellow; Paris Yellow; Pure Lemon Chrome L3GS	PbCrO$_4$	>11(1980)[c]	C	--	--	L:--/S: 0.1 mg/m^3 Ceiling (USA) 0.05-0.75 mg/m^3 TWA (I,N) 0.05-0.5 mg/m^3 TWA as chromium (SWED,USA-A) 0.45 mg/m^3 STEL as chromium (USA-A)

Name and CAS Reg. No.	Synonyms and Trade Names	Structural Formula	US Production -Thousand Kg (Year)	Use Class [a]	Indus-tries	Pro-cesses	Reported Workplace Levels(L)/Occupational Standards(S)[b,q,r,s]
Lead oxide (litharge) 1335-25-7	Chem. Abstr.: lead oxide [PbO] IUPAC: lead oxide (PbO) Chem I Sorb - BLT-06-90; CSD-8095; CSP-8080	PbO	>4.5(1977)[d]	A	II	1-2	L:--/S:--
Lithopone (barium sulphate and zinc sulphide) 7727-43-7 and 1314-98-3	Chem. Abstr.: barium sulphate (1:1) and zinc sulphide [ZnS] IUPAC: barium sulphate (1:1) and zinc sulphide Lithopone	$BaSO_4 + ZnS$	1,800 (1978)[c]	F	I II III IV	1-3 1-3 1-2 1-2	L:--/S:--
Magnesium carbonate 546-93-0	Chem. Abstr.: magnesium carbonate IUPAC: magnesium carbonate C.I. 77713 DCI Light Magnesium Carbonate; Magcarb L; Stan-Mag Magnesium Carbonate	$MgCO_3$	13.2(1980)[c]	F	I II III IV	1-3 1-3 1-2 1-2	L:--/S: 20 mg/m^3 (S)[1]
Magnesium oxide 1309-48-4	Chem. Abstr.: magnesium oxide [MgO] IUPAC: magnesium oxide calcined magnesia; C.I. 77711; magnesia Anscor P; Elastomag; Kyowamag 100; KM 40; Magcal; Maglite; Marmag; Seasorb; SLO 366; 469; Stanmag bars	MgO	>752,450 (1977)[d]	A	I II III IV	1-3 1-3 1-2 1-2	L:--/S: Fumes 15 mg/m^3 Ceiling(P,Y) 8-10 mg/m^3 TWA (A, BEL, DDR, BRD, N, S, USA, USA-A) 20 mg/m^3 STEL (DDR)
Magnesium silicate 14987-04-3	Chem. Abstr.: silicic acid [$H_4Si_3O_8$].magnesium salt (1:2) IUPAC: magnesium silicate ($Mg_2Si_3O_8$) magnesium trisilicate Dicarbocalm; Embal Talc; Glacier 325; Loomite; Magnosil; Mistron Frost, Vapor; Trisilicalm	$Mg_2Si_3O_8$	8.8(1980)[c]	F	I II III IV	1-3 1-3 1-2 1-2	L:--/S:--

Name and CAS Reg. No.	Synonyms and Trade Names	Structural Formula	US Production –Thousand Kg (Year)	Use Class [a]	Indus-tries	Pro-cesses	Reported Workplace Levels(L)/Occupational Standards(S)[b,q,r,s]
Mica 12001-26-2	Chem. Abstr.: mica; IUPAC: mica; C.I. 77019; Abhrak; Davenite; C 1000; HX 610; Micatex; Micromica; P 80 P; Suzorite	Complex mixture	--	F	I II III IV	1-3 1-3 1-2 1-2	L:--/S: .2-8 mg/m^3 Ceiling (CZ, USSR) 2.5-20 mg/m^3(A,I) 20 mg/m^3 TWA (F,USA, USA-A)
Pumice 1332-09-8	Chem. Abstr.: pumice; IUPAC: pumice	60-75% SiO_2 10-20% Al_2O_3	--	F, LA	I II III IV	1-3 1-3 1-2 1-2	L:--/S:--
Red lead 1314-41-6	Chem. Abstr.: lead oxide $[Pb_3O_4]$; IUPAC: lead oxide (Pb_3O_4); CI 77578; CI Pigment Red 105; gold satinobre; lead orthoplumbate; lead tetroxide; mennige; mineral orange; mineral red; minium; orange lead; Paris red; red lead oxide; trilead tetroxide	Pb_3O_4	14,000 (1979)[c]	A,C	I II III IV	1-3 1-3 1-2 1-2	L:--/S:--
Silica 7631-86-9	Chem. Abstr.: silica; IUPAC: silica silicon dioxide; diatomite; Aerosil; Armospheres; Carbosils; Cataloid; Cabosil; HDK-N, V, S; Himasil; Imsil; Ludox; Minusil; Neosyl; Positive Sol; Quso; Santocel; Snowtex; Ultrasil; Vulcasil; Zeofree; Zeosyl; Zeotex; Zorbax	SiO_2	>428,253[d] (1977)	F,M	I II III IV	1-3 1-3 1-2 1-2	L:--/S: 0.1-10 mg/m^3 (CZ,F,I,P,S)[1] 50-100 µg/m^3 TWA (respir-able) (SWED, USA-N) 1-2 mg/m^3 Ceiling (USSR) $\frac{1}{2}-1\left(\dfrac{30 \text{ mg/m}^3}{\% SiO_2 + 2}\right)$ TWA (USA) $\frac{1}{2}-1\left(\dfrac{30 \text{ mg/m}^3}{\% SiO_2 + 3}\right)$ (BEL,USA-A)[1] $\left(\dfrac{25 \text{ mg/m}^3}{\% \text{ respirable free}}\right)$ (A)[1] silica + 5 100-800 ppcm^3 TWA (BEL,DDR) 300-1500 ppcm^3 STEL (DDR)

Name and CAS Reg. No.	Synonyms and Trade Names	Structural Formula	US Production -Thousand Kg (Year)	Use Class [a]	Indus-tries	Pro-cesses	Reported Workplace Levels(L)/Occupational Standards(S) [b,q,r,s]
Sodium bicarbonate 144-55-8	Chem. Abstr.: sodium hydrogen carbonate; IUPAC: sodium hydrogen carbonate monosodium carbonate; baking soda; Celtone; Meylon; Soludal	$NaHCO_3$	> 414,054 (1977)[d]	BA	I II III IV	1-3 1-3 1-2 1-2	L:--/S:--
Sodium carbonate 497-19-8	Chem. Abstr.: disodium carbonate; IUPAC: disodium carbonate; soda; soda ash; Na-X	Na_2CO_3	7,427,515 (1979)[e,n]	A	--	--	L:--/S: 2 mg/m^3 Ceiling (USSR)
Sodium silicofluoride 16893-85-9	Chem. Abstr.: disodium hexafluorosilicate (2-); IUPAC: disodium hexafluorosilicate sodium fluorosilicate; sodium fluosilicate	Na_2SiF_6	54,149 (1979)[e]	LM	IV	1-2	L:--/S: 3 mg/m^3 Ceiling (CZ) 1.5 mg/m^3 TWA (CZ)
Sulphur 7704-34-9	Chem. Abstr.: sulphur; IUPAC: sulphur; Asulfasupra; Bensulfoid; Cosan; Elosal; Hexasul; Kolo 100; Kolloid-schwefel; Polsulkol Extra; Microthiol; Micowetsulf; Netzschwefel; Svovl; Sulkol; Sultaf; Sulfex; Sulfidal; Thiovit; Sufran; Shreesul, Wettasul	S	3,663,000 (1979)[e,p]	A	I II III IV	1-3 1-3 1-2 1-2	L:--/S:--
Talc 14807-96-6	Chem. Abstr.: talc $[Mg_3H_2(SiO_3)_4]$; IUPAC: talc; Agalite; Asbestine; Desertalc 57; Emtal; Fibrene C 400; Glacier 325; ITX; Loomite; Mistron Vapor; Supreme; Steawhite	$Mg_3H_2(SiO_3)_4$	>4500 (1977)[d]	F	I II III IV	1-3 1-3 1-2 1-2	L:--/S: 4-5 mg/m^3 Ceiling (CZ, USSR) 5 fibers less than 5 um long/cm^3 (fibrous) (F)[1] 2.5-5 mg/m^3 (A, CZ, I, F)[1] 5 mg/m^3 TWA (USA, USA-A)

Name and CAS Reg. No.	Synonyms and Trade Names	Structural Formula	US Production -Thousand Kg (Year)	Use Class[a]	Indus-tries	Pro-cesses	Reported Workplace Levels(L)/Occupational Standards(S)[b,q,r,s]
Titanium dioxide 13463-67-7	Chem. Abstr.: Titanium oxide (TiO2) IUPAC: titanium dioxide or titanium oxide (TiO2) C.I. Pigment White 6; titania A-Fil; Austiox; Bayertitan; Cab-O-Ti; Flamenco; Hombitan; Kronos; Rayox; Runa; Rutiox; Tioxide; Tipaque; Ti-Pure; Titan; Titanox; Tronox; Unitane; Zopaque	TiO_2	667,319 (1979)[e]	C	I II III IV	1-3 1-3 1-2 1-2	L:--/S: 10-20 mg/m^3 TWA (F,I,S,USA, USA-A)[1]
Zinc carbonate 3486-35-9	Chem. Abstr.: zinc carbonate IUPAC: zinc carbonate C.I. 77950	$ZnCO_3$	> 90(1977)[d]	A	II	1-2	L:--/S:--
Zinc nitrate 7779-88-6	Chem. Abstr.: zinc nitrate IUPAC: zinc nitrate zinc dinitrate Aerotex Accelerator No. 5; Celloxan; X4	$Zn(NO_3)_2$	--	LM	IV	1-2	L:--/S:--
Zinc oxide 1314-13-2	Chem. Abstr.: zinc oxide IUPAC: zinc oxide C.I. Pigment White 4; zinc white Actox; Amalox; Azo 11, 55; Azodox; Cadox; Eagle-Picher; Emar; Greenseal 8; Horse Head; Kadox; Permanent White; Protox; Red Seal 9; St. Joe; Vandem; White Seal 7; Zinca 20; Zincoid;	ZnO	>213,084 (1977)[d]	A,LM	I II III IV	1-3 1-3 1-2 1-2	L:--/S: dust: 6 mg/m^3 Ceiling (USSR) fumes: 5-6 mg/m^3 Ceiling (BUL, CZ, P, S, USSR, Y) 1-5 mg/m^3 TWA (A, BEL, CZ, F, DDR, BRD, H, I, J, N, SWED, S, USA) 10 mg/m^3 STEL (DDR, USA-N, USA-A)

TABLE 2

IDENTIFICATION, WORKPLACE OCCURRENCE AND STANDARDS

FOR CHEMICALS FOUND AS BY-PRODUCTS

IN THE RUBBER INDUSTRY

(For footnotes, see pp. 243-245)

Name and CAS Reg. No.	Synonyms and Trade Names	Structural Formula	Industries	Processes	Reported Workplace Levels(L)/Occupational Standards(S)[b],[q],[r],[s]

Benzo[a]pyrene 50-32-8	Chem. Abstr.: benzo(a)pyrene
	IUPAC: benzo(a)pyrene
	B(a)P: benzo(d,e,f)chrysene; 3,4-benzopyrene; 6,7-benzopyrene; 3,4-benzpyrene
			I	3	L: 32.3 µg/m³ [gg]
					   8.8 µg/m³ [gg]
					   15.3 µg/m³ [gg]
					S: 0.00015 mg/m³ Ceiling (USSR)
					   0.005 mg/m³ TWA (SWED)

Benzothiazole 95-16-9	Chem. Abstr.: benzothiazole IUPAC: benzothiazole 1-thia-3-azaindene Vangard BT		I	5	L:--/S:-- [ii]
1,3-Butadiene, trimer 16422-75-6	Chem. Abstr.: 1,3 butadiene, trimer IUPAC: 1,3-butadiene, trimer linear butadiene trimer	[CH₂=CHCH=CH₂]₃	I	5	L:--/S:-- [ii]
N-sec-Butylaniline 6068-69-5	Chem. Abstr.: N-(1-methylpropyl)-benzenamine IUPAC: N-sec-butylaniline		I	5	L:--/S:-- [ii]
tert-Butyl isothiocyanate 590-42-1	Chem. Abstr.: 2-isothiocyanato-2-methylpropane IUPAC: tert-butyl isothiocyanate	(CH₃)₃CN=C=S	I	5	L:--/S:-- [ii]

Name and CAS Reg. No.	Synonyms and Trade Names	Structural Formula	Industries	Processes	Reported Workplace Levels(L)/Occupational Standards(S)[b,q,r,s]
1,5,9-Cyclododecatriene 4904-61-4	Chem. Abstr.: 1,5,9-Cyclododecatriene IUPAC: 1,5,9-Cyclododecatriene CDT	$CH=CH(CH_2)_2CH=CH(CH_2)_2CH=CH(CH_2)_2$	I	5	L: 16.4 ppb[ii] S: --
1,5-Cyclooctadiene 111-78-4	Chem. Abstr.: 1,5-Cyclooctadiene IUPAC: 1,5-Cyclooctadiene	$CH=CH(CH_2)_2CH=CH(CH_2)_2$	I	5	L: 8.84 ppb[ii] S: --
Dimethylnaphthalene 28804-88-8	Chem. Abstr.: dimethylnaphthalene IUPAC: dimethylnaphthalene	$(CH_3)_2$	I	5	L:--/S:--[ii]
Ethylbenzene 100-41-4	Chem. Abstr.: ethylbenzene IUPAC: ethylbenzene ethylbenzol; phenylethane EB	CH_2CH_3	I	5	L:--/S: 100-435 mg/m^3[ii] Ceiling (CZ,P,Y) 200-435 mg/m^3 TWA (A,BEL, CZ,F,BRD,IrJ,N,R,S,SWED, USA,USA-A) 545 mg/m^3 STEL (USA-A)

Name and CAS Reg. No.	Synonyms and Trade Names	Structural Formula	Industries	Processes	Reported Workplace Levels(L)/Occupational Standards(S)[b,q,r,s]
Ethylnaphthalene 27138-19-8	Chem. Abstr.: ethylnaphthalene IUPAC: ethylnaphthalene 1-(or 2-)ethylnaphthalene	CH_2CH_3 (naphthalene)	I	5	ii L:--/S:--
Hydrogen sulphide 7783-06-4	Chem. Abstr.: hydrogen sulphide [H_2S] IUPAC: hydrogen sulphide dihydrogen monosulphide; hydrosulphuric acid; sulphur dihydride; Stink Damp	H_2S	I	2	hh L:--/S: 10 mg/m^3 Ceiling (BUL,CZ,P,R,Y,USSR, USA) 10-15 mg/m^3 TWA (A,BEL, CZ,F,DDR,BRD,H,I,J, N,R,SWED,S,USA-A) 15-21 mg/m^3 STEL (USA-A, DDR) 15 mg/m^3 10 min. STEL (USA-N) 70 mg/m^3 Peak 10 min. (USA)
Methylnaphthalene 1321-94-4	Chem. Abstr.: methylnaphthalene IUPAC: methylnaphthalene	CH_3 (naphthalene)	I	5	ii L:--/S:--
Nitrogen dioxide 10102-44-0	Chem. Abstr.: nitrogen oxide [NO_2] IUPAC: nitrogen dioxide nitrito; nitro	NO_2	I	5	hh L:--/S: 5-10 mg/m^3 Ceiling (A,BEL,BUL,CZ, I,N,P,SWED,S,USSR,USA, USA-A.Y) 5-10 mg/m^3 TWA (CZ,F, DDR,BRD,H,J) 1.8-10 mg/m^3 STEL (DDR,USA-N)

Name and CAS Reg. No.	Synonyms and Trade Names	Structural Formula	Industries	Processes	Reported Workplace Levels(L)/Occupational Standards(S)[b,q,r,s]
Nitrogen oxides --	Chem. Abstr.: -- IUPAC: --	NO_x	I II III IV	1-7 1-7 1-7 1-6	L:--/S: (measured as NO_2) 5-10 mg/m³ Ceiling (A,BEL,BUL,CZ,I,N,P,SWED,S,USSR,USA,USA-A,Y) 5-10 mg/m³ TWA (CZ,F,DDR,BRD,H,J) 1.8-10 mg/m³ STEL (DDR,USA-N)
N-Nitrosodibutylamine 924-16-3	Chem. Abstr.: N-butyl-N-nitroso-1-butanamine IUPAC: N-nitrosodibutylamine dibutyl nitrosamine	O=N—N with $(CH_2)_3CH_3$ / $(CH_2)_3CH_3$	--	--	L:--/S:--
N-Nitrosodiethylamine 55-18-5	Chem. Abstr.: N-ethyl-N-nitroso-ethanamine IUPAC: N-nitrosodiethylamine diethylnitrosamine; DEN; NDEA	O=N—N with CH_2CH_3 / CH_2CH_3	I	5	L: < 0.05-5 mg/m³ [mm] S: --
N-Nitrosodimethylamine 62-75-9	Chem. Abstr.: N-methyl-N-nitroso-methanamine IUPAC: N-nitrosodimethylamine; DMN; DMNA dimethylnitrosoamine; DMN; DMNA	O=N—N with CH_3 / CH_3	I I I I I I I	1 2 3 4 5 6 7	L: 0.38 µg/m³[ll]; 2.2 µg/m³[ll]; 64 µg/m³[ff] 27 µg/m³[jj]; 2.2 µg/m³[jj]; 7.1 µg/m³[jj]; 0.03 µg/m³[ff]; 0.24 µg/m³[ll]; 0.6 µg/m³[jj]; 2.5 µg/m³[jj]; 0.38 µg/m³[ll]; 2.9 µg/m³[ll] S: --
N-Nitrosomorpholine 59-89-2	Chem. Abstr.: 4-nitrosomorpholine IUPAC: 4-nitrosomorpholine nitrosomorpholine	morpholine ring, N—N=O	I I I I III II	1 3 5 7 2 3	L: 250 µg/m³[ff]; 3.7 µg/m³[ll] 9 µg/m³[ff]; 248 µg/m³[ll] 0.44 µg/m³[ff]; 1.5 µg/m³[ll] 1 µg/m³[jj]; 3.7 µg/m³[ll] 0.14 µg/m³[jj] 0.09 µg/m³[jj] S: --
N-Nitrosopiperidine 100-75-4	Chem. Abstr.: 1-nitrosopiperidine IUPAC: 1-nitrosopiperidine	piperidine ring, N—N=O	II	1-3,5	L: 2 µg/m³[oo] S:--

Name and CAS Reg. No.	Synonyms and Trade Names	Structural Formula	Industries	Processes	Reported Workplace Levels(L)/Occupational Standards(S)[b,q,r,s]
N-Nitrosopyrrolidine 930-55-2	Chem. Abstr.: 1-nitrosopyrrolidine IUPAC: 1-nitrosopyrrolidine N-nitroso-1-pyrrolidinamine	[structure: O=N-N ring]	I	3	L: 0.8 $\mu g/m^3$[ff]; 2.6 $\mu g/m^3$[11] S: --
Particulates --	Chem. Abstr.: -- IUPAC: -- inert dust; nuisance dust	Indefinite	I I I I I	2 3 5 2 3	L: 25.8 mg/m^3[gg] 32 mg/m³[gg] 10.3 mg/m³[gg] 20-50 mg/m³[hh] 11 mg/m³[hh] S: 8-20 mg/m³ Ceiling (CZ,BRD,DDR,S) 6-10 mg/m³ (A BEL F.H H SWED,I,P Y)[l] 5-15 mg/m³ TWA (DDR.USA USA-A)
Phthalimide 85-41-6	Chem. Abstr.: 1H-isoindole-1,3-(2H)-dione IUPAC: phthalimide 1,2-benzenedicarboximide; benzoimide; phenylimide	[structure]	I II	5 5	L:--/S:--
Styrene 100-42-5	Chem. Abstr.: ethenylbenzene IUPAC: styrene cinnamene; phenylethene; phenylethylene; styrol; styrolene; vinylbenzene Styropol SO	[structure: -CH=CH₂]	I	5	[ii] L:--/S: 5-920 mg/m³ Ceiling (BUL,CZ,P,R,Y,USSR, USA) 50-420 mg/m³ TWA (A,BEL, CZ,F,DDR,BRD,H,I,J,N, R,SWED,S,USA,USA-A) 400-525 mg/m³ STEL (USA-A, DDR) 2520 mg/m³ Peak 5 min./ 3 hours (USA)
Sulphur dioxide 7446-09-5	Chem. Abstr.: sulphur dioxide IUPAC: sulphur dioxide sulphurous acid anhydride; sulphurous anhydride; sulphurous oxide; sulphur oxide Fermenticide liquid	SO₂	I	2	L: 33 mg/m³[hh] S: 10 mg/m³ Ceiling (BUL,CZ,P,R,USSR,Y) 5-13 mg/m³ TWA (A,BEL, CZ,F,DDR,BRD,H,I,J,N, R,SWED,S,USA,USA-A, USA-N) 10-30 mg/m³ STEL (DDR, USA-A)

Name and CAS Reg. No.	Synonyms and Trade Names	Structural Formula	Industries	Processes	Reported Workplace Levels(L)/Occupational Standards(S)b,q,r,s
4-Vinylcyclohexene 100-40-3	Chem. Abstr.: 4-ethenylcyclohexene IUPAC: 4-vinylcyclohexene 1-vinyl-3-cyclohexene	CH=CH₂	1	5	L: 118 ppb[ii] S: --

Table 3. <u>Monomers and elastomers used in the rubber industry</u>

I.   <u>Monomers</u>

Acrylonitrile
1,3-Butadiene
Chloroprene (2-chloro-1,3-butadiene)
Chlorotrifluoroethylene
Dicyclopentadiene
Epichlorohydrin
Ethyl acrylate
Ethylene
Ethylene oxide
Ethylidene norbornen
1,4-Hexadiene
Hexafluoropropylene
Hexafluoropropylene/tetrafluoroethylene
Isobutylene
Isoprene (2-methyl-1,3-butadiene)
Methylene diphenyldiisocyanate[a]
Methylmethacrylate
Naphthalene-1,5-diisocyanate[a]
Polymethylene polyphenyl isocyanate[a]
Propylene
Propylene oxide
Styrene
Tetrafluoroethylene[a]
2,4-Toluenediisocyanate[a]
2,6-Toluenediisocyanate[a]
Vinyl acetate
Vinyl chloride
Vinylidene chloride

---

[a] Not technically monomers but used to make some elastomers

II. <u>Natural and synthetic rubber elastomers</u>

Natural rubber

Synthetic rubbers:
    Acrylic rubbers (NBR)
    Acrylonitrile-butadiene-styrene copolymer
    Chlorinated polyethylene
    Chlorobutyl rubber
    Chloroprene rubber
    Chlorosulphonated polyethylene (CSM)
    Epichlorohydrin elastomer (CO)
    Ethylene-propylene-diene terpolymer (EDPM)
    Fluoroelastomers (CFM)
    Isobutylene-isoprene elastomers (butyl rubber) (IIR)
    Isoprene-acrylonitrile elastomers
    Neoprene
    Nitrile elastomers (NBR)
    Polybutadienes (BR)
    Polybutenes
    Polychloroprenes (CR)
    Polyester
    Polyethylene
    Polyisobutylenes
    Polyisoprenes (MR)
    Polysulphides (T)
    Polytetrafluoroethene
    Polyvinyl chloride
    Resorcinol-formaldehyde latex
    Silicone elastomer (MQ)
    Styrene-butadiene rubbers (SBR)
    Oil-extended SBR
    Styrene-isoprene elastomers
    Thermoplastic polyester elastomers
    Thermoplastic polyolefin elastomers
    Urethane rubbers
    Vinyl acetate-ethylene copolymers

Table 4. Production of elastomers in member countries of the
          Council of Mutual Economic Assistance

Elastomer	Production (thousand kg)	Year
Natural rubber	3 855 000[a]	1979
Butyl rubber	453 000	1979
Ethylene-propylene-diene terpolymer and ethylene-propylene copolymers	319 000[b]	1978
Nitrile elastomers	226 000	1979
Polybutadienes	1 018 000	1979
Polychloroprenes	353 000	1979
Polyisoprenes	222 000[b]	1978
Styrene-butadiene rubber, including oil-extended	4 208 000	1979
Thermoplastic polyester elastomers	6 600	1979
Thermoplastic polyolefin elastomers	37 950	1979

[a] International Rubber Study Group (1981)

[b] Anon. (1979)

References

American Conference of Governmental Industrial Hygienists (1980) TLVs® Threshold Limit Values for Chemical Substances and Physical Agents in the Workroom Environment with Intended Changes for 1980, Cincinnati, OH

Anon. (1979) Global synthetic rubber output rises 3.1%. Oil and Gas Journal, 77,(19), p. 60

Borcherding, C.H., Salisbury, S.A. & Meyer, C.R. (1977) Health Hazard Evaluation Determination. The Goodyear Tire & Rubber Company Plant No. 1, Akron, Ohio (HHE 74-98-399), Cincinnati, OH, National Institute for Occupational Health & Safety

Burgess, W.A., DiBerardinis, L., Gold, A. & Treitman, R. (1977) Exposure to air contaminants in the tyre building (Abstract no. 39). Rubber Chem. Technol., 51, 379-381

Butler, G.J. & Taylor, J.S. (1973) Health Hazard Evaluation/-Toxicity Determination. Uniroyal Incorporated, Mishawaka, Indiana (HHE 72-13-27), Cincinnati, OH, National Institute for Occupational Safety & Health

Daniels, W.J. (1980) Health Hazard Evaluation Determination. Dearborn Rubber Corporation, Westmont, Illinois (HHE 79-151-657), Cincinnati, OH, National Institute for Occupational Safety & Health

Economic Research Service (1977) US Fats and Oils Statistics, 1961-76 (Statistical Bulletin No. 574), Washington DC, US Department of Agriculture, p. 20

Fajen, J.M. (1980) Industrial Hygiene Study of Workers Exposed to Nitrosamines. In: Proceedings of the First NCI/EPA/NIOSH Collaborative Workshop: Progress on Joint Environmental and Occupational Cancer Studies, Sheraton/Potomac, Rockville, Maryland, Cincinnati, OH, National Institute for Occupational Safety & Health, pp. 121-139

Fajen, J.M., Carson, G.A., Rounbehler, D.P., Fan, T.Y., Vita, R., Goff, U.E., Wolf, M.H., Edwards, G.S., Fine, D.H., Reinhold, V. & Biemann, K. (1979) N-Nitrosamines in the rubber and tire industry. Science, 205, 1262-1264

Gunter, B.J. & Lucas, J.B. (1975) Health Hazard Evaluation/-Toxicity Determination. Gates Rubber Company, Denver, Colorado (HHE 74-73-233), Cincinnati, OH, National Institute for Occupational Safety & Health

Hollett, B.A. & Schloemer, J. (1978) Hazard Evaluation and Technical Assistance Report. Newport Industrial Products, Firestone Tire & Rubber Co., Newport, Tennessee (TA 76-90), Cincinnati, OH, National Institute for Occupational Safety & Health

International Labour Office (1980) Occupational Exposure Limits for Airborne Toxic Substances, 2nd (rev.) ed. (Occupational Safety & Health Series No. 37), Geneva

International Rubber Study Group (1981) Production of natural rubber. Rubber Statistical Bulletin, 35(4), 7

Levy, B.S.B. (1975) Health Hazard Evaluation/Toxicity Determination. Converse Rubber Company, Malden, Massachusetts (HHE 75-15-250), Cincinnati, OH, National Institute for Occupational Safety & Health

Maier, A., Ruhe, R., Rosensteel, R. & Lucas, J.B. (1974) Health Hazard Evaluation/Toxicity Determination. Arco Polymer Incorporated, Monaca, Pennsylvania (HHE 72-90-107), Cincinnati, OH, National Institute for Occupational Safety & Health

McGlothlin, J.D. & Wilcox, T.G. (1980) Interim Report No. 3, Health Hazard Evaluation Project No. HE 79-109, Kelly-Springfield Tire Company, Cumberland, Maryland, Cincinnati, OH, National Institute for Occupational Safety & Health

National Board of Occupational Safety & Health (1981) Hygieniska Gransvarden (Limit Values) (Directions Concerning Limit Values for Air Contaminants at Places of Work, AFS 1981:8), Stockholm

National Institute for Occupational Safety & Health (1974) Criteria for a Recommended Standard...Occupational Exposure to Benzene, Cincinnati, OH, US Department of Health, Education, & Welfare, pp. 42-44, 57-58, 83, 129-131

National Institute for Occupational Safety & Health (1976) Criteria for a Recommended Standard...Occupational Exposure to Ethylene Dichloride (1,2-Dichloroethane), Washington DC, US Government Printing Office, pp. 55-56, 118

National Institute for Occupational Safety & Health (1980) Summary of NIOSH Recommendations for Occupational Health Standards, Cincinnati, OH

Noweir, M.H., El-Dakhakhny, A.-A. & Osman, H.A. (1972) Exposure to chemical agents in rubber industry. J. Egypt. publ. Health Assoc., 47, 182-201

Pagnotto, L.D., Elkins, H.B. & Brugsch, H.G. (1979) Benzene exposure in the rubber coating industry - a follow-up. Am. ind. Hyg. Assoc. J., 40, 137-146

Preussmann, R., Spiegelhalder, B. & Eisenbrand, G. (1980) Reduction of human exposure to environmental N-nitroso carcinogens. Examples of possibilities for cancer prevention. In: Pullman, B., Ts'o, P.O.P. & Gelboin, H., eds, Carcino-genesis: Fundamental Mechanisms and Environmental Effects, Dordrecht, D. Reidel, pp. 273-285

Preussmann, R., Spiegelhalder, B. & Eisenbrand, G. (1981) Reduction of human exposure to environmental N-nitroso compounds. In: Scanlan, R.A. & Tannenbaum, F.R., eds, N-Nitroso Compounds (ACS Symposium Series No. 174), Washington DC, American Chemical Society, pp. 217-228

Rappaport, S.M. & Fraser, D.A. (1977) Air sampling and analysis in a rubber vulcanization area. Am. ind. Hyg. Assoc. J., 38, 205-210

SRI International (1980a) 1980 Directory of Chemical Producers - USA, Menlo Park, CA, Chemical Information Services, pp. 853-861

SRI International (1980b) Directory of Chemical Producers – Western Europe, Vol. 2, Menlo Park, CA, Chemical Information Services, pp. 1669-1678

US Department of Commerce (1980a) US Imports for Consumption and General Imports (FT 246, Annual 1979), Washington DC, US Government Printing Office, pp. 273, 275

US Department of Commerce (1980b) Current Industrial Reports, Inorganic Chemicals, 1979 (MA28A), Washington DC, Bureau of the Census, pp. 3, 5, 7, 9, 10, 12, 15, 18

US Department of the Interior (1980) Mineral Industry Surveys, Asbestos in 1980, Washington DC, Bureau of Mines

US Environmental Protection Agency (1980) Chemicals in Commerce Information Systems (CICIS), Washington DC, Office of Pesticides and Toxic Substances, Chemical Information Division

US International Trade Commission (1977a) Synthetic Organic Chemicals, US Production and Sales, 1976 (USITC Publication 833), Washington DC, US Government Printing Office, pp. 193-194

US International Trade Commission (1977b) Synthetic Organic Chemicals, US Production and Sales, 1975 (USITC Publication 804), Washington DC, US Government Printing Office, p. 131

US International Trade Commission (1977c) Imports of Benzenoid Chemicals and Products, 1976 (USITC Publication 828), Washington DC, US Government Printing Office, pp. 25-26

US International Trade Commission (1978a) Synthetic Organic Chemicals, US Production and Sales, 1977 (USITC Publication 920), Washington DC, US Government Printing Office, pp. 233-242

US International Trade Commission (1978b) Imports of Benzenoid Chemicals and Products, 1977 (USITC Publication 900), Washington DC, US Government Printing Office, pp. 27-28, 385

US International Trade Commission (1979a) <u>Synthetic Organic Chemicals, US Production and Sales, 1978</u>   (<u>USITC Publication 1001</u>), Washington DC, US Government Printing Office, pp. 211–219

US International Trade Commission (1979b) <u>Imports of Benzenoid Chemicals and Products, 1978</u>   (<u>USITC Publication 990</u>), Washington DC, US Government Printing Office, pp. 26–28

US International Trade Commission (1980a) <u>Synthetic Organic Chemicals, US Production and Sales, 1979</u>   (<u>USITC Publication 1099</u>), Washington DC, US Government Printing Office, pp. 9, 15, 25, 26, 55–57, 131, 173, 175–182, 191, 238, 245, 255, 265–269, 271, 274, 276, 283, 294, 299, 301

US International Trade Commission (1980b) <u>Imports of Benzenoid Chemicals and Products, 1979</u>   (<u>USITC Publication 1083</u>), Washington DC, US Government Printing Office, pp. 29–31

US Occupational Safety & Health Administration (1980) <u>Air contaminants, lead</u>. <u>US Code fed. Regul.</u>, <u>Title 29</u>, 1910–1025

Van Ert, M.D., Arp, E.W., Harris, R.L., Symons, M.J. & Williams, T.M. (1980) Worker exposures to chemical agents in the manufacture of rubber tires: Solvent vapor studies. <u>Am. ind. Hyg. Assoc. J.</u>, <u>41</u>, 212–219

Williams, T.M., Harris, R.L., Arp, E.W., Symons, M.J. & Van Ert, M.D. (1980) Worker exposure to chemical agents in the manufacture of rubber tires and tubes: Particulates. <u>Am. ind. Hyg. Assoc. J.</u>, <u>41</u>, 204–211

Yeager, F.W., Van Gulick, N.N. & Lasoski, B.A. (1980) Dialkylnitrosamines in elastomers. <u>Am. ind. Hyg. Assoc. J.</u>, <u>41</u>, 148–150

CHEMICALS USED OR PRODUCED IN THE RUBBER INDUSTRY
THAT WERE PREVIOUSLY EVALUATED IN THE
IARC MONOGRAPHS SERIES

Chemical	Evaluation of carcinogenicity
Acrylic rubber (Polyacrylic acid)	No data on humans or animals (Vol. 19, pp. 62-71)
Acrylonitrile	Probably carcinogenic in humans; sufficient evidence in animals (Vol. 19, pp. 73-113; Supplement 1, p. 21)
4-Aminobiphenyl	Carcinogenic in humans (Vol. 1, pp. 74-79; Supplement 1, p. 22)
Asbestos	Carcinogenic in humans; (Vol. 14; Supplement 1, p. 23)
Benzene	Carcinogenic in humans (Vol. 7, pp. 203-221; Supplement 1, p. 23)
Benzidine	Carcinogenic in humans (Vol. 1, pp. 80-86; Supplement 1, p. 25)
Benzo[a]pyrene	No data on humans; sufficient evidence in animals (Vol. 3, pp. 91-136)
para-Benzoquinone dioxime	No data on humans; limited evidence in animals (Vol. 29, in press)

Bis(diethyldithiocarbamoyl)-
disulphide (Disulfiram)

No data on humans; inadequate data
on animals (Vol. 12, pp. 85-95)

Bis(dimethylthiocarbamoyl)-
disulphide (Thiram)

Inadequate data on humans and
animals (Vol. 12, pp. 225-236)

Cadmium sulphide
Cadmium yellow

Cadmium and certain cadmium
compounds are probably carcinogenic for humans; sufficient
evidence in animals for cadmium
sulphide (Vol. 11, pp. 39-74;
Supplement 1, pp. 27-28)

Carbon tetrachloride

Probably carcinogenic in humans;
sufficient evidence in animals
(Vol. 20, pp. 371-399; Supplement
1, p. 28)

Chloroform

No data on humans; sufficient
evidence in animals (Vol. 20,
pp. 401-417)

Chloroprene

Inadequate data on humans and
animals (Vol. 19, pp. 131-156;
Supplement 1, p. 29)

Chromium oxide

Chromium and certain chromium
compounds: carcinogenic in humans;
Cr[III]: inadequate data on animals
(Vol. 23, pp. 205-323; Supplement
1, pp. 29-30)

ortho-Dichlorobenzene

Inadequate data on humans and
animals (Vol. 7, pp. 231-241; to be
reevaluated in October 1981)

Dichloromethane
(Methylene chloride)

No data on humans; inadequate data
on animals (Vol. 20, pp. 449-465)

Diethyldithiocarbamic acid,
sodium salt (Sodium
diethyldithiocarbamate)

No data on humans; inadequate data
on animals (Vol. 12, pp. 217-223)

Diethyldithiocarbamic acid,   No data on humans; inadequate data
telluric salt (Ethyl   on animals (Vol. 12, pp. 115-129)
tellurac)

Di(2-ethylhexyl) adipate   No data on humans; limited evidence
                                     in animals (Vol. 29, in press)

Di(2-ethylhexyl) phthalate   No data on humans; sufficient
                                     evidence in animals (Vol. 29, in
                                     press)

Dimethyldithiocarbamic acid,   No data on humans; inadequate data
lead salt (Ledate)   on animals (Vol. 12, pp. 131-135)

Dimethyldithiocarbamic   No data on humans; inadequate data
selenium salt (Methyl   on acid, animals (Vol. 12, pp.
selenac)   161-166)

Dimethyldithiocarbamic   No data on humans; inadequate data
acid, zinc salt (Ziram)   on animals (Vol. 12, pp. 259-270)

Dinitrosopentamethylene-   No data on humans; inadequate data
tetramine   on animals (Vol. 11, pp. 241-245)

1,4-Dioxane   No data on humans; sufficient
                                     evidence in animals (Vol. 11, pp.
                                     247-256)

Epichlorohydrin   Inadequate data on humans; limited
                                     evidence in animals (Vol. 11, pp.
                                     131-139; Supplement 1, p. 33)

Ethyl acrylate   No data on humans; inadequate data
                                     on animals (Vol. 19, pp. 57-71)

Ethylene   No data on humans or animals (Vol.
                                     19, pp. 157-186)

Ethylene dichloride   No data on humans; sufficient
(1,2-Dichloroethane)   evidence in animals (Vol. 20, pp.
                                     429-448)

Ethylene oxide

Probably carcinogenic in humans; inadequate data on animals (Vol. 11, pp. 157-167; Supplement 1, p. 34)

1,3-Ethylene-2-thiourea

No data on humans; sufficient evidence in animals (Vol. 7, pp. 45-52)

Formaldehyde gas

Inadequate data on humans; sufficient evidence in animals (Vol. 29, in press)

Hydrazine

No data on humans; sufficient evidence in animals (Vol. 4, pp. 127-136)

Hydroquinone

No data on humans; inadequate data on animals (Vol. 15, pp. 155-175)

Iron oxide

Underground haematite mining is carcinogenic to humans; not carcinogenic in animals (Vol. 1, pp. 29-39; Supplement 1, p. 34)

Isopropyl alcohol

Manufacture of isopropanol using the strong-acid process is carcinogenic in humans; inadequate data on animals (Vol. 15, pp. 223-243; Supplement 1, p. 36)

Lead chromate

Inadequate data on humans; sufficient evidence in animals (Vol. 23, pp. 325-415)

Lead oxide (litharge)

Inadequate data on humans and animals (Vol. 23, pp. 325-415)

N-Methyl-N,4-dinitroso-aniline

No data on humans; limited evidence in animals (Vol. 1, pp. 141-142)

4,4'-Methylenebis(2-chloro-aniline) (MOCA)

Inadequate data on humans; sufficient evidence in animals (Vol. 4, pp. 65-71)

4,4'-Methylenedianiline	No data on humans; inadequate data in animals (Vol. 4, pp. 79-85)
4,4'-Methylenediphenyl-diisocyanate	No data on humans; inadequate data on animals (Vol. 19, pp. 314-340)
Methyl methacrylate	No data on humans; inadequate data on animals (Vol. 19, pp. 187-211)
Mineral oils	Carcinogenic in humans (Vol. 3, pp. 30-33; Supplement 1, p. 43)
Naphthalene-1,5-diisocyanate (1,5-Naphthalenediiso-cyanate)	No data on humans or animals (Vol. 19, pp. 311-340)
1-Naphthylamine	Inadequate data on humans; limited evidence in animals (Vol. 4, pp. 87-96)
2-Naphthylamine	Carcinogenic in humans (Vol. 4, pp. 97-111; Supplement 1, p. 39)
N-Nitrosodimethylamine	No data on humans; sufficient evidence in animals (Vol. 17, pp. 125-175)
N-Nitrosodiphenylamine	No data on humans; limited evidence in animals (Vol. 27, in press)
N-Nitrosomorpholine	No data on humans; sufficient evidence in animals (Vol. 17, pp. 263-286)
N-Nitrosopyrrolidine	No data on humans; sufficient evidence in animals (Vol. 17, pp. 313-326)
Perchloroethylene (Tetrachloroethylene)	No data on humans; limited evidence in animals (Vol. 20, pp. 491-514)
meta-Phenylenediamine	No data on humans; inadequate data on animals (Vol. 16, pp. 111-124)

N-Phenyl-2-naphthylamine   Inadequate data on humans and
                                 animals (Vol. 16, pp. 325-341)

Polychloroprene   Inadequate data on humans and
                                 animals (Vol. 19, pp. 141-156)

Polyethylene   Inadequate data on humans and
                                 animals (Vol. 19, pp. 144-186)

Polymethylene polyphenyl   No data on humans or animals (Vol.
isocyanate   19, pp. 314-340)

Polypropylene   No data on humans; inadequate data
                                 on animals (Vol. 19, pp. 218-230)

Propylene   No data on humans or animals (Vol.
                                 19, pp. 213-230)

Propylene oxide   No data on humans; limited evidence
                                 in animals (Vol. 11, pp. 191-199)

Resorcinol   No data on humans; inadequate data
                                 on animals (Vol. 15, pp. 155-175)

Selenium   Available evidence indicates no
                                 carcinogenic effect in humans;
                                 inadequate data on animals (Vol. 9,
                                 pp. 245-260)

Soots and tars   Carcinogenic in humans (Vol. 3, pp.
                                 22-42; Supplement 1, p. 43)

Styrene   Inadequate data on humans; limited
                                 evidence in animals (Vol. 19, pp.
                                 231-274; Supplement 1, p. 43)

Styrene-butadiene copolymers   Inadequate data on humans; no data
                                 on animals (Vol. 19, pp. 252-274)

Tetrafluoroethylene   No data on humans or animals (Vol.
                                 19, pp. 285-301)

Toluene-2,4-diamine (2,4-Diaminotuoluene)	No data on humans; <u>sufficient evidence</u> in animals (Vol. 16, pp. 83-95)
Toluene-2,5-diamine) (2,5-Diaminotoluene)	No data on humans; inadequate data on animals (Vol. 16, pp. 97-109)
2,4-Toluene diisocyanate	No data on humans or animals (Vol. 19, pp. 303-340)
2,6-Toluene diisocyanate	No data on humans or animals (Vol. 19, pp. 303-340)
1,1,1-Trichloroethane	No data on humans; inadequate data on animals (Vol. 20, pp. 515-531)
Trichloroethylene	No data on humans; <u>limited evidence</u> in animals (Vol. 11, pp. 263-276)
Tris(2,3-dibromopropyl) phosphate	No data on humans; <u>sufficient evidence</u> in animals (Vol. 20., pp. 575-588)
Urethane rubbers (Polyurethane)	Polyurethane foams (flexible and rigid): no data on humans; inadequate data on animals (Vol. 19, pp. 320-340)
Vinyl acetate	No data on humans; inadequate data on animals (Vol. 19, pp. 341-366)
Vinyl chloride	Carcinogenic in humans (Vol. 19, pp. 377-348; Supplement 1, p. 45)
4-Vinylcyclohexene	No data on humans; inadequate data on animals (Vol. 11, pp. 277-280)

CHEMICALS USED IN THE PRODUCTION OF SYNTHETIC RUBBER THAT WERE PREVIOUSLY EVALUATED IN THE <u>IARC MONOGRAPHS</u> SERIES

Chemical	Evaluation of carcinogenicity
Acrylic rubbers (Polyacrylic acid)	No data on humans or animals (Vol. 19, pp. 62-71)
Acrylonitrile	Probably carcinogenic in humans; <u>sufficient evidence</u> in animals (Vol. 19, pp. 73-113; Supplement 1, p. 21)
Chloroprene	Inadequate data on humans and animals (Vol. 19, pp. 131-156; Supplement 1, p. 29)
Epichlorohydrin	No data on humans; <u>limited evidence</u> in animals (Vol. 11, pp. 131-139)
Ethyl acrylate	No data on humans; inadequate data on animals (Vol. 19, pp. 57-71)
Ethylene	No data on humans or animals (Vol. 19, pp. 157-186)
Methylenediphenyl diisocyanate (4,4'-Methylenediphenyl diisocyanate)	No data on humans or animals (Vol. 19, pp. 314-340)

Chemical	Evaluation of carcinogenicity
Naphthalene-1,5-diisocyanate (1,5-Naphthalene diisocyanate)	No data on humans or animals (Vol. 19, pp. 311-340)
Polychloroprene	Inadequate data on humans and animals (Vol. 19, pp. 141-156)
Polyethylene	Inadequate data on humans and animals (Vol. 19, pp. 144-186)
Polymethylene polyphenyl isocyanate	No data on humans or animals (Vol. 19, pp. 314-340)
Polypropylene	No data on humans; inadequate data on animals (Vol. 19, pp. 218-230)
Propylene	No data on humans or animals (Vol. 19, pp. 213-230)
Styrene	Inadequate data on humans; limited evidence in animals (Vol. 19, pp. 231 -274; Supplement 1, p. 43)
Styrene-butadiene copolymers	Inadequate data on humans; no data on animals (Vol. 19, pp. 252-274)
2,4-Toluene diisocyanate	No data on humans or animals (Vol. 19, pp. 303-340)

Chemical	Evaluation of carcinogenicity
2,6-Toluene diisocyanate	No data on humans or animals (Vol. 19, pp. 303–340)
Urethane rubbers (Polyurethane)	Polyurethane foams (flexible and rigid): No data on humans; inadequate data on animals (Vol. 19, pp. 320–340)
Vinyl acetate	No data on humans; inadequate data on animals (Vol. 19, pp. 341–366)

CROSS INDEX OF CHEMICALS

2(3H)-Benzothiazolethione and zinc chloride
  See 2-Mercaptobenzothiazole, zinc chloride, 285

2(3H)-Benzothiazolethione, copper (2+) salt
  See 2-Mercaptobenzothiazole, copper salt, 285

2(3H)-Benzothiazolethione, sodium salt
  See 2-Mercaptobenzothiazole, sodium salt, 285

2(3H)-Benzothiazolethione, zinc salt
  See 2-Mercaptobenzothiazole, zinc salt, 286

2-Benzothiazolyl diethyldithiocarbamate
  See 2-Benzothiazyl-N,N-diethylthiocarbamoyl sulphide, 284

4-(2-Benzothiazolylthio)morpholine
  See N-Oxydiethylene-2-benzothiazolesulphenamide, 283

2-Benzothiazyl-N,N-diethylthiocarbamoyl sulphide, 284

Benzoyl peroxide, 316

para-Benzyloxyphenol, 308

para-(Benzyloxy)phenol
  See para-Benzyloxyphenol, 308

4-Biphenylamine
  See 4-Aminobiphenyl, 265

(1,1'-Biphenyl)-4-amine
  See 4-Aminobiphenyl, 265

(1,1'-Biphenyl)-4,4'-diamine
  See Benzidine, 266

Bis(4-aminocyclohexyl)methane carbamate, 264

Bis(4-aminocyclohexyl)methyl carbamate
  See Bis(4-aminocyclohexyl)methane carbamate, 264

1,3-Bis(2-benzothiazolylmercaptomethyl)urea, 284

N,N'-Bis(1,4-dimethylpentyl)-1,4-benzenediamine
  See N,N'-Bis(1,4-dimethylpentyl)-para-phenylene diamine, 249

N,N'-Bis(1,4-dimethylpentyl)-para-phenylenediamine, 249

Bis(dimethylphenyl) disulphide
  See Dixylyl disulphides, mixed, 295

2,5-Bis(1,1-dimethylpropyl)-1,4-benzenediol
  See 2,5-Di(1,1-dimethylpropyl)hydroquinone, 308

Bis(dimethylthiocarbamoyl) disulphide, 291

Bis(dimethylthiocarbamoyl)sulphide, 291

Bis(dimethylthiocarbamoyl) tetrasulphide, 291

Bis(dipentylcarbamodithioato-S,S')lead
  See Dipentyldithiocarbamic acid, lead salt, 280

Bis(dipentylcarbamodithioato-S,S')zinc
  See Diamyldithiocarbamic acid, zinc salt, 274

Bis(dipentyldithiocarbamato)lead
  See Dipentyldithiocarbamic acid, lead salt, 280

Bis(dipentyldithiocarbamato)zinc
  See Diamyldithiocarbamic acid, zinc salt, 274

Bis(N-ethyldithiocarbanilato)zinc
  See Ethylphenyldithiocarbamic acid, zinc salt, 280

Bis(2-ethylhexyl) adipate
  See Di-2-ethylhexyl adipate, 314

Bis(2-ethylhexyl)-1,2-benzenedicarboxylate
  See Di-2-ethylhexyl phthalate, 314

Bis(2-ethylhexyl) hexanedioate
  See Di-2-ethylhexyl adipate, 314

Bis(2-ethylhexyl) phthalate
  See Di-2-ethylhexyl phthalate, 314

Decyl diphenyl phosphite
  See Diphenyl decyl phosphite, 324

Dialkylamines, 100
  See Alkyl amines, 263

Dialkyl dithiocarbamates, 111
  See Thiocarbamates, 274

Dialkylthioruea, 296

Dialkyl thiuram sulphides, 111
  See, e.g., Tetrabutylthiuram disulphide, 293

4,4'-Diaminodiphenylmethane, 152, 160
  See 4,4'-Methylenedianiline, 257

2,4-Diaminotoluene, 160, 170
  See Toluenediamines, 253

2,5-Diaminotoluene, 160
  See Toluenediamines, 253

Diammonium sulphate
  See Ammonium sulphate, 341

Diamyldithiocarbamic acid, diamylammonium salt, 274

Diamyldithiocarbamic acid, zinc salt, 274

Diantimony trioxide
  See Antimony trioxide, 341

Diarylamines, 100
  See, e.g., Diphenylamines, 254

Diarylamine-ketone-aldehyde condensate, 259

Diarylamine-ketone condensate, 259

Diaryl and alkylaryl para-phenylenediamine, blended, 250

Diarylenediamines, mixed, 250

Hydrogen bis[pyrocatecholato(2-)]borate(1-) compound with
  1,3-di-<u>ortho</u>-tolylguanidine (1:1)
    See Dicatechol borate, di-<u>ortho</u>-tolylguanidine salt, 262

Hydrogen chloride, 79

Hydrogen peroxide, 85, 151, 170, 229, 346

Hydrogen peroxide [H_2O_2]
  See Hydrogen peroxide, 346

Hydrogen sulphide, 71, 134, 136, 354

Hydrogen sulphide [H_2S]
  See Hydrogen sulphide, 354

α-Hydro-ω-hydroxypoly(oxy-1,2-ethanediyl)
  See Polyethylene glycol(s), 321

Hydroperoxide, 103

Hydroquinone, 164, 308, 370

Hydroquinone monobenzylether, 165
  See <u>para</u>-Benzyloxyphenol, 308

Hydroquinones, 308

2-Hydroxybenzoic acid
  See Salicylic acid, 313

3-Hydroxybutanal reaction product with 1- and 2-naphthylamines
  See Aldol-(mixed α- and β-)naphthylamine condensate, 258

3-Hydroxybutanal reaction product with 1-naphthylamine
  See Aldol-α-naphthylamine condensate, 258

3-Hydroxybutyraldehyde reaction product with 1- and
  2-naphthylamines
  See Aldol-(mixed α- and β-)napthylamine condensate, 258

3-Hydroxybutyraldehyde reaction product with 1-naphthylamine
  See Aldol-α-naphthylamine condensate, 258

Lead oxide (litharge), 70, 347, 370

Lead oxide (PbO)
  See Lead oxide (litharge), 347

Lead oxide [Pb$_3$O$_4$]
  See Red lead, 348

Ledate
  See Dimethyldithiocarbamic acid, lead salt, 278

Lime, 34

Limestone, 71
  See Calcium carbonate, 343

Litharge, 34, 40, 101
  See Lead oxide (litharge), 347

Lithopone (barium sulphate and zinc sulphide), 347

Magnesium carbonate, 107, 347

Magnesium oxide, 72, 101, 347

Magnesium oxide [MgO]
  See Magnesium oxide, 347

Magnesium silicate, 347

Magnesium silicate [Mg$_2$Si$_3$O$_8$]
  See Magnesium silicate, 347

para-Mentha-1,8-diene
  See Dipentene, 333
Mercaptans, 104, 271

Mercaptoacetic acid, 1,2-ethanediyl ester
  See Ethylene glycol bis(thioglycolate), 272

Mercaptoacetic acid, 2-ethylhexyl ester
  See 2-Ethylhexyl mercaptoacetate, 272

2-Mercaptobenzimidazole, 165, 300

Tetrakis(diethylcarbamodithioato-S,S')tellurium
  See Diethyldithiocarbamic acid, tellurium salt, 277

Tetrakis(diethyldithiocarbamato)selenium
  See Diethyldithiocarbamic acid, selenium salt, 277

Tetrakis(diethyldithiocarbamato)tellurium
  See Diethyldithiocarbamic acid, tellurium salt, 277

Tetrakis(dimethylcarbamodithioato-S,S')selenium
  See Dimethyldithiocarbamic acid, selenium salt, 279

Tetrakis(dimethyldithiocarbamato)selenium
  See Dimethyldithiocarbamic acid, selenium salt, 279

(1,1,4,4-Tetramethyl-1,4-butanediyl)bis(1,1-dimethyl-
  ethyl)peroxide
  See 2,5-Dimethyl-2,5-di(tert-butylperoxy)hexane, 317

Tetramethyl succinodinitrile, 108

(1,1,4,4-Tetramethyltetramethylene)bis(tert-butyl peroxide)
  See 2,5-Dimethyl-2,5-di(tert-butylperoxy)hexane, 317

Tetramethylthiodicarbonic diamide {[(H$_2$N)C(S)]$_2$S}
  See Bis(dimethylthiocarbamoyl)sulphide, 291

Tetramethylthioperoxydicarbonic diamide {[(H$_2$N)C(S)]$_2$S$_2$}
  See Bis(dimethylthiocarbamoyl) disulphide, 291

Tetramethylthiourea, 153, 297

1,1,3,3-Tetramethyl-2-thiourea
  See Tetramethylthiourea, 297

Tetramethylthiuram disulphide, 94, 109, 115, 151, 165
  See Bis(dimethylthiocarbamoyl) disulphide, 291

Tetramethylthiuram monosulphide, 151, 165
  See Bis(dimethylthiocarbamoyl)sulphide, 291

1,1'-(Tetrathiodicarbonothioyl)bis(piperidine)
  See Di-N,N'-pentamethylenethiuram tetrasulphide, 293

Trichloroethene
  See Trichloroethylene, 331

Trichloroethylene, 107, 153, 331, 373

Trichloromethane
  See Chloroform, 328

1-Tridecanethiol
  See Tridecyl mercaptan, 273

Tridecyl mercaptan, 273

1,3,5-Triethylhexahydro-s-triazine
  See Triethyltrimethylene triamine, 264

1,3,5-Triethylhexahydro-1,3,5-triazine
  See Triethyltrimethylene triamine, 264

Triethyltrimethylene triamine, 264

4,4',4''-[(2,4,6-Trimethyl-1,3,5-benzenetriyl)tris(methylene)]-
  tris[2,6-bis(1,1-dimethylethyl)phenol]
  See 1,3,5-Trimethyl-2,4,6-tris(3,5-di-tert-butyl-
  4-hydroxybenzyl)benzene, 304

(3,3,5-Trimethylcyclohexylidine)bis(tert-butyl peroxide)
  See 1,1-Di-tert-butylperoxy-3,3,5-trimethylcyclohexane, 317

(3,3,5-Trimethylcyclohexylidene)bis[(1,1-dimethylethyl)peroxide]
  See 1,1-Di-tert-butylperoxy-3,3,5-trimethylcyclohexane, 317

2,2,4-Trimethylpentane
  See Isooctane, 333

2,4,4-Trimethyl-2-pentanethiol
  See tert-Octyl mercaptan, 272

α,α',α''-(2,4,6-Trimethyl-s-phenenyl)tris(2,6-di-tert-
  butyl-para-cresol)
  See 1,3,5-Trimethyl-2,4,6-tris(3,5-di-tert-butyl-4-
  hydroxybenzyl)benzene, 304

Numbers in bold indicate volume, and other numbers indicate page. References to corrigenda are given in parentheses. Compounds marked with an asterisk (*) were considered by the working groups, but monographs were not prepared because adequate data on carcinogenicity were not available.

A

Cholesterol   <u>10</u>, 99

Chromium and chromium compounds   <u>2</u>, 100
                                                     <u>23</u>, 205

    Barium chromate
    Basic chromic sulphate
    Calcium chromate
    Chromic acetate
    Chromic chloride
    Chromic oxide
    Chromic phosphate
    Chromite ore
    Chromium carbonyul
    Chromium potassium sulphate
    Chromium sulphate
    Chromium trioxide
    Cobalt-chromium alloy
    Ferrochromium
    Lead chromate
    Lead chromate oxide
    Potassium chromate
    Potassium dichromate
    Sodium chromate
    Sodium dichromate
    Strontium chromate
    Zinc chromate
    Zinc chromate hydroxide
    Zinc potassium chromate
    Zinc yellow

Chrysene   <u>3</u>, 159

Chrysoidine   <u>8</u>, 91

C.I. Disperse Yellow 3   <u>8</u>, 97

Cinnamyl anthranilate   <u>16</u>, 287

Cisplatin   <u>26</u>, 151

Citrus Red No. 2   <u>8</u>, 101 (corr.
                                                     <u>19</u>, 495)

Luteoskyrin   <u>10</u>, 163

Lynoestrenol   <u>21</u>, 407

Lysergide*

M

Magenta   <u>4</u>, 57 (corr. <u>7</u>,
                                                      320)

Maleic hydrazide   <u>4</u>, 173 (corr.
                                                      <u>18</u>, 125)

Maneb   <u>12</u>, 137

Mannomustine and its dihydrochloride   <u>9</u>, 157

Medphalan   <u>9</u>, 168

Medroxyprogesterone acetate   <u>6</u>, 157
                                               <u>21</u>, 417 (corr.
                                                      <u>25</u>, 391)

Megestrol acetate   <u>21</u>, 431

Melphalan   <u>9</u>, 167

6-Mercaptopurine   <u>26</u>, 249

Merphalan   <u>9</u>, 169

Mestranol   <u>6</u>, 87
                                               <u>21</u>, 257 (corr.
                                                      <u>25</u>, 391)

Methacrylic acid*

Methallenoestril*

Methotrexate   <u>26</u>, 267

Methoxsalen   <u>24</u>, 101